Current Topics in
Occupational Epidemiology

D1332639

Current Topics in Occupational Epidemiology

Edited by

Katherine M. Venables

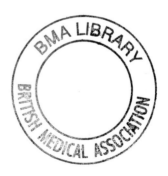

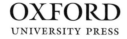

OXFORD
UNIVERSITY PRESS

OXFORD
UNIVERSITY PRESS

Great Clarendon Street, Oxford, OX2 6DP,
United Kingdom

Oxford University Press is a department of the University of Oxford.
It furthers the University's objective of excellence in research, scholarship,
and education by publishing worldwide. Oxford is a registered trade mark of
Oxford University Press in the UK and in certain other countries

Published in the United States of America by Oxford University Press
198 Madison Avenue, New York, NY 10016, United Sates of America

British Library Cataloguing in Publication Data

Data available

Library of Congress Control Number: 2013936568

ISBN 978–0–19–968390–1

Printed and bound by
CPI Group (UK) Ltd, Croydon, CR0 4YY

Oxford University Press makes no representation, express or implied, that the
drug dosages in this book are correct. Readers must therefore always check
the product information and clinical procedures with the most up-to-date
published product information and data sheets provided by the manufacturers
and the most recent codes of conduct and safety regulations. The authors and
the publishers do not accept responsibility or legal liability for any errors in the
text or for the misuse or misapplication of material in this work. Except where
otherwise stated, drug dosages and recommendations are for the non-pregnant
adult who is not breast-feeding

Links to third party websites are provided by Oxford in good faith and
for information only. Oxford disclaims any responsibility for the materials
contained in any third party website referenced in this work.

To the memory of Harry Walker.

Preface

Occupational epidemiology is the study of the distribution and determinants of illness and injury related to the work environment. These illnesses and injuries are preventable, and studying their epidemiology allows an evidence-based approach to prevention by policymakers. Furthermore, harmful work exposures can be conceptualized as a 'natural experiment' in the causation of illness and injury, because the workplace usually has much better-defined levels and timing of exposure than in the general community. Their study can therefore illuminate the causes and prevention of ill health in general. Work is also beneficial, and worklessness harmful, and occupational psychosocial 'exposures' and outcomes are increasingly studied.

This book brings together experts in occupational epidemiology to cover topics of current interest. Traditional methods can be used to study 'new' occupational diseases, as well as increase our understanding of the 'old'. New populations have come under study recently, such as the military, historically a group studied mainly by specialist researchers. Major secular trends in society mean that occupational epidemiological methods are now applied to issues such as the ageing workforce, return to work after illness, and migration of workers. The epidemiological approach can be extended to new data sources, such as surveillance systems. The high value of data from occupational epidemiology is shown in large-scale efforts to make the best use of data by pooling and by systematic reviews, and by their use in burden of disease studies. New paradigms and concepts underpin and sharpen statistical analyses, and the increasing application of health economic analyses will strengthen communication with policymakers.

The book is not a textbook of occupational epidemiology, nor does it aim to provide a fully comprehensive account of all possible current topics in occupational epidemiology. We hope that it will bring to a readership of specialists and non-specialists just some of the interesting areas in which occupational epidemiologists are active today.

Acknowledgement

The editor and authors wish to acknowledge the influence of the EPICOH conferences on occupational epidemiology over the last 30 years. These small, focused, international conferences bring together epidemiologists, statisticians, exposure assessment scientists, physicians, and policymakers in a lively forum for the discussion of new methods and findings. The EPICOH conferences are run by individual scientists (<http://www.epicoh.org>) under the aegis of the International Commission on Occupational Health (<http://www.icohweb.org>).

Contents

Part 7 **Making full use of the findings**

List of contributors

Raymond Agius
University of Manchester, UK

Fernando G. Benavides
University Pompeu Fabra, Barcelona,
Spain

Vincent Bonneterre
Université Joseph Fourier, Grenoble,
France

Marian Bos
Institute for Risk Assessment Sciences,
Utrecht University, The Netherlands

Alex Burdorf
Erasmus Medical Centre, Rotterdam,
The Netherlands

Harvey Checkoway
University of Washington, Seattle, USA

David Coggon
University of Southampton, UK

Robert A. Cohen
Stroger Hospital of Cook County and
University of Illinois, Chicago, USA

Marine Corbin
Massey University, Wellington, New
Zealand, and University of Turin, Italy

Stefania Curti
University of Bologna, Italy

Wietske Dohmen
Institute for Risk Assessment Sciences,
Utrecht University, The Netherlands

Tim Driscoll
University of Sydney, Australia

Andrea Farioli
University of Bologna, Italy

Nicola T. Fear
King's Centre for Military Health
Research at King's College London, UK

Emily Felt
University Pompeu Fabra, Barcelona,
Spain

Judith M. Graber
University of Illinois, Chicago, USA

Dick Heederik
Institute for Risk Assessment Sciences,
Utrecht University, The Netherlands

Magnus Helgesson
Uppsala University, Sweden

Sally Hutchings
Imperial College London, UK

Sharea Ijaz
Cochrane Occupational Safety and
Health Review Group, Finnish Institute
of Occupational Health

Bo Johansson
Uppsala University, Sweden

Sue Jowett
University of Birmingham, UK

David Kriebel
University of Massachusetts Lowell, USA

Hans Kromhout
Institute for Risk Assessment Sciences,
Utrecht University, The Netherlands

Ingvar Lundberg
Uppsala University, Sweden

Stefano Mattioli
University of Bologna, Italy

Brian G. Miller
Institute of Occupational Medicine,
Edinburgh, UK

Ann Olsson
International Agency for Research on
Cancer, Lyon, France

Keith T. Palmer
University of Southampton, UK

Neil Pearce
London School of Hygiene and Tropical
Medicine, UK, and Massey University,
Wellington, New Zealand

Susan Peters
Institute for Risk Assessment Sciences,
Utrecht University, The Netherlands, and
University of Western Australia

Brad A. Racette
Washington University, St Louis,
Missouri, USA

Oliver Rivero-Arias
University of Oxford, UK

Elena Ronda
University of Alicante, Spain

Lesley Rushton
Imperial College London, UK

Marc Schenker
University of California Davis, USA

Susan Searles Nielsen
University of Washington, Seattle, USA

Harry S. Shannon
McMaster University, Hamilton,
Ontario, Canada

Malcolm R. Sim
Monash University, Melbourne,
Australia

Thomas J. Smith
Harvard School of Public Health,
Boston, Massachusetts, USA

Leslie T. Stayner
University of Illinois, Chicago, USA

Kurt Straif
International Agency for Research on
Cancer, Lyon, France

Josefin Sundin
King's Centre for Military Health
Research at King's College London, UK

Katherine M. Venables
University of Oxford, UK

Jos Verbeek
Cochrane Occupational Safety and
Health Review Group, Finnish Institute
of Occupational Health, Finland

Eva Vingård
Uppsala University, Sweden

Francesco S. Violante
University of Bologna, Italy

Marjolein de Weerd
TNO, The Netherlands

Simon Wessely
King's Centre for Military Health
Research at King's College London, UK

List of abbreviations

AMSTAR	Assessment of Multiple SysTemAtic Reviews	ICD	International Classification of Diseases
BC	benefit/cost ratio	ICER	incremental cost-effectiveness ratio
BMDL	benchmark dose lower 95% confidence limit	Ig	immunoglobulin
BMI	body mass index	ILO	International Labour Organization
CAREX	database on CARcinogen EXposure in the European Union	INPV	incremental net present value
		ISCO	International Standard Classification of Occupations
CC	clonal complex		
CE	cumulative exposure	ISIC	International Standard Industrial Classification
CEP	cost-effectiveness plane		
CI	confidence interval	ITSAL	Inmigración, Trabajo y Salud project
COPD	chronic obstructive pulmonary disease		
		JEM	job-exposure matrix
Cr VI	chromium VI	KCMHR	King's Centre for Military Health Research
CWP	coal workers' pneumoconiosis		
		LBP	low back pain
DALY	disability-adjusted life year	lnOR	natural logarithm of the odds ratio
DASA	Defence Analytical Services and Advice		
		LOEL	lowest observed effect level
DEE	diesel engine exhaust	ML	maximum likelihood
EB	empirical Bayes	MLST	multilocus sequence typing
EDC	electrostatic dust cloth	MODERNET	Monitoring trends in Occupational Diseases and tracing new and Emerging Risks
EQUATOR	Enhancing the QUAlity and Transparency Of health Research		
		MOOSE	Meta-analysis Of Observational Studies in Epidemiology
ESBL	extended-spectrum beta-lactamase		
		MPP+	active metabolite of MPTP, 1-methyl-4-phenylpyridinium
ETS	environmental tobacco smoke		
GP	general practitioner	MPTP	1-methyl-4-phenyl-1,2,3,6-tetrahydropyridine
GRADE	Grading of Recommendations, Assessment, Development, and Evaluation		
		MRSA	methicillin-resistant Staphylococcus aureus
		MSSA	methicillin-sensitive Staphylococcus aureus
HR	hazard ratio or hierarchical regression		
		NCS	National Coal Study
IARC	International Agency for Research on Cancer		

NIOSH	National Institute for Occupational Safety and Health
NOAEL	no observed adverse effect level
NOCCA	Nordic Occupational Cancer Study
OECD	Organisation for Economic Co-operation and Development
OHS	occupational health and safety *or* occupational health service
OR	odds ratio
PAF	population attributable fraction
PAFR	platelet activating factor receptor
PAH	polycyclic aromatic hydrocarbon
PCR	polymerase chain reaction
PD	Parkinson disease
p(E)	proportion of the population exposed
PEROSH	partnership for European Research in Occupational Safety and Health
PICO	*Participants, Intervention/ Exposure, Comparison, and Outcome*
PFR	Pneumoconiosis Field Research
PMF	progressive massive fibrosis
PRISMA	Preferred Reporting Items for Systematic Reviews and Meta-Analyses

PTSD	post-traumatic stress disorder
PPV	pneumococcal polysaccharide vaccine
QALY	quality-adjusted life year
qPCR	real-time polymerase chain reaction
RCT	randomized controlled trial
RD	retinal detachment
RNV3P	Réseau National de Vigilance et de Prévention des Pathologies Professionnelles
RR	relative risk *or* risk ratio
RRD	rhegmatogenous retinal detachment
RTW	return to work
SB	semi-Bayes
SENSOR	Sentinel Event Notification System for Occupational Risks
SMR	standardized mortality ratio
SWORD	Surveillance of Work-related and Occupational Respiratory Disease
TCDD	2,3,7,8- tetrachlorodibenzo-p-dioxin
THOR	The Health and Occupation Reporting network
WAI	Work Ability Index
WEL	workplace exposure limit
YLD	years lived with disability
YLL	years of life lost

Part 1

Understanding old occupational diseases and evaluating the new

Chapter 1

Increased morbidity and mortality among coal workers: lessons learned from well-designed epidemiological research programmes

Judith M. Graber, Robert A. Cohen,
Brian G. Miller, and Leslie T. Stayner

Background

Coal workers were amongst the first occupational groups to be systematically studied in well-designed epidemiological research programmes. As a result, the causes and spectrum of non-malignant respiratory disease among coal workers have been rigorously explored and characterized.[1,2] While respirable silica (quartz) in mining has long been accepted as a cause of lung disease, the important contributing role of coal mine dust was questioned until the middle of the twentieth century.[3]

Occupational exposure to coal mine dust has now been shown unequivocally to cause excess mortality and morbidity from non-malignant respiratory disease, including coal workers' pneumoconiosis (CWP) and chronic obstructive pulmonary disease (COPD). The presence of respirable quartz, often a component of coal mine dust, contributes to disease incidence and severity, increasing the risk of morbidity and mortality in exposed workers. Respirable quartz may also cause silicosis and contribute to mixed dust pneumoconiosis. In addition, coal workers may be at increased risk for malignancies, including lung cancer, but evidence on this has been inconsistent.

Long-term studies of coal workers

Prior to the 1950s, studies of respiratory disease in coal miners were limited by the use of crude exposure measures, such as coal mining (or not) as an occupation,[4] duration of work as a miner or at the coalface, and age.[4–6] Many contemporary studies of coal workers continue to use these proxies for cumulative dust exposure[7,8] which are prone to severe misclassification as to the degree of exposure.

Great Britain

One of the first large-scale systematic studies of coal workers' health was the British Medical Research Council investigation into the prevalence of CWP in workers from

16 coal mines in South Wales in 1937–42.[9] Coal is classified into three major coal ranks: lignite, bituminous, and anthracite from lowest to highest carbon content and heating value. Coal in South Wales is primarily anthracite which, at the time, was believed to be the only form of coal that might cause respiratory disease. The results of the investigation led to a number of important milestones in the protection of miners under British law including the setting of dust exposure limits and the establishment in 1945 of the Pneumoconiosis Research Unit of the Medical Research Council in Cardiff, Wales.

The newly nationalized British coal industry established the Pneumoconiosis Field Research (PFR) programme in 1952[10] with the objective of determining how much and what types of coal caused pneumoconiosis and what dust levels should be maintained in order to prevent miners from becoming disabled by the air they breathed (Figure 1.1). Implied was a requirement to measure both exposures and health outcomes in a large cohort of miners over a prolonged period.

The PFR initially recruited coal miners from a representative 25 collieries across Britain and started a programme of airborne coal dust measurement combined with 5-yearly assessments of the miners by symptom and smoking questionnaires, lung function testing, and chest radiography. Three rounds of cross-sectional health surveys of working miners were completed in 24 mines, and another two or three in ten of these, ending in the early 1980s.[11,12] Innovatively, the PFR included estimates of individual workers' cumulative dust exposure. Dust concentrations and silica percentages were measured regularly in a wide range of occupational groups representing different working conditions. Time worked in those groups was obtained from each worker's pay records.[13] These were combined to produce cumulative exposure estimates for respirable coal mine and silica dust; exposures experienced before entry to the study were estimated based on work history questionnaires collected at recruitment.

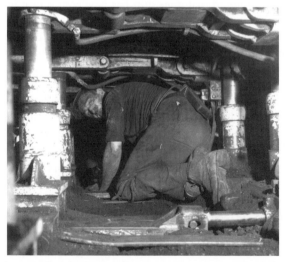

Figure 1.1 Underground coal miner working in a narrow seam in the UK.
Image reproduced by kind permission of the Institute of Occupational Medicine.

For the study of mortality, the cohort members were flagged in national record systems, which provide date and cause of death.[12]

United States of America

In the US, the Bureau of Mines and the Public Health Service actively studied anthracite and bituminous coal mines and miners throughout the mid-1900s.[3] These studies showed significant disease among workers with minimal silica exposure, suggesting that coal dust itself was toxic; however, these results were suppressed and not widely distributed. It was not until the 1960s that a popular movement of striking coal miners and their advocates demanded legislation to prevent, study, and compensate miners for respiratory diseases caused by coal dust exposure. This resulted in the enactment of the 1969 Federal Coal Mine Health and Safety Act, which included the first legally mandated permissible exposure limit for coal mine dust in the US. The provisions therein were a large step forward towards improving conditions for coal workers and establishing systems to monitor and study coal miners' respiratory health. The permissible exposure limit for coal mine dust (2 mg/m^3 since 1973 for dust of less than 5% silica) was chosen based on information produced by the PFR.[14]

In 1969, the National Institute for Occupational Safety and Health (NIOSH) initiated the National Coal Study (NCS), with data collection and methods based on those of the PFR.[15] Study mines were selected to be representative of those across major US coalfields. The NCS comprised three cross-sectional surveys (1969–81), and one follow-up study (1985–9).[15] Approximately 9000 miners were enrolled in the first survey.[14]

Estimates of cumulative coal mine dust exposure for each participant from beginning work as a miner until enrolment were constructed based on detailed work histories. Compliance data processed by the Mine Safety and Health Administration were used for 1969–70 dust levels.[16] Pre-1969 exposures were estimated using a ratio of Mine Safety and Health Administration compliance data to 1968-9 dust measurements collected for research purposes by the Bureau of Mines.

Coal mine dust lung diseases and lessons from the cohorts

The PFR and NCS have made major contributions to understanding the role of occupational dust exposure and respiratory health outcomes in coal workers. Additional detail can be found in extensive reviews on the subject.[1,2,17] Coal mine dust causes a variety of pulmonary diseases in susceptible hosts. This includes classic CWP,[1,2] the more recently described dust-related diffuse fibrosis,[18] and COPD.[1,2]

Coal workers' pneumoconiosis

CWP is an interstitial lung disease resulting from the accumulation of coal mine dust in miners' lungs and the tissue reaction to its presence.[19] CWP is assessed in living miners by chest radiograph acquired by analogue and, more recently, digital techniques.[20] It is classified using the International Labour Organization (ILO) standards[21] as simple or complicated; the latter is also known as progressive massive fibrosis (PMF) (Figure 1.2). Simple CWP is identified in coal workers radiographically by the

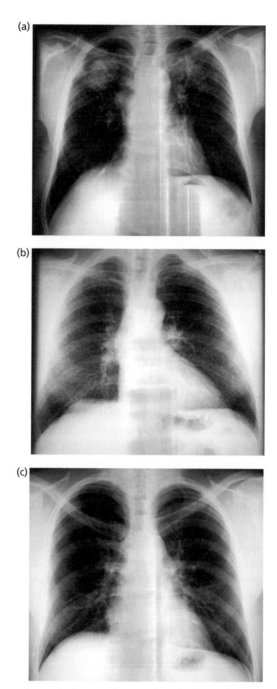

Figure 1.2 Chest radiographs from underground coal miners who took part in the Pneumoconiosis Field Research in the UK, (a) progressive massive fibrosis, (b) simple pneumoconiosis, (c) normal.

Images reproduced by kind permission of the Institute of Occupational Medicine.

presence of small opacities of less than 10 mm in diameter. One or more opacity of at least 10 mm in diameter is indicative of PMF. PMF is classified as to increasing severity by categories A, B, and C. Rapidly progressive CWP is defined as the development of PMF and/or an increase in small opacity profusion greater than one subcategory over 5 years. Coal workers may also develop silicosis and mixed dust pneumoconiosis. These may be distinguished on radiograph by opacity distribution and shape.[22]

While PMF is a progressive, debilitating disease which is predictive of disability and mortality,[19] simple CWP has also been associated with elevated mortality from pneumoconioses.[23–26] A causal exposure-response relationship has been established between cumulative coal mine dust exposure and risk of developing both CWP and PMF,[27–31] and with mortality from pneumoconiosis and PMF.[23–26,30] Incidence, the stage of CWP, and progression to PMF, as well as mortality, are positively associated with increasing proportion of respirable silica in the coal mine dust[32] and higher coal rank.[17,33]

Chronic obstructive pulmonary disease

COPD is a progressive disease characterized by chronic irreversible airway obstruction.[34] People with COPD may have chronic bronchitis (cough and sputum production) or emphysema (loss of lung tissue), or features of both. Epidemiological studies define chronic bronchitis using standardized questionnaires to elicit symptoms.[35] Respiratory impairment and the pattern of airway obstruction are determined from spirometry. Emphysema can be diagnosed in some circumstances by chest radiographs, but is definitively diagnosed by autopsy studies.[18] Tobacco smoking is the major risk factor for COPD.

Not only do coal workers experience occupational mortality from CWP and PMF,[12,23–26] they also have excess mortality from COPD compared to the general population. Cross-sectional and longitudinal studies from the PFR and NCS have demonstrated an exposure-response relationship between cumulative coal mine dust exposure and chronic bronchitis,[36–40] respiratory symptoms,[41] and pulmonary function even in the presence of normal radiographic findings.[42] The relationship between the rate of decline of lung function and coal mine dust exposure is not linear, the greatest reduction occurring in the first few years of exposure.[43]

Occupational coal mine dust exposure is also associated with increased risk of emphysema, and this has been demonstrated in studies that controlled for the effects of cigarette smoking and age.[44,45]

Exposure-response relationships for excess mortality from non-malignant respiratory disease

Studies from the PFR and NCS provide ample evidence for an exposure-response relationship between cumulative coal mine dust exposure and mortality from both the pneumoconioses and COPD. The most recent of many mortality studies of the miners enrolled in the PFR was conducted with follow-up to 2006.[26] This study included 17 820 miners with almost 11 000 confirmed deaths. Standardized mortality ratios (SMRs) increased in later follow-up periods for non-malignant respiratory disease, consistent with the healthy worker effect, which decreases with length of follow-up.[46] A strong positive exposure-response relationship was seen for pneumoconiosis-related mortality with coal mine dust, with a relative risk (RR) of lifetime cumulative exposure of 100 ghm^{-3} ($RR_{100\ ghm^{-3}}$) 1.55; 95% confidence interval (95% CI) 1.43–1.69, the cumulative exposure being equal to approximately 30 years of 1740 working hours in a mean concentration of 2 mg/m^3. The strong relationship was also seen with respirable quartz dust exposure (risk of lifetime cumulative exposure of 5 ghm^{-3} ($RR_{5\ ghm^{-3}}$) 1.21; 95% CI 1.12–1.31) and with a 15-year lag in single-exposure models. In models with both exposures the effect of coal mine dust was stronger ($RR_{100\ ghm^{-3}}$ 1.92; 95% CI 1.71–2.15) and that of quartz was eliminated ($RR_{5\ ghm^{-3}}$ 0.74; 95% CI 0.65–0.80). However, in a study of respirable coal mine and quartz dust as predictors of pulmonary inflammation and fibrosis in US coal miners, the potency of quartz per unit of exposure was approximately 20 times higher than that of coal mine dust.[47]

A positive and significant exposure-response relationship was also seen in the PFR between COPD mortality and coal mine dust exposure with a 15-year lag ($RR_{100\ ghm^{-3}}$ 1.17; 95% CI 1.11–1.24) in models controlling for major potential confounders including smoking.[26] Respirable quartz was not significantly associated with COPD in a model containing both exposures ($RR_{5\ ghm^{-3}}$ 0.96; 95% CI 0.88–1.04), but coal mine dust remained a strong and significant predictor of COPD ($RR_{100\ ghm^{-3}}$ 1.21; 95% CI 1.11–1.32).

An update of the mortality data from the NCS was completed to 31 December 2007; 9033 miners were followed and 5907 deaths observed.[25] The findings were similar to those from the PFR study: significant exposure-response relationships were seen for silica exposure (log-transformed variable) and mortality ($RR_{2.6\ mg/m^3}$ 1.23; 95% CI 1.00–1.52) but not in the model which included both silica and coal mine dust exposures ($RR_{2.6\ mg/m^3}$ 1.12; 95% CI 0.88–1.42). The association between coal mine dust exposure and COPD was significant among never smokers (RR 1.93; 95% CI 1.12–3.34) and former smokers (RR 1.61; 95% CI 1.06–2.44), but not current smokers (RR 1.04; 95% CI 0.81–1.34).

Excess mortality among coal workers who had severe declines in lung function has been observed in studies from both the PFR and NCS.[48,49]

Lung cancer

The relationship between coal mine dust exposure and lung cancer mortality has been examined extensively in the epidemiological literature. Kennaway and Kennaway first reported an apparent deficit of lung cancer among coal workers in 1936.[50] Several other early coal miner mortality studies reported similar findings,[6,51,52] while others did not.[53–55] In 1977, the International Agency for Research on Cancer (IARC) concluded that there was inadequate evidence to classify coal dust as to its carcinogenicity to humans (IARC Group 3).[56] It has been proposed that negative findings in early studies may be explained by the ban on smoking in underground mines because of the explosive nature of methane gas combined with coal mine dust, which reduces miners' exposure to the primary population risk factor for lung cancer.[57] Another hypothesis based on experimental evidence is that exposure to coal dust may inhibit the expression and activity of *CYP1A1* in the lung, a gene involved in lung carcinogenesis by promoting the activation of aromatic hydrocarbons in cigarette smoke to reactive intermediates.[58]

Findings from the most recent mortality follow-ups of the PFR and NCS may suggest a positive association between coal mining and lung cancer mortality. An overall excess of lung cancer mortality was observed from the NCS study[25] but not from the PFR study[26] (Table 1.1). However, summary rates can obscure underlying patterns[46] and both studies showed significant excesses in the last tertile of follow-up time.[25,26]

A significant exposure-response relationship between cumulative silica dust and lung cancer was reported from the PFR study, but not the NCS (Table 1.2). In contrast, the NCS study observed a positive and significant exposure-response relationship between coal mine dust exposure (log-transformed) and lung cancer mortality.

Table 1.1 SMRs for mortality due to lung cancer

Follow-up time	British PFR[26]		US NCS[25]	
	Years (deaths)	SMR (95% CI)	Years (deaths)	SMR (95% CI)
All	1959–2005 (958)	0.99 (0.93–1.06)	1969–2007 (568)	1.08 (1.00–1.18)
Last tertile	1990–2005 (395)	1.16 (1.05–1.28)	2000–2007 (127)	1.23 (1.02–1.45)

Sources: data from Miller BG and MacCalman L, Cause-specific mortality in British coal workers and exposure to respirable dust and quartz, *Occupational and Environmental Medicine*, Volume **67**, pp. 270–6, Copyright © 2010 by the BMJ Publishing Group Ltd and Graber JM, Morbidity and mortality among underground coal miners (dissertation) University of Illinois, Chicago, USA, Copyright © 2012.

Table 1.2 Estimated relative risks (RRs) for mortality due to lung cancer estimated in Cox proportional hazards models from PFR and NCS follow-up studies

Exposure	British PFR[26] RR[a] (95% CI)	US NCS[25] RR[a] (95% CI)
Coal mine dust	1.03 (0.96–1.10)	1.70 (1.02–2.83)
Quartz	1.07 (1.01–1.13)	1.05 (0.90–1.23)
Coal mine dust controlling for quartz	0.91 (0.82–1.01)	1.71 (1.03–2.85)
Quartz controlling for coal mine dust	1.14 (1.04–1.25)	0.99 (0.84–1.18)
Coal mine dust: 2000–7	–	1.41 (1.19–1.67)
Quartz: 2000–7	–	1.17 (1.11–1.23)

[a] RRs expressed for lifetime cumulative exposures for the PFR as 100 ghm^{-3} respirable dust or/and 5 ghm^{-3} respirable quartz with a 15-year lag; controlling for entry date, age (quadratic)×(smoking at entry), cigarettes at entry, and regional rates; for the NCS as cohort's mean cumulative exposure (coal mine dust = 64.6 mg/m^3-years; silica = 2.6 mg/m^3-years), models controlled age at study entry, race, coal rank, smoking frequency and status at entry, and year of birth

Sources: data from Miller BG and MacCalman L, Cause-specific mortality in British coal workers and exposure to respirable dust and quartz, *Occupational and Environmental Medicine*, Volume **67**, pp. 270–6, Copyright © 2010 by the BMJ Publishing Group Ltd and Graber JM, Morbidity and mortality among underground coal miners (dissertation) University of Illinois, Chicago, USA, Copyright © 2012.

However, in the later years of follow-up in the NCS study (2000–7), both coal mine dust and silica were significantly associated with lung cancer mortality.

The finding of excess lung cancer mortality after additional follow-up of both the PFR and NCS, as well as the increasing SMRs with follow-up time, are indicative of a strong healthy worker effect.[46] This effect may also in part be due to diminished protection from smoking with time, if miners were to resume or increase smoking frequency when they terminate mining employment.[26]

Selection biases in studies of coal workers: the healthy worker effect

Like most occupational cohort studies, those of coal workers are affected by the healthy worker effect. A strength of the PFR and NCS studies is the ability to use internal analysis (i.e. comparing workers by exposure level) which controls for selection bias at hire, one component of the effect.[59] However, internal analyses may not fully control for ongoing selection bias if symptoms of adverse health effects are related to exposure (referred to as the healthy worker survivor effect) and may bias findings towards the null hypothesis of no effect.[60]

Work status is a key component of the healthy worker survivor effect, as are length of time since entering the industry and employment duration.[61] Both the PFR and NCS studies have consistently found higher rates of symptoms and disease among former miners compared with current miners, consistent with a healthy worker survivor effect.[62,63] In Great Britain, the impact and evaluation of this effect are further complicated because many mines were closed beginning in the early 1980s, when the mining industry was severely reduced.

Current and future challenges and conclusions

In early studies from both the NCS and the PFR it became apparent that the mandatory exposure limits were not preventing debilitating disease in coal workers in either Britain or the US[11,64]

In the US, the prevalence of CWP is monitored by NIOSH's Coal Workers' X-ray Surveillance Program. After a steady decline in the tenure-specific prevalence of CWP and PMF from 1970 until 1995, the tenure-specific prevalence of CWP began to increase (Figure 1.3).[65,66,67] Perhaps most alarmingly, the CWP was also accompanied by increased rates of rapidly progressive CWP and silicosis.

Further investigations found that new cases of CWP and rapidly progressive CWP were occurring among miners whose work in coal mining began after the 2 mg/m^3 standard was enacted.[65] Reasons for the increased disease prevalence appear to be multifactorial and may include higher silica exposure due to mining of narrower coal seams (such as illustrated in Figure 1.1) and other changing work practices, such as longer working shifts, which would increase the amount of dust deposited in the lungs.[2,17,20,66-68] Studies conducted in coal mines in Scotland have demonstrated that miners exposed to relatively low levels of coal mine dust with a high level of quartz showed unexpectedly rapid progression of pneumoconiosis.[32,69]

The prevalence and severity of COPD related to coal mine dust exposure is not addressed by most surveillance programmes which rely almost entirely on chest

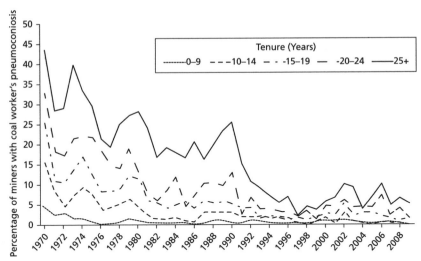

Figure 1.3 Percentage of examined underground miners in the US with coal workers' pneumoconiosis (ILO category 1/01) by tenure in mining, 1970–2009.
Adapted from Work-Related Lung Disease Surveillance System (eWoRLD), *Coal workers' pneumoconiosis: morbidity*, NIOSH, Atlanta, USA. Coal workers' pneumoconiosis data from NIOSH Coal Workers' X-ray Surveillance Program (CWXSP).

radiographs. Unfortunately NIOSH's recommendations that spirometry become an integral part of medical surveillance has yet to be fully implemented.[1]

The percentage of all miners who are surface coal workers has increased in the US from about a third (34.4%) in 1978 to almost half (47.4%) in 2007.[70] These miners are also at risk from disease and premature death due to respiratory disease, including CWP, PMF, and silicosis.[68]

Coal mining is rapidly expanding in the developing world. From 2007 to 2010 coal production declined in the US by 6% and Europe by 10% but increased in Eurasia by 9%, in Africa by 3%, and in Asia and Oceania by 19%.[71] China saw a dramatic increase of 39% from 2007 to 2011. There have been few epidemiological studies published that characterize the disease burden among coal workers during this expansion but, in one study conducted among miners in Liaoning Province, China, rates of CWP were high.[72] There are an estimated six million underground miners in China at present;[73] hence even low disease rates will cause a high burden of illness and excess premature mortality.

Conclusion

Studies conducted using the British and US coal workers' cohorts have made important contributions to our understanding of disease aetiology and prevalence as well as providing vital data for setting and evaluating dust control limits. The risks of CWP, PMF, and COPD increase with cumulative exposure to coal mine dust, and exposure to respirable silica brings additional risks. Some studies suggest that lung cancer risk may also be increased among coal miners.

Worldwide, ongoing exposure to coal mine dust presents an increased risk of morbidity and mortality from respiratory diseases for both underground and surface coal workers and, in some regions, the prevalence and severity of disease may be increasing. It is unclear to what degree these disturbing trends reflect a lack of enforcement, inadequacy of current dust control regulations, or changes in the characteristics of exposure related to changes in the processes used to mine coal.

Whatever the causes of ongoing disease, past studies provide sufficient knowledge to implement prevention activities. Exposures to coal mine dust and silica must be reduced. In addition, resources should be directed to building capacity for workplace surveillance, including of lung function, in both the developed and the developing world. New epidemiological investigations of disease risks among current and former miners could assist policymakers in devising strategies to prevent morbidity and mortality from respiratory disease among these workers.

Acknowledgements

The authors thank the following employees of US NIOSH for their thorough and insightful reviews, which greatly augmented the chapter's breadth and depth: Michael D. Attfield PhD, Eileen D. Kumpel PhD, and A. Scott Laney PhD.

References

1. **NIOSH.** *Criteria for a recommended standard: occupational exposure to respirable coal mine dust.* DHHS (NIOSH) publication number 95–106. Cincinnati, OH: US DHHS (NIOSH), 1995. Available at: <http://www.cdc.gov/niosh/docs/95-106/> (accessed 24 January 2013).

2. **NIOSH.** *Current intelligence bulletin 64: coal mine dust exposures and associated health outcomes—review of information published since 1995.* DHHS (NIOSH) Publication Number 2011–172. Cincinnati, OH: US DHHS (NIOSH), 2011. Available at: <http://www.cdc.gov/niosh/docs/2011-172/pdfs/2011-172.pdf> (accessed 24 January 2013).

3. **Derickson A.** *Black lung: anatomy of a public health disaster.* Ithaca, NY: Cornell University Press, 1998.

4. **Enterline PE, Lainhart WS.** The relationship between coal mining and chronic nonspecific respiratory disease. *Am J Public Health Nations Health* 1967;**57**:484–95.

5. **Rom WN, Kanner RE, Renzetti AD Jr,** *et al.* Respiratory disease in Utah coal miners. *Am Rev Respir Dis* 1981;**123**:372–7.

6. **Atuhaire LK, Campbell MJ, Cochrane AL, Jones M, Moore F.** Specific causes of death in miners and ex-miners of the Rhondda Fach 1950–80. *Br J Ind Med* 1986;**43**:497–9.

7. **Une H, Esaki H, Osajima K, Ikui H, Kodama K, Hatada K.** A prospective study on mortality among Japanese coal miners. *Ind Health* 1995;**33**:67–76.

8. **Graber JM, Cohen RA, Basanets A,** *et al.* Results from a Ukrainian-US collaborative study: prevalence and predictors of respiratory symptoms among Ukrainian coal miners. *Am J Ind Med* 2012;**55**:1099–109.

9. **Fay JWJ, Rae S.** The pneumoconiosis field research of the National Coal Board. *Ann Occup Hyg* 1959;**1**:149–61.

10. **Fay JW.** The National Coal Board's pneumoconiosis field research. *Nature* 1957;**180**:309–11.

11. **Jacobsen M, Rae S, Walton WH, Rogan JM.** New dust standards for British coal mines. *Nature* 1970;**227**:445–7.

12. **Miller BG, Jacobsen M.** Dust exposure, pneumoconiosis, and mortality of coalminers. *Br J Ind Med* 1985;**42**:723–33.

13. **Fay JW, Ashford JR.** A survey of the methods developed in the National Coal Board's pneumoconiosis field research for correlating environmental exposure with medical condition. *Br J Ind Med* 1961;**18**:175–96.

14. **Attfield M, Reger R, Glenn R.** The incidence and progression of pneumoconiosis over nine years in U.S. coal miners: I. Principal findings. *Am J Ind Med* 1984;**6**:407–15.

15. **Attfield MD.** Pneumoconiosis in coal miners: NIOSH research and surveillance. *Morb Mortal Wkly Rep Surveill Summ* 1983;**32**:39SS–42SS.

16. **Attfield MD, Morring K.** The derivation of estimated dust exposures for U.S. coal miners working before 1970. *Am Ind Hyg Assoc J* 1992;**53**:248–55.

17. **Attfield M, Castranova V, Kuempel E, Wagner G.** Coal. In: Bingham E, Cohrssen B (eds) *Patty's toxicology* (6th edn). Hoboken, NJ: Wiley, 2012, pp. 301–24.

18. **Green FHY, Brower PL, Vallyathan V, Attfield M.** Coal mine dust exposure and type of pulmonary emphysema in coal workers. In: Chiyotani K, Hosoda Y (eds) *Advances in the prevention of occupational respiratory diseases: proceedings of the 9th International Conference on Occupational Respiratory Diseases, Kyoto, 13–16 October 1997*. Amsterdam: Elsevier Science, 1988, pp. 948–53.

19. **Speizer, F.** Environmental lung disease. In: Fauci AS, Braunwald E, Isselbacher KJ, *et al.* (eds) *Harrison's principles of internal medicine* (14th edn). New York: McGraw-Hill, 1998, pp. 1430–2.

20. **Laney AS, Weissman DN.** The classic pneumoconioses: new epidemiological and laboratory observations. *Clin Chest Med* 2012;**33**:745–58.

21. **International Labour Organization.** *Guidelines for the use of the ILO international classification of radiographs of pneumoconioses (revised edition)*. Geneva: ILO, 2011. Available at <http://www.ilo.org/wcmsp5/groups/public/ – -ed_protect/ – -protrav/ – -safework/ documents/publication/wcms_168260.pdf> (accessed 24 January 2013).

22. **Cohen R, Velho V.** Update on respiratory disease from coal mine and silica dust. *Clin Chest Med* 2002;**23**:811–26.

23. **Attfield MD, Kuempel ED.** Mortality among U.S. underground coal miners: a 23-year follow-up. *Am J Ind Med* 2008;**51**:231–45. (Correction in *Am J Ind Med* 2010;**53**:550.)

24. **Kuempel ED, Stayner LT, Attfield MD, Buncher CR.** Exposure-response analysis of mortality among coal miners in the United States. *Am J Ind Med* 1995;**28**:167–84.

25. **Graber JM.** *Morbidity and mortality among underground coal miners* Dissertation. University of Illinois, Chicago, IL, 2012.

26. **Miller BG, MacCalman L.** Cause-specific mortality in British coal workers and exposure to respirable dust and quartz. *Occup Environ Med* 2010;**67**:270–6.

27. **Attfield M, Reger R, Glenn R.** The incidence and progression of pneumoconiosis over nine years in U.S. coal miners: II. Relationship with dust exposure and other potential causative factors. *Am J Ind Med* 1984;**6**:417–25.

28. **Hurley JF, Burns J, Copland L, Dodgson J, Jacobsen M.** Coalworkers' simple pneumoconiosis and exposure to dust at 10 British coalmines. *Br J Ind Med* 1982;**39**:120–7.

29. **Jacobsen M.** Evidence of dose-response relation in pneumoconiosis. 2. *Trans Soc Occup Med* 1972;**22**:88–94.

30. **Hurley JF, Alexander WP, Hazledine DJ, Jacobsen M, Maclaren WM.** Exposure to respirable coalmine dust and incidence of progressive massive fibrosis. *Br J Ind Med* 1987;**44**:661–72.

31. **Ashford JR, Fay JW, Smith CS.** The correlation of dust exposure with progression of radiological pneumoconiosis in British coal miners. *Am Ind Hyg Assoc J* 1965;**26**:347–61.

32. **Seaton A, Dick JA, Dodgson J, Jacobsen M.** Quartz and pneumoconiosis in coalminers. *Lancet* 1981;**2**:1272–5.

33. **Ruckley VA, Fernie JM, Chapman JS,** *et al.* Comparison of radiographic appearances with associated pathology and lung dust content in a group of coalworkers. *Br J Ind Med* 1984;**41**:459–67.

34. **Celli BR, MacNee W, ATS/ERS Task Force.** Standards for the diagnosis and treatment of patients with COPD: a summary of the ATS/ERS position paper. *Eur Respir J* 2004;**23**:932–46.

35. **Ferris BG.** Epidemiology Standardization Project (American Thoracic Society). *Am Rev Respir Dis* 1978;**118**(6 part 2):1–120.

36. **Rae S, Walker DD, Attfield MD.** Chronic bronchitis and dust exposure in British coalminers. *Inhaled Part* 1970;**2**:883–96.

37. **Kibelstis JA, Morgan EJ, Reger R, Lapp NL, Seaton A, Morgan WK.** Prevalence of bronchitis and airway obstruction in American bituminous coal miners. *Am Rev Respir Dis* 1973;**108**:886–93.

38. **Marine WM, Gurr D, Jacobsen M.** Clinically important respiratory effects of dust exposure and smoking in British coal miners. *Am Rev Respir Dis* 1988;**137**:106–12.

39. **Seixas NS, Robins TG, Attfield MD, Moulton LH.** Exposure-response relationships for coal mine dust and obstructive lung disease following enactment of the Federal Coal Mine Health and Safety Act of 1969. *Am J Ind Med* 1992;**21**:715–34.

40. **Henneberger PK, Attfield MD.** Respiratory symptoms and spirometry in experienced coal miners: effects of both distant and recent coal mine dust exposures. *Am J Ind Med* 1997;**32**:268–74.

41. **Cowie HA, Miller BG, Rawbone RG, Soutar CA.** Dust related risks of clinically relevant lung functional deficits. *Occup Environ Med* 2006;**63**:320–5.

42. **Attfield MD, Hodous TK.** Pulmonary function of U.S. coal miners related to dust exposure estimates. *Am Rev Respir Dis* 1992;**145**:605–9.

43. **Seixas NS, Robins TG, Attfield MD, Moulton LH.** Longitudinal and cross sectional analyses of exposure to coal mine dust and pulmonary function in new miners. *Br J Ind Med* 1993;**50**:929–37.

44. **Ruckley VA, Gauld SJ, Chapman JS,** *et al.* Emphysema and dust exposure in a group of coal workers. *Am Rev Respir Dis* 1984;**129**:528–32.

45. **Kuempel ED, Wheeler MW, Smith RJ, Vallyathan V, Green FH.** Contributions of dust exposure and cigarette smoking to emphysema severity in coal miners in the United States. *Am J Respir Crit Care Med* 2009;**180**:257–64.

46. **McMichael AJ.** Standardized mortality ratios and the 'healthy worker effect': Scratching beneath the surface. *J Occup Med* 1976;**18**:165–8.

47. **Kuempel ED, Attfield MD, Vallyathan V,** *et al.* Pulmonary inflammation and crystalline silica in respirable coal mine dust: dose-response. *J Biosci* 2003;**28**:61–9.

48. **Sircar K, Hnizdo E, Petsonk E, Attfield M.** Decline in lung function and mortality: implications for medical monitoring. *Occup Environ Med* 2007;**64**:461–6.

49. **Miller BG, Jacobsen M, Steele RC.** *Coalminers' mortality in relation to radiological category, lung function and exposure to airborne dust.* TM/81/10:1981. Edinburgh: Institute of Occupational Medicine, 1981. Available at: <http://www.iom-world.org/research/report_list.php?pageNum_listReports=25&totalRows_listReports=459> (accessed 6 February 2013).

50. **Kennaway NM, Kennaway EL.** A study of the incidence of cancer of the lung and larynx. *J Hyg (Lond)* 1936;**36**:236–7.

51. **Liddell FD.** Morbidity of British coal miners in 1961–62. *Br J Ind Med* 1973;**30**:1–14.

52. **Costello J, Ortmeyer CE, Morgan WK.** Mortality from lung cancer in U.S. coal miners. *Am J Public Health* 1974;**64**:222–4.

53. **Enterline PE.** A review of mortality data for American coal miners. *Ann N Y Acad Sci* 1972;**200**:260–72.

54. **Rockette HE.** Cause specific mortality of coal miners. *J Occup Med* 1977;**19**:795–801.

55. **Goldman KP.** Mortality of coal-miners from carcinoma of the lung. *Br J Ind Med* 1965;**22**:72–7.

56. **IARC Working Group on the Evaluation of Carcinogenic Risks to Humans.** *Silica, some silicates, coal dust and para-aramid fibrils.* IARC Monographs on the Evaluation of Carcinogenic Risks to Humans. Volume 68. Lyon: World Health Organization, 1997. Available at: <http://monographs.iarc.fr/ENG/Monographs/vol68/index.php> (accessed 24 January 2013).

57. **Stayner LT, Graber JM.** Does exposure to coal dust prevent or cause lung cancer? *Occup Environ Med* 2011;**68**:167–8.

58. **Ghanem MM, Porter D, Battelli LA,** *et al.* Respirable coal dust particles modify cytochrome P4501A1 (CYP1A1) expression in rat alveolar cells. *Am J Respir Cell Mol Biol* 2004;**31**:171–83.

59. **Arrighi HM, Hertz-Picciotto I.** Controlling the healthy worker survivor effect: an example of arsenic exposure and respiratory cancer. *Occup Environ Med* 1996;**53**:455–62.

60. **Robins JM, Blevins D, Ritter G, Wulfsohn M.** G-estimation of the effect of prophylaxis therapy for Pneumocystis carinii pneumonia on the survival of AIDS patients. *Epidemiology* 1992;**3**:319–36.

61. **Gilbert ES.** Some confounding factors in the study of mortality and occupational exposures. *Am J Epidemiol* 1982;**116**:177–88.

62. **Henneberger PK, Attfield MD.** Coal mine dust exposure and spirometry in experienced miners. *Am J Respir Crit Care Med* 1996;**153**:1560–6.

63. **Soutar CA, Hurley JF.** Relation between dust exposure and lung function in miners and ex-miners. *Br J Ind Med* 1986;**43**:307–20.

64. **Attfield MD, Morring K.** An investigation into the relationship between coal workers' pneumoconiosis and dust exposure in U.S. coal miners. *Am Ind Hyg Assoc J* 1992;**53**:486–92.

65. **Antao VC, Petsonk EL, Sokolow LZ,** *et al.* Rapidly progressive coal workers' pneumoconiosis in the United States: geographic clustering and other factors. *Occup Environ Med* 2005;**62**:670–4.

66. **Laney AS, Attfield MD.** Quartz exposure can cause pneumoconiosis in coal workers (letter). *J Occup Environ Med* 2009;**51**:867.

67. **CDC NIOSH.** Work-Related Lung Disease Surveillance System (eWoRLD). *Coal workers' pneumoconiosis: morbidity.* Atlanta, GA: CDC NIOSH. Available at: <http://www2a.cdc.gov/drds/WorldReportData/FigureTableDetails.asp?FigureTableID=2549&GroupRefNumber=F02-05> (accessed 24 January 2013).

68. **Centers for Disease Control and Prevention (CDC).** Pneumoconiosis and advanced occupational lung disease among surface coal miners—16 states, 2010–2011. *Morb Mortal Wkly Rep* 2012;**61**:431–4.

69. **Miller BG, Hagen S, Love RG,** *et al.* Risks of silicosis in coalworkers exposed to unusual concentrations of respirable quartz. *Occup Environ Med* 1998;**55**:52–8.

70. **Mine Safety and Health Administration.** *Table 03. Average number of employees at coal mines in the United States, by primary activity, 1978–2008.* Washington, DC: US Department of Labor, 2012. Available at: <http://www.msha.gov/stats/part50/wq/1978/wq78cl03.asp> (accessed 24 January 2013).

71. **US Energy Information Administration.** *International energy statistics, coal production, all countries by region.* Washington DC: US Department of Energy. Available at: <http://www.eia.gov/cfapps/ipdbproject/IEDIndex3.cfm?tid=1&pid=7&aid=1> (accessed 24 January 2013).

72. **Liu H, Tang Z, Weng D,** *et al.* Prevalence characteristics and prediction of coal workers' pneumoconiosis in the Tiefa Colliery in China. *Ind Health* 2009;**47**:369–75.

73. **Liu FD, Pan ZQ, Liu SL,** *et al.* The estimation of the number of underground coal miners and the annual dose to coal miners in China. *Health Phys* 2007;**93**:127–32.

Chapter 2

Microbial resistance in livestock farming: occupational and public health concerns

Dick Heederik, Marian Bos,
and Wietske Dohmen

Introduction

Staphylococcus aureus is a Gram-positive, coagulase-positive, coccus of the family Staphylococcaceae. Staphylococcal species are commensal colonizers of the skin of animals and humans. They are also found on mucous membranes of the upper respiratory tract and lower urogenital tract and, transiently, in the digestive tract. Staphylococci are resistant to dehydration and are stable for long periods in the environment.[1] Colonization with *S. aureus* may occur on mucous membranes of the respiratory or intestinal tract, or on other body surfaces, and is usually asymptomatic. Nasal colonization with *S. aureus* in the human population occurs among around 30% of individuals. Methicillin-resistant *S. aureus* (MRSA) are strains that have developed resistance to beta-lactam antibiotics, which include the penicillins (methicillin, dicloxacillin, nafcillin, oxacillin, etc.) and the cephalosporins and, as a result, may cause difficult-to-treat infections in humans. Nasal colonization with MRSA in the general population is low; the highest rate reported in a population-based survey was 1.5%.[2,3] Infections with MRSA are associated with treatment failure and increased severity of disease.[4,5] The continuing emergence of pathogens that are resistant to antimicrobials is a global concern.

In 2004 a case of, at that time non-typeable, MRSA was reported in a 6-month-old girl admitted to a hospital in the Netherlands. Despite several decolonization attempts, the girl remained MRSA positive. The girl's father was a pig farmer and she lived with her parents on the farm. Her parents were also found to be MRSA colonized.[6] This strain had been observed earlier in France, around the turn of the century, in a study among pig farmers and their animals.[7] Since neither the girl nor her family had a history of travelling, or of admission to a foreign hospital, further investigations began into the source of the MRSA.[8] Genotyping showed that the same MRSA strain was also found in the pigs on the farm, and also neighbouring pig farmers and their animals were carriers of this strain. The strain could not be typed by pulsed-field gel electrophoresis and was therefore initially labelled non-typeable MRSA (NT-MRSA). Later on, this strain and some related strains appeared strongly associated with livestock production, and were labelled livestock-associated MRSA (LA-MRSA) and are nowadays referred to as MRSA ST398.

Several aspects contributed to the rapid attention paid to the emergence of this new strain. Firstly, although MRSA is endemic in many hospitals around the world and has also emerged in the general community, the Netherlands is, together with Scandinavian countries, a low MRSA prevalence country (0.1%) due to its active 'search and destroy' policy.[9,10] Therefore, occurrence in a high rate in a specific population triggered immediate attention. Secondly, this LA-MRSA spread rapidly across Europe[11,12] and North America,[13] and the epidemiology differed considerably from hospital-acquired MRSA. MRSA was rarely isolated from animals before 2000. If isolated from animals, MRSA strains were generally supposed to be of human origin, especially when found in companion animals. The general opinion was that animal husbandry was of little relevance to MRSA which caused diseases in humans, and that MRSA was a problem caused by antimicrobial use in human medicine.[14] Finally, early prevalence studies among occupational risk groups, such as livestock farmers and veterinarians, had shown that their nasal carriage prevalence was high, varying between 20% and 70%. Because hospital strains of MRSA easily transmit from humans to humans, there was considerable concern that due to this high prevalence in high-risk occupationally exposed individuals, LA-MRSA might transmit to the general population through family members and other human-human contacts.

Thus, there was a particular context (low MRSA prevalence country), a remarkably rapid spread (probably because of farm-to-farm transmission due to (international) animal transports), and a high prevalence among livestock farmers. The MRSA case illustrates the rapid emergence, and transmission from animals to humans, of a new strain of resistant micro-organisms from an animal reservoir, creating risks for different occupational groups. Occupational health and public health aspects of this new emerging resistant strain are explained and discussed and put in a wider context by briefly touching upon another form of microbial resistance, related to extended-spectrum beta-lactamase (ESBL)-producing bacteria in livestock production which is attracting wider attention at present. This form of microbial resistance might be associated with comparable public health risks in the future.

Emergence of microbial resistance

It is common knowledge that the use of antimicrobial agents in humans, animals, and plants promotes the selection and spread of antimicrobial-resistant bacteria and resistance genes through genetic mutations and gene transfer.[15] Antimicrobial agents are widely used in veterinary medicine and modern food animal production depends on the use of large amounts of antimicrobials for disease control. Use of antimicrobials probably played an important role in the emergence of MRSA ST398.

Routine molecular typing methods, such as multilocus sequence typing (MLST) and spa-typing, helped to place the new strain in the context of other MRSA strains. However, these methods are not well able to characterize heterogeneity within the clonal complex 398 (CC398). A clonal complex is a group of strains with the same ancestral genotype and with minor genetic variation. As a result, the evolution and global epidemiology of CC398 has been clarified only in part. Microarray studies have shown that core genomes of CC398 isolates are distinctly different from common *S. aureus* isolates from humans.[16] Therefore it has been assumed that pigs or other animals are the natural host of CC398. In Europe and North America, MRSA strains in livestock farmers and their animals mainly belong to the new clonal complex CC398. In Asia another strain, ST9, seems to be dominant in pigs.[17] Although the time of the very first emergence of LA-MRSA is known only by approximation, a recent phylogenetic reconstruction study on the basis of CC398 collections from different years and from different countries suggests that MRSA CC398 originated in humans as methicillin sensitive *S. aureus* (MSSA). This MSSA probably lost phage-based human virulence genes when it jumped from humans to animals, where at the same time it acquired tetracycline and methicillin resistance.[18] Thus, a bidirectional zoonotic exchange seems to have led to the CC398 complex. The use of antimicrobials in veterinary practice very likely contributed. Although use of antimicrobial agents as growth promoters has been abolished in the European Union, antimicrobials are being used for treatment of animals, often at the herd level, leading to a high consumption for some animal species.

The methicillin resistance of *S. aureus* is determined by the *mecA* gene which codes for a variant of the penicillin-binding protein (PBP2a). The *mecA* gene resides on a mobile genetic element, the staphylococcal cassette chromosome *mec* (SCC*mec*).[19] The presence of the SSC*mec* types in LA-MRSA is shared with community-acquired MRSA types and this suggests transmission of genetic information between these MRSA lineages. ST398 strains generally do not contain the Panton-Valentine leucocidin (PVL) genes that code for a cytotoxin that determines to a large extent the virulence of community-acquired MRSA types. However, some anecdotal information exists about ST398 strains that have acquired PVL genes, probably from human MRSA types.[16,20]

Epidemiology of MRSA ST398

A case-control study showed that pig and cattle farming were risk factors for human acquisition of MRSA ST398. However, the risk estimates in this study should be viewed with care because the controls were hospital-acquired MRSA cases instead of general population controls, artificially inflating the odds ratios for associations between MRSA ST398 occurrence and farming-related exposures.[21] Since 2005 onwards, LA-MRSA has been increasingly frequently reported in different food production animals, including cattle, pigs, and poultry (see Table 2.1), in other European countries than the Netherlands, and in the Americas and Asia.[11,13] High animal-to-human transmission of ST398 has been reported in pig farming, leading to an elevated prevalence of nasal MRSA carriage ranging from a few per cent in Ireland up to 86% in German pig farmers (Table 2.1). One study showed a clear association between the prevalence of MRSA carriage among participants from farms with MRSA colonized pigs (50%) versus 3% on farms without colonized pigs (relative risk 16.5; 95% confidence interval 2.4–114.9; p <0.001).[22] A direct association between MRSA carriage in animals and humans was also observed in a cross-sectional study in veal calf farming.[23] This is remarkable, because the MRSA prevalence among animals is expected to vary

Table 2.1 Prevalence of nasal MRSA carriage found in different occupational group surveys across the world

Occupational group	Country	Population size	MRSA carrier %	ST398 carrier %	Comment
Pig farmers	Netherlands[6]	26	23	23	Captive sample
Pig farmers	Netherlands[25]	50	0.3		
Pig farmers	Belgium[22]	127	37.8	37.8	Relation with MRSA in animals
Pig farmers	Germany[26]	113		86	
Pig workers	US[13]	20	45	45	
Pig farmers, slaughterhouse workers, veterinarians	Ireland[27]	100	2	0	
Pig farmers	Netherlands[a]	110[b]	80	Predominant	
Pig farmers	Canada[28]	25	5		Relation with MRSA in animals
Veal farmers	Netherlands[23]	97	33	>29	Relation with MRSA in animals
Veal farmers	Netherlands[c]	58[b]	41		
Veterinarians	Mainly US[29]	345	7	0	
Veterinarians	Mainly Europe[30]	235	14	13.1	
Veterinarians, livestock farmers, veterinary students, assistants	Denmark[31]	725 total 231 vets	1.5 3.9	0.006 1.3	
Veterinarians	Czech Republic[32]	280	0.7	0	
Veterinarians	Belgium[33]	146	9.5	7.5	
Veterinarians	Denmark[33]	143	1.4	1.4	
Veterinarians, laboratory workers, meat inspection personnel	Germany[12]	86		23	
Pig slaughterhouse workers	Netherlands[34]	249	5.6		
Pig slaughterhouse workers	Netherlands[35]	341	3.2	2.4	Detailed exposure assessment included

(Continued)

Table 2.1 *(Continued)*

Occupational group	Country	Population size	MRSA carrier %	ST398 carrier %	Comment
Poultry slaughter house workers	Netherlands[36]	466	5.6	Predominant	
Hospital personnel	Netherlands[37]	853	0.23	0.12[d]	10-fold higher risk in individuals with direct animal contact (NS[e])

[a] data from Van Cleef BA et al., *Dynamics of MRSA carriage in pig farmers: a prospective cohort study*, unpublished paper, Copyright © 2013

[b] Sampled on multiple occasions, persistent and intermittent carriers grouped together

[c] data from Dorado-Garcia A et al., *Determinants for persistent livestock-associated MRSA carriage in veal calf farmers and their family members*, unpublished paper, Copyright © 2013

[d] Two positive samples were found, one was non-typeable, the other one did not survive storage and could not be typed

[e] NS = not statistically significant

due to the production system in which an all-in all-out system is applied, and thus all calves are replaced on a regular basis. Interestingly, the prevalence among veal calves was dependent on the contact intensity between animals, which varies with their age and development, and is low when young animals are brought in and housed in individual sections, compared to later in life when they have group housing.[24]

Veterinarians are also frequently in direct contact with livestock, and are clearly at elevated risk of LA-MRSA carriage when compared to the general population. The average nasal LA-MRSA carriage prevalence in slaughterhouse workers is lower than in livestock farmers, and decreases along the slaughter line.[34-36] Contact with live animals is the prominent risk factor for MRSA carriage among slaughterhouse personnel. Although meat samples may be MRSA positive, the level of contamination does not seem sufficient to lead to nasal carriage. Prevalence of MRSA-positive surface wipe samples and air levels are highest at the start of the slaughter process.[34] Thus, slaughterhouses are low LA-MRSA contamination working environments, when compared to livestock farms.

Of all LA-MRSA carrying individuals, a fraction appear to be persistent carriers.[38] After repeatedly sampling veal farmers and their family members before, during, and after a period of no animal contact (either a holiday or the empty-barn period between two production cycles) only 7% of the participants were persistent carriers, with the majority (58%) being intermittent carriers.[38] Among pig farmers, the number of persistent carriers is higher and estimated at around 40%, with a similar number of intermittent carriers.[30] According to a recent study which applied similar methodology, again the numbers appeared lower for veal farmers, 16% and 26% for persistent and intermittent carriage respectively.[29] LA-MRSA carriage was frequently detected in field workers immediately after short-term occupational exposure consisting of the collection of nasal samples from pigs and veal calves. The majority of these field workers tested negative 24 hours later.[39] These observations lead to the suggestion that carriage in farmers may, at least in part, be the result of repeated exposure instead of true colonization. A clear exposure-response relation has been observed between the number of hours of animal contact and nasal MRSA ST398 carriage.

Few studies have examined transmission from humans to humans. Generally, studies among family members of livestock farmers show a considerably lower prevalence than among the farmers with more intense animal contact. Nevertheless, a positive association between MRSA carrier status of family members and MRSA carriage of the farmer (highly exposed people) is demonstrated in veal farming.[40] LA-MRSA is approximately six times less transmissible than hospital-acquired MRSA.[41,42] However, human-to-human transmission rates outside hospital settings could be different. Farmers usually belong to a healthy population (as compared to hospitalized patients with non-ST398 MRSA) and they may therefore be less likely to transmit the pathogen to other individuals. Studies in pig- and poultry-dense areas show that transmission through air in the general environment is unlikely. Individuals who are ST398 carriers in the general population usually have direct animal contact.[43,44] On the other hand, the emergence of ST398 isolates without known risk factors for acquisition and without a link to livestock has been reported.[45] In addition, a human-specific ST398 clone has recently been identified and thus the spread of LA-MRSA from occupational populations to the general population cannot be ruled out.[46] Transmission dynamics, especially between humans not directly exposed to animals, remain unclear and might be changing. Recently, a meta-population model has been published which describes the capacity of MRSA ST398 to spread in humans, from occupationally exposed populations to the general population.[47] A stochastic, discrete-time meta-population model was used to explore the effect of varying both the probability of persistent carriage and that of acquiring MRSA due to contact with pigs on the transmission dynamics of MRSA ST398 in humans, using population structure information from Norfolk, UK. The key determinants of the basic reproduction ratio R_0 for MRSA ST398 were explored. Simulations showed that the presence of recurrent exposures to pigs in risk populations may allow MRSA ST398 to persist in the meta-population and transmission events to occur beyond the farming community, even when the probability of persistent carriage is low. When persistent carriage is below 10%, spread to the general population is not likely. These results indicate that implementing a control policy that only targets human carriers may not be sufficient to control MRSA ST398 in the community if it remains present in animals, especially against the background of recent observations of a high prevalence of (persistent) MRSA ST398 carriage in pig farmers. More refined modelling approaches are needed that include the most recent information from epidemiological association studies.

So far, MRSA ST398 does not appear to be highly infectious for humans, although the epidemiological information is limited so far, but several case reports have been published involving skin lesions, bacteraemia, endocarditis, and ventilator-associated pneumonia in hospital patients.[16,48–53] There is anecdotal information on skin infections in pig farmers, but the population studied is too small for firm conclusions.[22]

The role of LA-MRSA air exposure

Transmission through air seems an important route and might explain differences in prevalence between populations. Quantification of LA-MRSA exposure was first conducted in a study in three Dutch pig slaughterhouses, by means of a quantitative culture method on air filter samples and glove rinse samples.[35] Three quantitative polymerase chain reactions (PCRs) were used to measure three targets in these samples. Each individual marker has limitations and is not specific for MRSA ST398. The *mecA* gene determines methicillin resistance of MRSA, but can also be present in coagulase-negative staphylococcal species. The SSC*mec* real-time PCR (qPCR) detects both *S. aureus* and SCC*mec*, but the latter is highly variable and needs several probes. Lastly, the ST398-specific PCR does not distinguish between resistant and sensitive *S. aureus* ST398. Therefore, a combination of the three qPCRs was deemed necessary. Personal air samples were collected in the breathing zone with conventional personal sampling equipment. Exposure was detectable only in areas where the prevalence in workers was highest: lairage and scalding/dehairing areas.[35] Results were confirmed by culture results. Gloves were sampled as proxy for the hand-to-mouth transmission route. The higher glove qPCR results were mainly found in the lairage and slaughter areas, decreasing towards negative at the end of the slaughter line. The low environmental contamination at the end of the slaughterhouse process does not seem to contribute to carriage among the workers. And the fact that a negligible prevalence is found among workers at this stage of the process indicates that human-human transmission risk must be very low as well.

In studies among pig and veal farmers, LA-MRSA was detected in active air samples, collected in the sties or byres in parallel to measuring prevalence in the animals.[24] These repeated samples showed that the higher the LA-MRSA prevalence in veal calves, the higher the LA-MRSA load detected in air samples.

Most exposure information comes from studies in which LA-MRSA was detected in settled dust on veal and pig farms by means of electrostatic dust cloths (EDCs), a passive static sampling method for dust. Analysis of EDCs by qPCR has shown that the average amount of colony-forming unit equivalents per EDC on veal farms is much lower than on pig farms (Table 2.2).

Pig farmers on average have a considerably higher prevalence (~60%) of nasal MRSA carriage than veal farmers (~30%), which correlates with the difference in

Table 2.2 Average number of colony-forming unit equivalents per electrostatic dust collector (EDC) based on qPCR

Origin of EDCs	*S. aureus*	MRSA	MSSA ST398	MRSA ST398
Pig housing (n = 457)	441.9	386.5	1281.8	217.4
Veal calf housing (n = 391)	38.4	35.9	47.0	12.8

Source: data from Van Cleef BA et al., *Dynamics of MRSA carriage in pig farmers: a prospective cohort study*, unpublished paper, Copyright © 2013 and Dorado-Garcia A et al., *Determinants for persistent livestock-associated MRSA carriage in veal calf farmers and their family members*, unpublished paper, Copyright © 2013.

dust levels and MRSA dust exposure levels (unpublished data). This, together with the information from slaughterhouse studies and observations among family members, suggests that transmission through air (inhalation of dust particles containing MRSA) is the major transmission route for these highly exposed occupations. These results emphasize the need to keep exposure as low as possible by reducing the load at the source, livestock and their environment, by thorough cleaning and disinfection of animal housing and reducing the prevalence among animals.

ESBL microbial resistance in livestock farming

Enterobacteriaceae that produce ESBLs are an emerging concern in public health. ESBLs inactivate beta-lactam antimicrobials by hydrolysis and therefore cause resistance to various beta-lactam antimicrobials, including penicillins and cephalosporins.[54] The major ESBL-producing bacteria involved in human infections are *Escherichia coli* and *Klebsiella pneumoniae*.[55] Many different ESBL genes exist. The most common ESBL genes belong to the TEM, SHV, and CTX-M families.[56] CTX-M type ESBLs have been predominant in humans in the past 10 years. More specifically, CTX-M-15 is the most common type reported in humans globally, followed by CTX-M-14.[57] The genes encoding for ESBLs are often located on plasmids which can be transferred between different bacterial species. Also, coexistence with other types of antimicrobial resistance occurs. In humans, infections with ESBL-producing Enterobacteriaceae are associated with increased burden of disease and costs.[58]

A variety of ESBLs have been identified in bacteria derived from food-producing animals worldwide. The occurrence of different ESBL types depends on the animal species and the geographical area. In Europe, CTX-M-1 is common in poultry, cattle, and pigs but, in Asia, mainly CTX-M-14 is reported in poultry, and other types of the CTX-M family (CTX-M-2, CTX-M-14, and CTX-M-15) are reported in cattle and pigs.[57]

High use of antimicrobials and inappropriate use of cephalosporins in livestock production are considered to be associated with the emergence and high prevalence of ESBL-producers in the animals.[59,60] Food-producing animals can serve as a reservoir for ESBL producing Enterobacteriaceae and ESBL genes. Transmission from animals to humans can theoretically occur through different routes. ESBL genes have been determined in isolates from meat samples.[61,62] A degree of similarity in ESBL genes, plasmids, and *E. coli* genotypes found in humans and retail chicken is suggestive for transmission through the food chain.[8] Although it is known that antimicrobial-resistant Enterobacteriaceae can be transmitted from live animals to humans, there is only limited evidence for the transmission of ESBL-producing Enterobacteriaceae directly from animals to humans.[63] In Denmark, transmission from CTX-M-1 encoding plasmids was reported between pigs and farm workers.[64] In the Netherlands, a high prevalence of ESBL genes was found in all broiler farms studied and on one-third of farmers.[65] Compared to a reported 5% ESBL carriage in patients in the southern part of the Netherlands, a higher risk for people working with poultry is indicated.[62] These recent findings suggest that transmission from animals to humans may occur through (in)direct contact with livestock during work. This may thus pose an occupational health risk for farmers and potentially for other humans with regular contact with this working population. Currently, data on the distribution of ESBL genes in pigs and people working with pigs in the Netherlands are being collected. Preliminary results show that there is a strong association between ESBL carriage in pig farmers and ESBL occurrence on the farm. Also, ESBL gene types determined in farmers corresponded to those detected in pigs on their farm.

Compared to MRSA, the dynamics of ESBLs seem more complex. Hospitalization and international travel are known risk factors, as for MRSA.[66,67] There are many potential reservoirs of significance for humans which contribute to the risk of becoming an ESBL carrier. Besides ESBLs in livestock, ESBL-producing Enterobacteriaceae have been reported in companion animals[65] and wildlife.[68] Next to animal-derived food products, other food products such as vegetables may be contaminated with ESBLs. Another potential reservoir is the environment; ESBLs have been detected in drinking water[69] and sewage.[70] The variety of potential ESBL transmission routes makes it complex to determine the role of direct contact with livestock as an occupational risk for ESBL carriage. However, the increasing occurrence of ESBLs in livestock worldwide and the emerging insight into transmission through direct contact suggests that farmers have a higher risk of becoming a carrier of ESBLs. Until now, there have not been sufficient data available to quantify the relevant importance of this route of transmission. In addition, there are more possibilities for exchange of genetic information than have been described for MRSA because, for instance, plasmids, mobile genetic elements, can code for ESBLs. Identification of ESBL-producing Enterobacteriaceae, ESBL genes, and plasmids in humans and animals living in close contact should provide further insights. The health risk emerging from being an ESBL carrier has so far not been estimated for any working (farmer) population.

Conclusions

These examples show that microbial resistance is becoming a major issue for occupational health professionals. Occupational health and hygiene expertise can contribute to reducing the prevalence among livestock farmers and other exposed individuals. Vaccination of livestock has been suggested as a means to eradicate MRSA among livestock, but vaccines are not yet available. Other approaches have to be considered which contribute to a lower prevalence among animals, such as reduction of the use of antimicrobials in combination with reducing transmission from animals to humans. MRSA prevalence is low among animals from alternative breeding systems with low use of antimicrobials, also leading to low carriage rates in farmers.[71] There seems room for a contribution from the expertise of occupational health specialists in reducing airborne exposure as an important transmission route. In addition, present 'search and destroy' strategies may stigmatize and isolate livestock farming populations. Common occupational hygiene approaches may help to keep the farming community on board and reduce the prevalence which, in turn, reduces the risk for the general population. Integrated approaches are required to reduce the burden of antimicrobial resistance in occupationally exposed livestock-producing communities.

References

1. Quinn PJ, Markey BK, Carter ME, Donnelly WJ, Leonard FC. *Veterinary microbiology and microbial disease.* Oxford: Blackwell Science, 2002.

2. Scanvic A, Denic L, Gaillon S, Giry P, Andremont A, Lucet JC. Duration of colonization by methicillin-resistant Staphylococcus aureus after hospital discharge and risk factors for prolonged carriage. *Clin Infect Dis* 2001;**32**:1393–8.

3. Gorwitz RJ, Kruszon-Moran D, McAllister SK, *et al.* Changes in the prevalence of nasal colonization with Staphylococcus aureus in the United States, 2001–2004. *J Infect Dis* 2008;**197**:1226–34.

4. Finch R, Hunter PA. Antibiotic resistance—action to promote new technologies: report of an EU Intergovernmental Conference held in Birmingham, UK, 12–13 December 2005. *J Antimicrob Chemother* 2006;**58**(Suppl 1):i3–22.

5. Swartz MN. Human diseases caused by foodborne pathogens of animal origin. *Clin Infect Dis* 2002;**34**(Suppl 3):S111–22.

6. Voss A, Loeffen F, Bakker J, Klaassen C, Wulf M. Methicillin-resistant Staphylococcus aureus in pig farming. *Emerg Infect Dis* 2005;**11**:1965–6.

7. Armand-Lefevre L, Ruimy R, Andremont A. Clonal comparison of Staphylococcus aureus isolates from healthy pig farmers, human controls, and pigs. *Emerg Infect Dis* 2005;**11**:711–4.

8. Huijsdens XW, van Dijke BJ, Spalburg E, *et al.* Community-acquired MRSA and pig-farming. *Ann Clin Microbiol Antimicrob* 2006;**5**:26. doi: 10.1186/1476-0711-5-26.

9. Tiemersma EW, Bronzwaer SL, Lyytikäinen O, *et al.* Methicillin-resistant Staphylococcus aureus in Europe, 1999–2002. *Emerg Infect Dis* 2004;**10**:1627–34.

10. Kluytmans JA. Methicillin-resistant Staphylococcus aureus in food products: cause for concern or case for complacency? *Clin Microbiol Infect* 2010;**16**:11–5.

11. Guardabassi L, Stegger M, Skov R. Retrospective detection of methicillin resistant and susceptible Staphylococcus aureus ST398 in Danish slaughter pigs. *Vet Microbiol* 2007;**122**:384–6.

12. Meemken D, Cuny C, Witte W, Eichler U, Staudt R, Blaha T. [Occurrence of MRSA in pigs and in humans involved in pig production—preliminary results of a study in the northwest of Germany.] *Dtsch Tierarzt Wochensch* 2008;**115**:132–9. [Article in German, English abstract.]

13. Smith TC, Male MJ, Harper AL, *et al.* Methicillin-resistant Staphylococcus aureus (MRSA) strain ST398 is present in midwestern U.S. swine and swine workers. *PloS One* 2009;**4**:e4258. doi: 10.1371/journal.pone.0004258.

14. Catry B, Van Duijkeren E, Pomba MC, *et al.* Reflection paper on MRSA in food-producing and companion animals: epidemiology and control options for human and animal health. *Epidemiol Infect* 2010;**138**:626–44.

15. Aarestrup FM. Veterinary drug usage and antimicrobial resistance in bacteria of animal origin. *Basic Clin Pharmacol Toxicol* 2005;**96**:271–81.

16. van Belkum A, Melles DC, Peeters JK, *et al.* Methicillin-resistant and -susceptible Staphylococcus aureus sequence type 398 in pigs and humans. *Emerg Infect Dis* 2008;**14**:479–83.

17. Wagenaar JA, Yue H, Pritchard J, *et al.* Unexpected sequence types in livestock associated methicillin-resistant Staphylococcus aureus (MRSA): MRSA ST9 and a single locus variant of ST9 in pig farming in China. *Vet Microbiol* 2009;**139**:405–9.

18. Price LB, Stegger M, Hasman H, *et al*. Staphylococcus aureus CC398: host adaptation and emergence of methicillin resistance in livestock. *MBio* 2012;**3**. doi: 10.1128/mBio.00305-11.

19. Pinho MG, de Lencastre H, Tomasz A. An acquired and a native penicillin-binding protein cooperate in building the cell wall of drug-resistant staphylococci. *Proc Natl Acad Sci U S A* 2001;**98**:10886–91.

20. Welinder-Olsson C, Florén-Johansson K, Larsson L, Oberg S, Karlsson L, Ahrén C. Infection with Panton-Valentine leukocidin-positive methicillin-resistant Staphylococcus aureus t034. *Emerg Infect Dis* 2008;**14**:1271–2.

21. van Loo I, Huijsdens X, Tiemersma E, *et al*. Emergence of methicillin-resistant Staphylococcus aureus of animal origin in humans. *Emerg Infect Dis* 2007;**13**:1834–9.

22. Denis O, Suetens C, Hallin M, *et al*. Methicillin-resistant Staphylococcus aureus ST398 in swine farm personnel, Belgium. *Emerg Infect Dis* 2009;**15**:1098–101.

23. Graveland H, Wagenaar JA, Heesterbeek H, Mevius D, van Duijkeren E, Heederik D. Methicillin resistant Staphylococcus aureus ST398 in veal calf farming: human MRSA carriage related with animal antimicrobial usage and farm hygiene. *PloS One* 2010;**5**:e10990. doi: 10.1371/journal.pone.0010990.

24. Graveland H, Wagenaar JA, Verstappen KM, Oosting-van Schothorst I, Heederik DJ, Bos ME. Dynamics of MRSA carriage in veal calves: a longitudinal field study. *Prev Vet Med* 2012;**107**:180–6.

25. van den Broek IVF, van Cleef BAGL, Haenen A, *et al*. Methicillin-resistant Staphylococcus aureus in people living and working in pig farms. *Epidemiol Infect* 2009;**137**:700–8.

26. Cuny C, Nathaus R, Layer F, Strommenger B, Altmann D, Witte W. Nasal colonization of humans with methicillin-resistant Staphylococcus aureus (MRSA) CC398 with and without exposure to pigs. *PloS One* 2009;**4**:e6800. doi: 10.1371/journal.pone.0006800.

27. Horgan M, Abbott Y, Lawlor PG, *et al*. A study of the prevalence of methicillin-resistant Staphylococcus aureus in pigs and in personnel involved in the pig industry in Ireland. *Vet J* 2011;**190**:255–9.

28. Khanna T, Friendship R, Dewey C, Weese JS. Methicillin resistant Staphylococcus aureus colonization in pigs and pig farmers. *Vet Microbiol* 2008;**128**:298–303.

29. Hanselman BA, Kruth SA, Rousseau J, *et al*. Methicillin-resistant Staphylococcus aureus colonization in veterinary personnel. *Emerg Infect Dis* 2006;**12**:1933–8.

30. Wulf MW, Sørum M, van Nes A, *et al*. Prevalence of methicillin-resistant Staphylococcus aureus among veterinarians: an international study. *Clin Microbiol Infect* 2008;**14**:29–34.

31. Moodley A, Nightingale EC, Stegger M, Nielsen SS, Skov RL, Guardabassi L. High risk for nasal carriage of methicillin-resistant Staphylococcus aureus among Danish veterinary practitioners. *Scand J Work Environ Health* 2008;**34**:151–7.

32. Zemlicková H, Fridrichová M, Tyllová K, Jakubů V, Machová I. Carriage of methicillin-resistant Staphylococcus aureus in veterinary personnel. *Epidemiol Infect* 2009;**137**:1233–6.

33. Garcia-Graells C, Antoine J, Larsen J, Catry B, Skov R, Denis O. Livestock veterinarians at high risk of acquiring methicillin-resistant Staphylococcus aureus ST398. *Epidemiol Infect* 2012;**140**:383–9.

34. Van Cleef BA, Broens EM, Voss A, *et al*. High prevalence of nasal MRSA carriage in slaughterhouse workers in contact with live pigs in the Netherlands. *Epidemiol Infect* 2010;**138**:756–63.

35. Gilbert MJ, Bos ME, Duim B, *et al*. Livestock-associated MRSA ST398 carriage in pig slaughterhouse workers related to quantitative environmental exposure. *Occup Environ Med* 2012;**69**:472–8.

36. **Mulders MN, Haenen AP, Geenen PL,** *et al.* Prevalence of livestock-associated MRSA in broiler flocks and risk factors for slaughterhouse personnel in the Netherlands. *Epidemiol Infect* 2010;**138**:743–55.

37. **Wulf MW, Tiemersma E, Kluytmans J,** *et al.* MRSA carriage in healthcare personnel in contact with farm animals. *J Hosp Infect* 2008;**70**:186–90.

38. **Graveland H, Wagenaar JA, Bergs K, Heesterbeek H, Heederik D.** Persistence of livestock associated MRSA CC398 in humans is dependent on intensity of animal contact. *PloS One* 2011;**6**:e16830. doi: 10.1371/journal.pone.0016830.

39. **van Cleef BA, Graveland H, Haenen AP,** *et al.* Persistence of livestock-associated methicillin-resistant Staphylococcus aureus in field workers after short-term occupational exposure to pigs and veal calves. *J Clin Microbiol* 2011;**49**:1030–3.

40. **Graveland H, Duim B, van Duijkeren E, Heederik D, Wagenaar JA.** Livestock-associated methicillin-resistant Staphylococcus aureus in animals and humans. *Int J Med Microbiol* 2011;**301**:630–4.

41. **Bootsma MC, Wassenberg MW, Trapman P, Bonten MJ.** The nosocomial transmission rate of animal-associated ST398 meticillin-resistant Staphylococcus aureus. *J R Soc Interface* 2011;**8**:578–84.

42. **Wassenberg MW, Bootsma MC, Troelstra A, Kluytmans JA, Bonten MA.** Transmissibility of livestock-associated methicillin-resistant Staphylococcus aureus (ST398) in Dutch hospitals. *Clin Microbiol Infect* 2011;**17**:316–9.

43. **Bisdorff B, Scholhölter JL, Claussen K, Pulz M, Nowak D, Radon K.** MRSA-ST398 in livestock farmers and neighbouring residents in a rural area in Germany. *Epidemiol Infect* 2012;**140**:1800–8.

44. **van Cleef BA, Verkade EJ, Wulf MW,** *et al.* Prevalence of livestock-associated MRSA in communities with high pig-densities in the Netherlands. *PloS One* 2010;**5**:e9385. doi: 10.1371/journal.pone.0009385.

45. **Lekkerkerk WS, van de Sande-Bruinsma N, van der Sande MA,** *et al.* Emergence of MRSA of unknown origin in the Netherlands. *Clin Microbiol Infect* 2012;**18**:656–61.

46. **Uhlemann AC, Porcella SF, Trivedi S,** *et al.* Identification of a highly transmissible animal-independent Staphylococcus aureus ST398 clone with distinct genomic and cell adhesion properties. *MBio* 2012;**3**. doi: 10.1128/mBio.00027-12.

47. **Porphyre T, Giotis ES, Lloyd DH, Stärk KD.** A metapopulation model to assess the capacity of spread of meticillin-resistant Staphylococcus aureus ST398 in humans. *PloS One* 2012;**7**:e47504. doi: 10.1371/journal.pone.0047504.

48. **Ekkelenkamp MB, Sekkat M, Carpaij N, Troelstra A, Bonten MJ.** [Endocarditis due to meticillin-resistant Staphylococcus aureus originating from pigs.] *Ned Tijdschr Geneeskd* 2006;**150**:2442–7. [Article in Dutch, English abstract.]

49. **Yao D, Yu FY, Qin ZQ,** *et al.* Molecular characterization of Staphylococcus aureus isolates causing skin and soft tissue infections (SSTIs). *BMC Infect Dis* 2010;**10**:133. doi: 10.1186/1471-2334-10-133.

50. **Aspiroz C, Lozano C, Gilaberte Y, Zarazaga M, Aldea MJ, Torres C.** [Molecular characterisation of methicillin resistant Staphylococcus aureus strains ST398 in patients with skin infections and their relatives.] *Enferm Infecc Microbiol Clin* 2012;**30**:18–21. [Article in Spanish, English abstract.]

51. **Lozano C, Aspiroz C, Ara M, Gómez-Sanz E, Zarazaga M, Torres C.** Methicillin-resistant Staphylococcus aureus (MRSA) ST398 in a farmer with skin lesions and in pigs of his farm: clonal relationship and detection of lnu(A) gene. *Clin Microbiol Infect* 2011;**17**:923–7.

52. Lozano C, Aspiroz C, Charlez L, *et al.* Skin lesion by methicillin-resistant Staphylococcus aureus ST398-t1451 in a Spanish pig farmer: possible transmission from animals to humans. *Vector Borne Zoonotic Dis* 2011;**11**:605–7.

53. Witte W, Strommenger B, Stanek C, Cuny C. Methicillin-resistant Staphylococcus aureus ST398 in humans and animals, Central Europe. *Emerg Infect Dis* 2007;**13**:255–8.

54. Bush K, Jacoby GA. Updated functional classification of beta-lactamases. *Antimicrob Agents Chemother* 2010;**54**:969–76.

55. Pitout JD, Laupland KB. Extended-spectrum beta-lactamase-producing Enterobacteriaceae: an emerging public-health concern. *Lancet Infect Dis* 2008;**8**:159–66.

56. Smet A, Martel A, Persoons D, *et al.* Broad-spectrum beta-lactamases among Enterobacteriaceae of animal origin: molecular aspects, mobility and impact on public health. *FEMS Microbiol Rev* 2010;**34**:295–316.

57. Ewers C, Bethe A, Semmler T, Guenther S, Wieler LH. Extended-spectrum beta-lactamase-producing and AmpC-producing Escherichia coli from livestock and companion animals, and their putative impact on public health: a global perspective. *Clin Microbiol Infect* 2012;**18**:646–55.

58. Hawkey PM, Jones AM. The changing epidemiology of resistance. *J Antimicrob Chemother* 2009;**64**(Suppl 1):i3–10.

59. Dutil L, Irwin R, Finley R, *et al.* Ceftiofur resistance in Salmonella enterica serovar Heidelberg from chicken meat and humans, Canada. *Emerg Infect Dis* 2010;**16**:48–54.

60. Liebana E, Carattoli A, Coque TM, *et al.* The public health risks of enterobacterial isolates producing extended-spectrum beta-lactamases or AmpC beta-lactamases in food and food-producing animals: an EU perspective of epidemiology, analytical methods, risk factors, and control options. *Clin Infect Dis* 2013;**56**:1030–7.

61. Jouini A, Vinué L, Slama KB, *et al.* Characterization of CTX-M and SHV extended-spectrum beta-lactamases and associated resistance genes in Escherichia coli strains of food samples in Tunisia. *J Antimicrob Chemother* 2007;**60**:1137–41.

62. Overdevest I, Willemsen I, Rijnsburger M, *et al.* Extended-spectrum beta-lactamase genes of Escherichia coli in chicken meat and humans, the Netherlands. *Emerg Infect Dis* 2011;**17**:1216–22.

63. Levy SB, FitzGerald GB, Macone AB. Spread of antibiotic-resistant plasmids from chicken to chicken and from chicken to man. *Nature* 1976;**260**:40–2.

64. Moodley A, Guardabassi L. Transmission of IncN plasmids carrying blaCTX-M-1 between commensal Escherichia coli in pigs and farm workers. *Antimicrob Agents Chemother* 2009;**53**:1709–11.

65. Dierikx C, van der Goot J, Fabri T, van Essen-Zandbergen A, Smith H, Mevius D. Extended-spectrum-beta-lactamase- and AmpC-beta-lactamase-producing Escherichia coli in Dutch broilers and broiler farmers. *J Antimicrob Chemother* 2013;**68**:60–7.

66. Tängdén T, Cars O, Melhus A, Löwden E. Foreign travel is a major risk factor for colonization with Escherichia coli producing CTX-M-type extended-spectrum beta-lactamases: a prospective study with Swedish volunteers. *Antimicrob Agents Chemother* 2010;**54**:3564–8.

67. Ben-Ami R, Rodríguez-Baño J, Arslan H, *et al.* A multinational survey of risk factors for infection with extended-spectrum beta-lactamase-producing enterobacteriaceae in nonhospitalized patients. *Clin Infect Dis* 2009;**49**:682–90.

68. Guenther S, Ewers C, Wieler LH. Extended-spectrum beta-lactamases-producing E. coli in wildlife, yet another form of environmental pollution? *Front Microbiol* 2011;**2**:246. doi: 10.3389/fmicb.2011.00246.

69. **Xi C, Zhang Y, Marrs CF,** *et al.* Prevalence of antibiotic resistance in drinking water treatment and distribution systems. *Appl Environ Microbiol* 2009;**75**:5714–8.

70. **Mesa RJ, Blanc V, Blanch AR,** *et al.* Extended-spectrum beta-lactamase-producing Enterobacteriaceae in different environments (humans, food, animal farms and sewage). *J Antimicrob Chemother* 2006;**58**:211–5.

71. **Cuny C, Friedrich AW, Witte W.** Absence of livestock-associated methicillin-resistant staphylococcus aureus clonal complex CC398 as a nasal colonizer of pigs raised in an alternative system. *Appl Environ Microbiol* 2012;**78**:1296–7.

Chapter 3

The search for environmental risk factors for Parkinson disease

Harvey Checkoway, Susan Searles Nielsen, and Brad A. Racette

Introduction

Parkinson disease (PD), initially described by James Parkinson in 1817,[1] is a debilitating neurodegenerative disorder with motor, cognitive, and autonomic nervous system involvement. PD represents the most common severe form of the clinical syndrome of parkinsonism. The characteristic motor signs of PD are bradykinesia, muscle rigidity, gait disturbance, and postural instability.[2] These signs are due to loss of dopaminergic neurons predominantly in the midbrain substantia nigra, evidenced by Lewy bodies and neurites, which are the signature features detected at autopsy.[3] The vast majority of cases are diagnosed clinically; several accepted disease classification schemes, such as the UK Brain Bank criteria,[4] are commonly invoked for diagnostic accuracy in epidemiological research. A 30–50% excess incidence in men compared to women has been a consistent observation in most populations. PD is very rare under age 50, but incidence rates increase dramatically up to the eighth decade of life. PD incidence and prevalence vary considerably by race, ethnicity, and geography, with highest rates observed among Caucasians and Hispanics.[5,6] PD prevalence is approximately 2% among persons aged 65 and older, and is expected to increase in many countries as the world population ages.[7]

Despite extensive toxicological and epidemiological research, the causes of PD remain largely unexplained. Mendelian inheritance accounts for a very small fraction of cases (~5–10%).[8] Consequently, environmental factors, including those in the workplace and the ambient environment, various medications, and lifestyle factors, such as smoking and diet, are presumed to account for the vast majority of PD incidence.[9] Environmental exposures may interact with genetic factors, but very few specific gene/environment interactions have been observed consistently.

One of the first aetiological clues regarding an environmental risk factor came from Couper's 1837 case series description of five Scottish ore crushers who developed clinical parkinsonism associated with overexposure to manganese.[10] An association between manganese poisoning and signs of parkinsonism was subsequently corroborated by Rodier[11] in his survey of Moroccan miners. We will return to possible causal links between manganese and PD later in this chapter in the discussion of metals as potential risk factors. Virtually no other aetiological insights emerged following Parkinson's initial clinical description until the recognition of a parkinsonian-like syndrome (Von Economo's encephalitis) among survivors of the Spanish influenza in 1917.[12] It was even thought that PD would disappear once the survivor cohort had died. However, it was eventually determined that Von Economo's encephalitis was not, in fact, PD, but rather a reversible encephalitic condition that shared some similar features. In the late 1970s, convincing evidence for a role of environmental determinants of PD derived from a cluster of six cases of irreversible parkinsonism among Northern California intravenous drug abusers who had injected a meperidine analogue contaminated with 1-methyl-4-phenyl-1,2,3,6-tetrahydropyridine (MPTP).[13] Experimental research subsequently established that the active metabolite of MPTP, 1-methyl-4-phenylpyridinium (MPP+), induced parkinsonism in rodents and non-human primates. Those observations, coupled with the recognition of the structural similarity of MPP+ to the herbicide paraquat, prompted extensive toxicological and epidemiological research on pesticides.[14]

Epidemiological associations with PD

Lifestyle factors

Epidemiological research on aetiological factors has involved investigations of factors that appear either to increase or reduce risk. Among the latter, cigarette smoking has been the most prominent and consistently observed 'protective' factor. PD risk among ever smokers is roughly half that of never smokers, and numerous studies have detected dose-response relations with duration, intensity, and pack-years smoked.[15] The explanation for the inverse risk relation with smoking remains elusive, however. Selective survival to older ages among non-smokers does not explain this phenomenon.[16] Alternative hypotheses that remain to be confirmed or refuted include neuroprotection due to nicotine and perhaps other components of cigarette smoke, or a 'premorbid personality' type related to risk avoidance among persons who eventually develop PD. Some additional support for a direct neuroprotective effect of nicotine is provided by observations that environmental tobacco smoke is also associated with reduced PD risk, especially among persons who were never active smokers.[17] Caffeine intake and use of non-steroidal anti-inflammatory medications have also been associated with reduced PD risks, although not as consistently as smoking.[9] No other dietary factors are clearly associated with PD.

Environmental exposures

Characterizing underlying pathogenesis mechanisms remains an important area of toxicological research, findings from which are clearly helpful in guiding epidemiological research and interpreting observations. Although no one predominant mechanism has been established, there is strong evidence that nigral system toxicity that ultimately culminates in PD results from the complex interactions between oxidative stress, inflammation, and abnormal aggregation and removal of various proteins, especially alpha synuclein, a major component of Lewy bodies.[18]

In the following sections, we will summarize epidemiological evidence for associations with environmental exposures. We will focus on the exposures that, owing to their widespread occurrence and biological plausibility, have been investigated most often: pesticides, metals, and solvents. The intention is not to be comprehensive, but rather to highlight important epidemiological findings, especially those for which there is supportive clinical or toxicological evidence.

Pesticides

The MPTP episode focused considerable attention on pesticides, starting with paraquat. Animal models of PD induction have been established for the combination of the herbicide paraquat and the manganese-containing fungicide maneb,[19] and for rotenone, an 'organic' insecticide.[20] A summary of findings from some of the major epidemiological investigations of pesticides and PD conducted since 2000 is provided in Table 3.1. Associations with insecticides and herbicides have been examined most frequently, largely in the context of population-based case-control studies[21–27]; there have also been some cohort studies.[28,29] As can be seen from Table 3.1, the findings are heterogeneous, no doubt due to great variability in the chemical specificity that was permitted by various approaches to assess exposures. The majority of studies have been population-based case-control studies in which pesticide exposures were based on questionnaire self-reports, and were categorized into broad groupings of insecticides, herbicides, or other (e.g. fungicides). There are, however, some studies in which chemical-specific exposure data were derived to test toxicologically based hypotheses, suggesting elevated risks related to a combination of paraquat and maneb[25] and to rotenone.[27] There is limited evidence for other specific pesticides, although exposure misclassification may contribute to under-estimated associations.

Metals

Some metals, including manganese, lead, and mercury, are widespread occupational and environmental exposures with well-established neurotoxic properties.[30] Consequently, metals have been a focus of PD aetiological research. Manganese has been of particular concern as a potential PD risk factor, largely prompted by the long recognition of the clinical similarities of manganism and PD. Metals have been examined as risk factors in numerous population-based case-control studies, several community surveys, and in cohort studies of welders. Associations with manganese and other metals from population-based case-control studies have been mostly weak or null,[31] in large part due to the relative infrequency of exposures in the general population and ambiguities of exposure assessment. An exception is a study from Michigan[32] that indicated relative risks in the range of 2.5–10.6 for manganese and various combinations of metals (e.g. lead with copper), although statistical precision was low. Several ecological studies of manganese levels in air emissions or soil concentrations also suggest associations with PD.[33–35]

Welders have been a target study group because of their common and relatively high exposures to manganese. The evidence for a causal relation from studies of welders has been mixed[36–42] (see Table 3.2 for a summary). It is noteworthy that diagnostic methods and exposure assessment approaches among welder studies have been

Table 3.1 Epidemiological studies of PD and pesticide exposures

Study (year)	Location	Design No. of subjects	Exposure assessment method	Main findings
Ascherio et al. (2006)[28]	US	Cohort 143 325 (413 PD cases)	Questionnaire	Pesticides: 1.7 (1.2–2.3)[a]
Kamel et al. (2007)[29]	US	Cohort 55 931 (78 PD cases)	Questionnaire for specific pesticides (type, frequency, duration of use)	Cumulative use all pesticides >397 days: 2.3 (1.2–4.5)
Dick et al. (2007)[21]	5 European countries	Case-control 767 cases, 1989 controls	Job/exposure matrix applied to questionnaire data	'high' vs.no pesticide exposure: 1.4 (1.0–1.9)
Brighina et al. (2008)[22]	US	Case-control 833 cases, 833 controls	Questionnaire	Age <60: Pesticides: 1.8 (1.1–2.9) Herbicides: 2.5 (1.3–4.5)
Hancock et al. (2008)[23]	US	Case-control 319 cases, 296 controls	Questionnaire for specific pesticides (type, frequency, duration of use)	Negative family history of PD: Pesticides cumulative use >179 days: 3.3 (1.8–5.7)
Elbaz et al. (2009)[24]	France	Case-control 224 cases, 557 controls	Questionnaire for specific pesticides (type, frequency, duration of use); expert assessment	Men: Organochlorine insecticides: 2.4 (1.2–5.0)
Costello et al. (2009)[25]	US	Case-control 368 cases, 341 controls	Graphical Information System mapping of pesticide use reporting data	Age <60: Paraquat + maneb: 5.1 (1.8–14.7)
Tanner et al. (2009)[26]	US, Canada	Case-control 511 cases, 511 controls	Questionnaires, Classification of Standard Occupational Job Codes	Pesticides: 1.9 (1.1–3.2) 2,4 Dichlorophenoxyacetic acid: 2.6 (1.0–6.5) Paraquat: 2.8 (0.8–9.7)
Tanner et al. (2011)[27]	US	Nested case-control study	Questionnaire for specific pesticides (type, frequency, duration of use)	Rotenone: 2.5 (1.3–4.7) Paraquat: 2.5 (1.4–4.7)

[a] Relative risk estimate (95% confidence interval)

heterogeneous, which precludes simple conclusions regarding manganese specifically, or welding occupation more broadly. Although PD and manganism share some clinical features, pathological and neuroimaging studies suggest that they may be different phenotypes.[43]

Table 3.2 Cohort studies of PD and parkinsonism among welders

Study (year)	Location	Cohort size	PD outcome	Exposure assessment; reference group	Main findings
Racette et al. (2005)[36]	US	1423	Neurological examination	Welder occupation type; community survey in Alabama	Overall: 7.6 (3.3–17.7)[a] Boilermakers: 10.3 (2.6–40.5)
Fryzek et al. (2005)[37]	Denmark	6163	Hospitalization	Welder occupation; national rates	Overall: 0.9 (0.4–1.8) Employed >20 yrs: 0.8 (0.2–2.0)
Fored et al. (2006)[38]	Sweden	49 488	Hospitalization, mortality	Welder occupation; national rates	0.9 (0.8–1.0)
Marsh and Gula (2006)[39]	US	12 595[b]	Medical insurance claims	Welding job title; controls without PD	Overall: 1.0 (0.3–2.3) >30 yrs welding: 1.0 (0.3–1.6)
Park et al. (2006)[40]	S. Korea	38 560	Hospitalization billing claims	Welding job title classified by airborne manganese levels; non-exposed white collar workers	Low exposure: 3.6 (0.7–18.6) High exposure: 2.0 (0.3–12.5)
Stampfer et al. (2009)[41]	US	107 773	Mortality	Welder occupation on death certificate; other occupations	0.9 (0.8–0.9)
Racette et al. (2012)[42]	US	811	Neurological examination	Weighted welding hours; non-welders	16% welders, 0% non-welders; Highest exposed: 1.0 (0.6–1.6)

[a] Relative risk estimate (95% confidence interval)
[b] Nested case-control study of 66 incident cases and 660 controls

Solvents

Solvents are another class of compounds that are commonly used in industry, are widespread workplace and environmental contaminants, and have a range of neurotoxic properties. Here again, findings from most epidemiological studies have indicated weak or null associations[44–49] (see Table 3.3 for a summary) that often fail to

Table 3.3 Epidemiological studies of PD and solvent exposures

Study	Location	Design No. of subjects	Exposure assessment method	Main findings
McDonnell et al. (2003)[44]	UK	Nested case-control 182 cases, 423 controls	Job title	Overall: 1.5 (0.8–2.9)[a] >30 yrs welded: 3.6 (1.3–10.3)
Park et al. (2005)[45]	US	Proportional mortality 33 678	Usual occupation on death certificate	1.1 (1.0–1.1)
Ascherio et al. (2006)[28]	US	Cohort 143 325 (413 cases)	Questionnaire	0.8 (0.5–1.2)
Dick et al. (2007)[21]	5 European countries	Case-control 767 cases, 1089 controls	Job-exposure matrix applied to questionnaire data	Low: 1.2 (0.9–1.6) High: 0.9 (0.7–1.2)
Petersen et al. (2008)[46]	Faroe Islands	Case-control 79 cases, 154 controls	Questionnaire	1.7 (0.8–3.5)
Firestone et al. (2010)[47]	US	Case-control 404 cases, 526 controls	Questionnaire, classified by industrial hygienists	Men: 1.0 (0.7–1.3) Women: 1.7 (1.0–3.0)
Feldman et al. (2011)[48]	Sweden	Cohort (Swedish twin registry)	Questionnaire, classified by job-exposure matrix	Any: 0.9 (0.7–1.3) Highest exposed: 1.4 (0.6–2.9)
Goldman et al. (2012)[49]	US	Nested case-control study (twin registry) 99 cases, 99 controls	Questionnaire, classified by industrial hygienists	Trichloroethylene: 6.1 (1.2–33) Perchloroethylene: 10.5 (1.0–113) Toluene: 1.3 (0.5–3.3)

[a] Relative risk estimate (95% confidence interval)

identify exposures to either specific compounds or classes (e.g. aliphatic versus aromatic). A notable exception is a study of twins demonstrating apparently elevated risks associated with exposures to trichloroethylene and tetrachloroethylene.[49] Some prior case reports of PD among trichloroethylene-exposed workers also provide support for a possible aetiological link.[50]

Discussion and recommendations

The aetiology of PD continues to be elusive, suggesting that multiple environmental exposures may play aetiological roles individually or synergistically. It seems quite likely that no single factor, with the exception of cigarette smoking, accounts for a substantial portion of PD incidence. It should also be appreciated that PD is a complex disease and, in fact, may represent multiple distinct diseases that share common clinical and pathological features. Consequently, identifying environmental risk factors with large attributable risks may not be a realistic goal.

Selection of risk factors

Toxicological research that elucidates disease pathogenesis mechanisms has helped to sharpen epidemiological research focus, exemplified by relatively strong epidemiological results for paraquat[25] and rotenone,[27] and suggestive findings for some chlorinated solvents.[49] Guidance from mechanistically based toxicological research should continue to be valuable, but should not constrain exploration of other risk factors. The emergence of the exposome concept, wherein biochemical assays of biospecimens can reveal a broad spectrum of current and past environmental exposures may have applicability in PD epidemiological research, especially where sequential biospecimens have been obtained at critical life junctures.[51]

There are environmental agents, other than those highlighted here, that deserve further consideration due to their widespread occurrence, and plausible aetiological links with PD. For example, there is some epidemiological evidence for elevated risks related to exposures to various persistent organic pollutants, such as polychlorinated biphenyls, which are widespread in many environmental settings.[30] Another agent deserving of more investigation is endotoxin (lipopolysaccharide), which is produced by Gram-negative bacteria. There is a relatively convincing animal model of endotoxin-induced parkinsonism in which the underlying mechanism is considered to be neuroinflammation leading to nigral system damage.[52] Endotoxin is a contaminant of particulates in indoor and outdoor environments, especially in some occupational settings involving exposures to cotton dust, animal farming, and sewage treatment. Epidemiological research explicitly testing the hypothesis that endotoxin causes or contributes to PD risk has thus far been very limited, but could be a productive area for further investigation.

Study design considerations

The majority of epidemiological research on PD and environmental exposures has been conducted in the context of population-based case-control studies. This design has the well-known advantages of convenient accrual of large case numbers and, typically, direct contact with study subjects or proxy respondents to conduct interviews, and opportunities to obtain biological specimens for molecular studies. However, these advantages can be offset by severe limitations. In some instances, environmental factors have not been the principal focus, and consequently, the quality of exposure data is inadequate for hypothesis testing. Often, exposures to specific agents are rare in the general population or not identifiable by study subjects. Case-control studies conducted in areas with relatively high frequency of exposures of interest, such as the study of pesticides in the Central Valley of California,[25] are most appropriate for testing specific hypotheses.

Identifying incident, rather than prevalent, PD cases is a desirable goal, but can be complicated because PD, like many chronic disorders, can have a prolonged pre-diagnostic interval. Moreover, diagnostic accuracy will vary greatly depending on access to medical care and availability of movement disorder specialists. Another challenge in population-based case-control studies is careful selection of appropriate controls from the same study base that generated the cases. This basic validity requirement is too often ignored in PD studies (although this problem is hardly unique to PD research). Selection of convenience controls (e.g. spouses or friends) is arguably acceptable for purely genetic association studies, but is clearly inappropriate for investigations of environmental and lifestyle factors for well-known reasons that need not be articulated here.

Occupational cohorts with well characterized exposures are a suitable alternative choice of study populations for PD research. There are some challenges in studying worker populations, however. Except in extremely large cohorts, case numbers, and hence statistical power, will be low. Reliance on mortality may be required for some cohorts, given that PD incidence typically occurs at post-retirement ages. However, PD mortality data can suffer from incomplete or inaccurate reporting. A feasible alternative is to investigate for clinical signs of PD among active and, where accessible, former workers. Clinical signs are far more frequent than PD diagnoses, ranging up to 20–40% in some worker groups.[36,42] Standardized protocols for assessing parkinsonian signs are available, and have been used successfully among welders, for example. Prevalence surveys can then be extended into longitudinal assessments that can address disease progression in relation to environmental exposures, lifestyle factors, and medication use.

Incorporation of molecular or imaging biomarkers into epidemiological PD research has potential for refining exposure assessment, and for improving diagnostic and disease severity classification. The advantages and limitations of exposure biomarker measurement, especially for assessing long-term exposures, are well known. One important application of neuroimaging is to estimate brain region-specific exposures, as suggested from imaging findings in a recent study of manganese deposition in actively employed welders' brains.[53] Imaging patterns may ultimately assist in characterizing agent-specific PD phenotypes. The limited feasibility of conducting large-scale imaging studies is a current constraint, but this may be overcome in the future.

Studies of gene/environment interactions to identify potential susceptibility subgroups have been undertaken in PD research. Thus far, the results have mostly been disappointing. Pooling data among studies is one method to enhance statistical power to detect interactions, and deserves further consideration. Following common protocols for genetic assays is a relatively straightforward exercise, whereas harmonizing exposure assessment among epidemiological studies can only be ensured in the planning stages of the research; pooling exposure data in a post hoc manner, although conceptually worthwhile, can introduce exposure misclassification. We would therefore encourage epidemiologists to develop common protocols that ensure some homogeneity in diagnostic accuracy and exposure assessment validity and specificity for both environmental agents of interest and important covariates, such as smoking, medication use, and family history of PD.

Conclusion

Although identification of modifiable environmental exposures that are strongly related to PD risk has not yet been achieved, the potential gains in disease prevention in a world with an aging population clearly justify ongoing future epidemiological research.

References

1. **Parkinson J.** *An essay on the shaking palsy.* London: Sherwood, Neely and Jones, 1817. Reprinted in: Neuropsychiatric classics. *J Neuropsychiatry Clin Neurosci* 2002;**14**:223–36.

2. **Samii A, Nutt JG, Ransom BR.** Parkinson's disease. *Lancet* 2004;**363**:1783–93.

3. **Agid Y.** Parkinson's disease: pathophysiology. *Lancet* 1991;**337**:1321–4.

4. **Hughes AJ, Daniel SE, Kilford L, Lees AJ.** Accuracy of clinical diagnosis of idiopathic Parkinson's disease: a clinico-pathological study of 100 cases. *J Neurol Neurosurg Psychiatry* 1992;**55**:181–4.

5. **Van Den Eeden SK, Tanner CM, Bernstein AL,** *et al.* Incidence of Parkinson's disease: variation by age, gender, and race/ethnicity. *Am J Epidemiol* 2003;**157**:1015–22.

6. **Wright Willis A, Evanoff BA, Lian M, Criswell SR, Racette BA.** Geographic and ethnic variation in Parkinson disease: a population-based study of US Medicare beneficiaries. *Neuroepidemiology* 2010;**34**:143–51.

7. **Elbaz A, Bower JH, Maraganore DM,** *et al.* Risk tables for parkinsonism and Parkinson's disease. *J Clin Epidemiol* 2002;**55**:25–31.

8. **Martin I, Dawson VL, Dawson TM.** Recent advances in the genetics of Parkinson's disease. *Annu Rev Genomics Hum Genet* 2011;**12**:301–25.

9. **Wirdefeldt K, Adami HO, Cole P, Trichopoulos D, Mandel J.** Epidemiology and etiology of Parkinson's disease: a review of the evidence. *Eur J Epidemiol* 2011;**26**(Suppl 1):S1–58.

10. **Couper J.** On the effects of black oxide of manganese when inhaled into the lungs. *British Annals of Medicine, Pharmacy, Vital Statistics, and General Science* 1837;**1**:41–2.

11. **Rodier J.** Manganese poisoning in Moroccan miners. *Br J Ind Med* 1955;**12**:21–35.

12. **von Economo C.** *Encephalitis lethargica: its sequelae and treatment.* Translated and adapted by Newman KO. London: Oxford University Press, 1931.

13. **Langston JW, Ballard P, Tetrud JW, Irwin I.** Chronic Parkinsonism in humans due to a product of meperidine-analog synthesis. *Science* 1983;**219**:979–80.

14. **Langston JW, Irwin I, Ricaurte GA.** Neurotoxins, parkinsonism and Parkinson's disease. *Pharmacol Ther* 1987;**32**:19–49.

15. **Ritz B, Ascherio A, Checkoway H,** *et al.* Pooled analysis of tobacco use and risk of Parkinson disease. *Arch Neurol* 2007;**64**:990–7.

16. **Morens DM, Grandinetti A, Davis JW, Ross GW, White LR, Reed D.** Evidence against the operation of selective mortality in explaining the association between cigarette smoking and reduced occurrence of idiopathic Parkinson disease. *Am J Epidemiol* 1996;**144**:400–4.

17. **Searles Nielsen S, Gallagher LG, Lundin JI,** *et al.* Environmental tobacco smoke and Parkinson's disease. *Mov Disord* 2012;**27**:293–6.

18. **Cannon JR, Greenamyre JT.** The role of environmental exposures in neurodegeneration and neurodegenerative diseases. *Toxicol Sci* 2011;**124**:225–50.

19. Manning-Bog AB, McCormack AL, Li J, Uversky VN, Fink AL, Di Monte DA. The herbicide paraquat causes up-regulation and aggregation of alpha-synuclein in mice: paraquat and alpha-synuclein. *J Biol Chem* 2002;**277**:1641–4.

20. Betarbet R, Sherer TB, MacKenzie G, Garcia-Osuna M, Panov AV, Greenamyre JT. Chronic systemic pesticide exposure reproduces features of Parkinson's disease. *Nat Neurosci* 2000;**3**:1301–6.

21. Dick FD, De Palma G, Ahmadi A, *et al*. Environmental risk factors for Parkinson's disease and parkinsonism: the Geoparkinson study. *Occup Environ Med* 2007;**64**:666–72.

22. Brighina L, Frigerio R, Schneider NK, *et al*. Alpha-synuclein, pesticides, and Parkinson disease: a case-control study. *Neurology* 2008;**70**:1461–9.

23. Hancock DB, Martin ER, Mayhew GM, *et al*. Pesticide exposure and risk of Parkinson's disease: a family-based case-control study. *BMC Neurol* 2008;**8**:6. doi:10.1186/1471-2377-8-6.

24. Elbaz A, Clavel J, Rathouz PJ, *et al*. Professional exposure to pesticides and Parkinson disease. *Ann Neurol* 2009;**66**:494–504.

25. Costello S, Cockburn M, Bronstein J, Zhang X, Ritz B. Parkinson's disease and residential exposure to maneb and paraquat from agricultural applications in the central valley of California. *Am J Epidemiol* 2009;**169**:919–26.

26. Tanner CM, Ross GW, Jewell SA, *et al*. Occupation and risk of parkinsonism: a multicenter case-control study. *Arch Neurol* 2009;**66**:1106–13.

27. Tanner CM, Kamel F, Ross GW, *et al*. Rotenone, paraquat, and Parkinson's disease. *Environ Health Perspect* 2011;**119**:866–72.

28. Ascherio A, Chen H, Weisskopf MG, *et al*. Pesticide exposure and risk for Parkinson's disease. *Ann Neurol* 2006;**60**:197–203.

29. Kamel F, Tanner C, Umbach D, *et al*. Pesticide exposure and self-reported Parkinson's disease in the Agricultural Health Study. *Am J Epidemiol* 2007;**165**:364–74.

30. Caudle WM, Guillot TS, Lazo CR, Miller GW. Industrial toxicants and Parkinson's disease. *Neurotoxicology* 2012;**33**:178–88.

31. Mortimer JA, Borenstein AR, Nelson LM. Associations of welding and manganese exposure with Parkinson disease: review and meta-analysis. *Neurology* 2012;**79**:1174–80.

32. Gorell JM, Johnson CC, Rybicki BA, *et al*. Occupational exposure to manganese, copper, lead, iron, mercury and zinc and the risk of Parkinson's disease. *Neurotoxicoloy* 1999;**20**:239–47.

33. Lucchini RG, Albini E, Benedetti L, *et al*. High prevalence of Parkinsonian disorders associated to manganese exposure in the vicinities of ferroalloy industries. *Am J Ind Med* 2007;**50**:788–800.

34. Finkelstein MM, Jerrett M. A study of the relationships between Parkinson's disease and markers of traffic-derived and environmental manganese air pollution in two Canadian cities. *Environ Res* 2007;**104**:420–32.

35. Wright Willis A, Evanoff BA, Lian M, *et al*. Metal emissions and urban incident Parkinson disease: a community health study of Medicare beneficiaries by using geographic information systems. *Am J Epidemiol* 2010;**172**:1357–63.

36. Racette BA, Tabbal SD, Jennings D, Good L, Perlmutter JS, Evanoff B. Prevalence of parkinsonism and relationship to exposure in a large sample of Alabama welders. *Neurology* 2005;**64**:230–5.

37. Fryzek JP, Hansen J, Cohen S, *et al*. A cohort study of Parkinson's disease and other neurodegenerative disorders in Danish welders. *J Occup Environ Med* 2005;**47**:466–72.

38. **Fored CM, Fryzek JP, Brandt L,** *et al*. Parkinson's disease and other basal ganglia or movement disorders in a large nationwide cohort of Swedish welders. *Occup Environ Med* 2006;**63**:135–40.

39. **Marsh GM, Gula MJ.** Employment as a welder and Parkinson disease among heavy equipment manufacturing workers. *J Occup Environ Med* 2006;**48**:1031–46.

40. **Park J, Yoo CI, Sim CS,** *et al*. Occupations and Parkinson's disease: a multi-center case-control study in South Korea. *Neurotoxicology* 2006;**26**:99–105.

41. **Stampfer MJ.** Welding occupations and mortality from Parkinson's disease and other neurodegenerative diseases among United States men, 1985–1999. *J Occup Environ Hyg* 2009;**6**:267–72.

42. **Racette BA, Criswell SR, Lundin JI,** *et al*. Increased risk of parkinsonism associated with welding exposure. *Neurotoxicology* 2012;**33**:1356–61.

43. **Lucchini RG, Martin CJ, Doney BC.** From manganism to manganese-induced parkinsonism: a conceptual model based on the evolution of exposure. *Neuromolecular Med* 2009;**11**:311–21.

44. **McDonnell L, Maginnis C, Lewis S,** *et al*. Occupational exposure to solvents and metals and Parkinson's disease. *Neurology* 2003;**61**:716–7.

45. **Park RM, Schulte PA, Bowman JD,** *et al*. Potential occupational risks for neurodegenerative diseases. *Am J Ind Med* 2005;**48**:63–77

46. **Petersen MS, Halling J, Bech S,** *et al*. Impact of dietary exposure to food contaminants on the risk of Parkinson's disease. *Neurotoxicology* 2008;**29**:584–90.

47. **Firestone JA, Lundin JI, Powers KM,** *et al*. Occupational factors and risk of Parkinson's disease: a population-based case-control study. *Am J Ind Med* 2010;**53**:217–23.

48. **Feldman AL, Johansson AL, Nise G, Gatz M, Pedersen NL, Wirdefeldt K.** Occupational exposure in parkinsonian disorders: a 43-year prospective cohort study in men. *Parkinsonism Relat Disord* 2011;**17**:677–82.

49. **Goldman SM, Quinlan PJ, Ross GW,** *et al*. Solvent exposures and Parkinson disease risk in twins. *Ann Neurol* 2012;**71**:776–84.

50. **Zaheer F, Slevin JT.** Trichloroethylene and Parkinson disease. *Neurol Clin* 2011;**29**:657–65.

51. **Wild CP.** The exposome: from concept to utility. *Int J Epidemiol* 2012;**41**:24–32.

52. **Qin L, Wu X, Block ML,** *et al*. Systemic LPS causes chronic neuroinflammation and progressive neurodegeneration. *Glia* 2007;**55**:453–62.

53. **Criswell SR, Perlmutter JS, Huang JL,** *et al*. Basal ganglia intensity indices and diffusion weighted imaging in manganese-exposed welders. *Occup Environ Med* 2012;**69**:437–43.

Chapter 4

Infectious pneumonia in workers exposed to metal fume

Keith T. Palmer and David Coggon

Introduction

Siderosis, the accumulation of ferric oxide particles in the lung, was described over a century ago by Zenker.[1] Enquiries subsequently focused on the effect of this pneumoconiotic process on lung function, generally concluding that it was benign.[2] More recently, however, it has become apparent that iron and perhaps other elements in metal fume influence the risk of lower respiratory tract infection. The evidence accrued has been sufficient to trigger mechanistic investigations, a reappraisal of health risks in workers exposed to metal fume, and recommendations for risk control. In this chapter we review the emerging evidence, with a focus on epidemiological enquiries.

Mortality data

Welders die more often from pneumonia than do their social class peers. This much has been revealed by successive analyses of occupational mortality for England and Wales. The pattern can now be traced back more than seven decades. During 1930–32, 285 deaths were observed with 171 expected;[3] in 1949–53, 70 deaths versus 31 expected;[4] in 1959–63, 101 deaths as compared with 54.9 expected;[5] and in 1970–72, 66 deaths with 42.0 expected.[6]

A more recent analysis, covering the periods 1979–80 and 1982–90, offered greater statistical power to explore potential determinants.[7] This confirmed the association with welding, but went further in clarifying that the excess applied also to several other occupations entailing exposure to metal fume, such as moulders and coremakers, and furnacemen in foundries. The excess was attributable largely to deaths from pneumonias other than bronchopneumonia, principally lobar pneumonia, but also covering a range of other less common pneumonias (Table 4.1). Moreover, the effect was limited to men below the normal retirement age of 65 years (Table 4.2).

The finding that risks decline after retirement is an argument against confounding by lifestyle variables such as smoking, as is the specificity of effect to lobar rather than bronchopneumonia. Additionally, in the various national analyses of occupational mortality, at-risk occupations did not have comparable excesses of lung cancer or of mortality from non-respiratory infections.

The most recent analysis of occupational mortality for England and Wales, covering 1991–2000,[8] reaffirmed the pattern: excesses of mortality at ages 20–64 years were

Table 4.1 Mortality from pneumonia in metal-working occupations in England and Wales, 1979–80 and 1982–90

Occupation	Pneumococcal and unspecified lobar pneumonia			Bronchopneumonia			Other and unspecified pneumonia		
	Deaths observed	PMR[a]	(95% CI)	Deaths observed	PMR[a]	(95% CI)	Deaths observed	PMR[a]	(95% CI)
Welders	55	255	(192–332)	68	126	(98–159)	29	211	(141–303)
Furnacemen	6	154	(57–336)	12	117	(61–205)	4	186	(51–477)
Rollermen	3	418	(86–1223)	2	106	(13–385)	0	0	(0–948)
Moulders and coremakers (metal)	18	292	(173–461)	18	111	(66–176)	4	117	(32–300)
Annealers, hardeners, temperers (metal)	4	392	(107–1003)	4	138	(38–352)	0	0	(0–655)
Galvanizers and tin platers	1	142	(4–790)	2	115	(14–414)	2	428	(52–1547)
Sheet-metal workers	21	190	(117–290)	29	101	(68–146)	9	127	(58–242)

[a] Proportional mortality ratio (95% confidence interval), standardized for age and social class

Source: data from *The Lancet*, Volume 344, Coggon D et al., Lobar pneumonia: an occupational disease in welders, pp. 41–3, Copyright © 1994, Published by Elsevier Ltd

Table 4.2 Mortality from pneumonia among male welders in England and Wales, 1979–80 and 1982–90

Type of pneumonia (ICD-9 code)	Welders					
	Ages 20–64			Ages 65–74		
	Deaths observed	PMR[a]	(95% CI)	Deaths observed	PMR[a]	(95% CI)
Viral (480)	6	199	(73–433)	0	0	(0–409)
Pneumococcal and unspecified lobar (481)	55	255	(192–332)	20	107	(65–165)
Other bacterial (482)	4	160	(44–409)	0	0	(0–297)
Other specified (483)	3	548	(113–1603)	0	0	(0–2209)
Unspecified (486)	16	209	(119–339)	5	60	(20–141)

[a] Proportional mortality ratio (95% confidence interval), standardized for age and social class

Source: data from *The Lancet*, Volume 344, Coggon D et al., Lobar pneumonia: an occupational disease in welders, pp. 41–3, Copyright © 1994, Published by Elsevier Ltd

found for pneumococcal and lobar pneumonia (54 deaths vs 27.3 expected) and for pneumonias other than bronchopneumonia (71 vs 52.4) but no excess was apparent for these causes of death at older ages, or for bronchopneumonia at any age. Again, risks were evident across a range of occupations which have in common their exposure to metal fumes. Thus, in the UK, a hazard has remained manifest for a long period up to the present day, despite any improvements over time in the control of exposure to metal fume at work.

The findings in this series of national mortality statistics are compatible with several studies of occupational mortality in specific industries. In 1980, Beaumont and Weiss reported on the mortality experience of 8679 male members of a US metal trades union employed in shipyards, metal fabrication shops, and small boat yards, recording a significant excess of deaths from pneumonia in welders relative to what would have been expected from rates in all American men.[9] Five years later, Newhouse et al. found a significant excess death rate from pneumonia among welders employed at a shipyard in North East England, relative to platers and electricians from the same work site.[10] More recently, Torén et al. described the mortality experience of a large Swedish cohort of construction workers, which included over 30 000 men with exposure to metal fume. Risk of death from pneumonia was raised more than twofold among this group and was higher still when lobar pneumonia and pneumococcal pneumonia were analysed specifically (raised 3.7- and 5.8-fold respectively).[11] However, the risk of pneumonia in retired workers with former exposure to metal fume was little different from that in other retired workers (raised 1.16-fold). In apparent contrast, no cases of fatal pneumonia were found in a cohort of welders from a Naval dockyard in England during the 1950s to 1970s,[12] although only 0.4 deaths from pneumonia were expected. The rarity of fatal pneumonia in a working-aged population means that many studies of metal workers will have lacked statistical power to explore the question adequately.

Morbidity data

Analyses of death certificates therefore support a case for a hazard that is reversible when exposure stops. However, they do not clarify whether the additional risk applies to all categories of pneumonia or only to those caused by certain specific micro-organisms, whether the risk is the same for all types of metal or specific to certain metal(s), and whether the effect is on the incidence of infections or on their case fatality, or both.

To confirm the hazard and to characterize it further, the authors conducted a hospital-based case-control study,[13] set in five metropolitan districts (Sandwell, Dudley, Walsall, Wolverhampton, and Birmingham) of the English county of West Midlands, an area selected because of its relatively high prevalence of metal-working occupations. During a 31-month period, interviews were completed with 525 cases (men aged 20–64 years admitted to one of 11 hospitals with community-acquired pneumonia) and 1122 age matched controls (men admitted to the same hospital wards under the same consultants with acute non-respiratory illnesses). Information was collected on lifetime occupational history, including exposure at work to metal fume and a selection of 'dummy' particulate substances, and on smoking habits and other potential confounding factors.

In line with the mortality data, hospitalized pneumonia proved to be more common among welders and other workers with exposure to metal fume than in workers from non-exposed jobs. Moreover, risks were confined to exposures in the previous 12 months (adjusted odds ratio (OR) 1.6; 95% confidence interval (CI) 1.1–2.4), and not evident if the most recent exposure was more than 12 months before admission (OR 1.1). (It should be noted that most workers exposed in the previous 12 months were also exposed in the previous week, limiting capacity to define the time of elevated risk more closely.)

Also consistent with the mortality data, risks were higher when radiographic images (read blind to occupational history) displayed shadowing in a lobar, segmental, or subsegmental pattern than when the appearance was one of bronchopneumonia. Risks were highest when recent exposure was to ferrous fumes (Table 4.3), although few subjects were exposed solely to non-ferrous metals or alloys, leaving open the question as to whether other kinds of metal fume carry a risk.

Many cases of lobar pneumonia are caused by infection by *Streptococcus pneumoniae* and, in 43 cases where this organism was recovered from blood or sputum, the OR for exposure to metal fume was almost doubled while that for exposure to ferrous fume was elevated over threefold.

A heightened risk of pneumococcal infection was also established bacteriologically in a study from Alberta, Canada,[14] which estimated the rate of invasive pneumococcal disease as some 2.7 times higher in welders than in adults of working age from the general population.

In the West Midlands study, however, effects were not restricted to the pneumococcus.[13] Another microbiological diagnosis was made in 88 men, including 22 infected by *Legionella*, 12 by *Mycoplasma*, and 12 by *Haemophilus influenzae*: risks of infection with these were roughly doubled by exposure to welding fume. A relationship

Table 4.3 Associations with occupational exposure to metal fume in the year before the effective date according to the radiological pattern of pneumonia

Exposure relative to the effective date	Controls (n = 1122)	All men with pneumonia (n = 525)		Lobar pneumonia (n = 158)		Segmental/subsegmental pneumonia (n = 142)		Bronchopneumonia (n = 225)	
	No.	No.	OR[a] (95% CI)	No.	OR[a] (95% CI)	No.	OR[a] (95% CI)	No.	OR[a] (95% CI)
Never exposed to metal fume	742	325	1.0	97	1.0	89	1.0	139	1.0
Exposed to metal fume in the year before the effective date:									
any metal	71	58	1.6 (1.1–2.4)	20	1.8 (1.0–3.3)	18	1.8 (1.0–3.3)	20	1.3 (0.8–2.3)
ferrous metal with or without other metals/alloys	46	46	2.0 (1.3–3.1)	17	2.3 (1.2–4.3)	14	2.4 (1.2–4.7)	15	1.6 (0.8–3.0)
ferrous metal, but not other metals/ alloys	24	28	2.2 (1.2–4.0)	12	3.0 (1.4–6.7)	8	2.4 (1.0–5.9)	8	1.6 (0.7–3.7)
other metals or alloys, but not ferrous metal	19	8	0.8 (0.4–2.0)	2	0.7 (0.2–3.2)	2	0.7 (0.2–3.2)	4	1.0 (0.3–3.2)

[a] Odds ratio (95% confidence interval)

Reproduced from Palmer KT et al., Exposure to metal fume and infectious pneumonia, *American Journal of Epidemiology*, Volume **157**, pp. 227–33, Copyright © 2003 Johns Hopkins Bloomberg School of Public Health, published by Oxford University Press

to a broader range of micro-organisms would also be consistent with mortality data from the UK, which repeatedly indicate elevated risk for 'pneumonias other than lobar or bronchopneumonia' (ICD-9 480, 482, 483, 486: viral pneumonia and pneumonia attributed to various specified organisms, such as *Klebsiella*, *Pseudomonas*, *H. influenzae*, *Streptococcus*, and *Legionella*).[7,8]

Case reports

Supplementing a relatively small pool of epidemiological studies are several case reports on infective risk in workers exposed to metal fume. In 2001, the Norwegian Labour Inspection Authority received three independent reports of deaths from pneumonia with septicaemia among previously healthy middle-aged men, all exposed to welding fumes immediately prior to their illness; and the Authority identified nine cases of non-fatal pneumonia—three in workers exposed to fumes from cutting, grinding, and welding, and hospitalized with lobar pneumonia, and six in workers engaged in ship repair, who were treated as outpatients. In consequence the Authority issued a warning about the potentially lethal risk of fumes from thermal metal work.[15] Published case reports also exist linking fatal pneumonia in metal fume-exposed occupations with atypical micro-organisms, such as *Acinetobacter*[16] and *Bacillus cereus*.[17]

Animal experiments

Recently, inhalation experiments have confirmed that welding fume can promote bacterial growth in animals. Antonini et al., for example, compared rats exposed to fume from mild steel welding with those exposed only to air.[18] Fumes, mostly composed of iron and manganese oxides (81% iron by weight), were freshly generated by gas metal arc welding. They were presented to the rats in an exposure chamber in a regimen which lasted 3 hours per day for several days. A standard intratracheal inoculum of *Listeria monocytogenes* was then delivered to the animals, which were sacrificed 3 days later. Fume-exposed rats had a higher lung burden of the organism, there being a 27-fold increase in lung colony-forming units on sacrifice.

Possible mechanisms

A coherent body of evidence thus indicates that metal fume is a hazard for pneumonia. The next important research question concerns how this hazard translates into risk in everyday circumstances of exposure. Presently, knowledge is lacking on the exposure-response relationship and what constitutes a 'safe' or 'unsafe' level or pattern of exposure to metal fume. Given the rarity of pneumonia, exposures in epidemiological studies have been estimated in retrospect, typically using surrogate measures, such as job title, and this is crude for risk characterization.

An alternative approach would draw on an understanding of mechanisms: with better knowledge, a biomarker of susceptibility might be developed with which to characterize dose-response and monitor the effect of workplace exposures. A mechanistic understanding could even shed light on options for protection more specific than the general imperative to reduce workplace exposure to all metal fumes as a class.

In this section we review some current theories on causation and some of the ongoing mechanistic work that we have followed and in which we have shared.

The pattern of epidemiological evidence, while not ruling out other possibilities, is generally compatible with a hazard from iron in metal fume. Iron could promote infective risk in at least one of two ways: by acting as a growth nutrient for micro-organisms, or as a cause of free radical injury.

The growth nutrient hypothesis

We have reviewed elsewhere the hypothesis that iron promotes infection by acting as a growth nutrient.[19] In brief, most body iron is stored intracellularly (in ferritin, haemosiderin, and haem), the extracellular fraction being bound to high-affinity iron-binding proteins (transferrin and lactoferrin) which keep the concentration of free iron in equilibrium as low as 10^{-18} M. There is competition for free iron between host and micro-organisms, and the balance of this may be disturbed if exogenous iron exceeds the capacity of the iron-binding protein system. Several strategies for iron withholding by hosts, and iron liberation and scavenging by micro-organisms, are recognized.[20]

Consistent with the idea that excess iron promotes infection are a range of experiments involving iron dosing *in vitro* and *in vivo*,[21,22] and observations in patients with clinical disorders involving iron overload (e.g. haemochromatosis, sickle cell disease, accidental iron overdose, lactoferrin deficiency).[19] Also compatible with the hypothesis is the inhalation experiment mentioned by Antonini et al., demonstrating heightened infection in rats breathing an aerosol of predominantly ultra-fine iron-rich particulate matter generated by welding mild steel.[18]

The defence injury hypothesis

Alternatively, iron or metal fume particulates of other compositions could injure or impair host defence mechanisms.

Several mechanisms may be relevant, including the iron-dependent reduction of hydrogen peroxide, to generate toxic hydroxyl radicals.[23] Metal particles, or carbon coated with metals, have proved cytotoxic to macrophages in animals at ambient concentrations as low as 0.1 mg/m^3.[24] Precise details of mechanism remain elusive at present, however. Thus, in Antonini's experiment, no important differences were found in several markers of lung injury or inflammation (lactic dehydrogenase, albumin polymorphonuclear count, macrophage count) or in profile of cytokines and chemokines. In contrast, the same group previously reported a transient influx of polymorphs into rats' lungs, although in response to a less physiological dosing regimen involving one large intratracheal bolus of welding fume.[25] Some evidence exists that aged fumes are less inflammatory than freshly generated ones,[26] which may contribute to the difference in findings.

In keeping with some of the animal observations, in a cross-sectional comparison of welders and other matched blue-collar workers we found no indication of a generalized inflammatory response (cell counts in blood and sputum, C-reactive protein in blood, and tumour necrosis factor α, interleukin-8, matrix metallopeptidase-9, myeloperoxidase, α2-macroglobulin levels in sputum);[26] nor were there important differences in markers of immunocompetence (respiratory burst of blood neutrophils, circulating pneumococcal immunoglobulin (Ig)G, sputum IgA), although the welders had higher iron levels and a substantially lower unsaturated iron-binding capacity in sputum, indicating a greater lung burden of iron.

More recently, another avenue of enquiry has opened up which may help to explain the infective risk of metal fume. Many cases of bacterial pneumonia arise from strains of pneumococci that have the capacity to adhere firmly to, and invade, bronchial epithelium.[27] They act by co-opting host proteins, including the platelet activating factor receptor (PAFR), which can be stimulated by a bacterial phospholipid that mimics the natural ligand platelet activating factor. Expression of PAFR promotes adhesion of micro-organisms, while chemical blockade of the receptor attenuates the effect.[28] By the same token, mice that are deficient in PAFR are resistant to pneumococcal pneumonia.[29] Recently, Mushtaq et al. have demonstrated that this pathway may be instrumental in the effect of urban particulate matter on pneumonic risk. In their *in vitro* experiment, particles of PM_{10}, when incubated with airways epithelial (A549) cells, promoted pneumococcal adhesion in a dose-dependent way via a PAFR-dependent pathway which was also mediated in part by oxidative stress.[30]

With this research group, we are currently exploring the scope of metal fume to affect pneumococcal adhesion. Early findings offer promise. In one experiment, monolayers of A549 were treated with particulate matter generated by hyperbaric welding, with and without a PAFR blocker (CV3988). Cells were then incubated with a standard aliquot of pneumococcus and adherent and internalized bacteria assessed by quantitative culture. Welding fume significantly increased pneumococcal adhesion to A549 cells in a dose-dependent manner (p <0.01 vs medium control), while PAFR blockade with CV3988 attenuated this particulate-stimulated adhesion (p <0.005).[31] These findings require replication and their relation to real-life exposures and *in vivo* responses in workers also requires elaboration. However, scope exists to explore how effects vary by composition of particulate and by dose in the hunt for a better mechanistic understanding and a practical biomarker of risk.

Prevention

Continuing uncertainties about dose-response and the range of metals that may confer risk limit the practical advice that can be given on control of fume at source. In some circumstances (e.g. well-enclosed automated laser welding and cutting, plastic, electron beam, and friction stir welding, work on laser metal or powder bed deposition, and cold spray technologies) exposures should be minimal or absent. Otherwise, welders should always use appropriate and effective local exhaust ventilation, keeping the exhaust hood near the work-piece, not placing their face in the plume, wearing appropriate personal protective equipment (using an 'improved' rather than a 'standard' helmet), always cleaning the work-piece prior to welding to remove contaminants, and undertaking other tasks, such as grinding, away from the area in which welding is taking place if possible. These measures should help to minimize exposure to welding fume and metal particulates; but how much this will mitigate infective risk is unclear given the limited exposure information for affected cases.

In view of this uncertainty and the continuing toll of excess deaths in recent mortality statistics,[8] the Joint Committee on Vaccination and Immunisation, on behalf of the Department of Health in England, decided in November 2011 to recommend that 'welders who have not received the pneumococcal polysaccharide vaccine (PPV23) previously should be offered a single dose of 0.5ml of PPV23 vaccine' and that 'employers should ensure that provision is in place for workers to receive PPV23'.[32] The advice was subsequently modified, encouraging extension of use to a broader range of workers with regular exposure to metal fume.[33] The vaccine cost about £30 per dose at 2011 prices.

PPV23, although a safe vaccine which generates a good antibody response following a single injection, is not a panacea for risk reduction. Rather, the 23 capsular serotypes it includes account for 96% of the pneumococcal isolates that cause serious infection in the UK, and PPV has been estimated by a Cochrane review to be 74% effective (95% CI 56–85%) in preventing invasive pneumococcal disease, and similarly effective in preventing pneumococcal pneumonia.[34] Following a single injection, post-immunization antibody levels begin to wane after about 5 years, the length of sufficient protection being uncertain. However, assuming the incidence of invasive pneumococcal disease in welders reported in Alberta[14] and that immunity lasts at least 10 years, we estimate that 588 welders (95% CI 363–1551) would need to be vaccinated to prevent one case of this disease per 10 years,[35] a return that compares reasonably with other respected public health interventions.

Waning immunity matters because a booster dose of the present vaccine is not recommended. This creates a dilemma regarding the optimal timing of vaccination: as the incidence of invasive pneumococcal disease climbs at older ages from a low base, a bigger absolute risk reduction may be enjoyed by older welders than younger ones. Set against this, withholding vaccination requires a judgement about the likelihood a welder will remain exposed at older ages and would deny protection in the interim. The Department of Health in England did not recommend an age restriction, and there is hope that a polyvalent pneumococcal conjugate vaccine, currently under testing in adults, will provide a more lasting immune memory and be used for re-vaccination, circumventing the problem.

It should also be recognized that PPV23 can only hope to prevent that part of the excess risk which is pneumococcal—probably a majority of cases, but not those caused by other micro-organisms. And that some uncertainty exists regarding whom to vaccinate, as many workers will undertake welding or be exposed to metal fumes as an infrequent part of their job.

These limitations, and the challenge of ensuring good uptake of the vaccine, have encouraged a few commentators from the UK to argue for a postponement of vaccination programmes, pending a better vaccine and more knowledge.[36] We think this is wrong-minded in the same way that an argument not to use a face mask or exhaust ventilation would be wrong if based on the case that protection is sometimes imperfect—partial controls are better than none at all, while estimates of benefit recognize that not all cases in welders are pneumococcal in origin.[35,36] Certainly, workers exposed to metal fume have been dying in excess of pneumonia for some eight decades, with an attributable mortality which bears comparison with that from occupational asthma;[8] and latest mortality statistics in England and Wales give no grounds for optimism regarding the efficacy of fume control in the workplace. Measures to combat this relatively neglected occupational disease are long overdue.

Acknowledgements

Parts of the work described in this chapter were supported by the Medical Research Council, the Health and Safety Executive, the Colt Foundation, and the Worshipful Company of Blacksmiths.

References

1. **Zenker FA.** Ueber Staublinhalationskrankheiten der lung. *Dtsch Arch Klin Med* 1866;**2**:116.

2. **Seaton A.** Pneumoconioses. In: Warrell DA, Cox TM, Firth JD (eds) *Oxford textbook of medicine* (5th edn). Oxford: Oxford University Press, 2010, pp. 3414–24.

3. **Registrar General.** *Decennial supplement England and Wales 1931.* London: HMSO, 1938.

4. **Registrar General.** *Decennial supplement England and Wales 1951. Occupational mortality part II vol 1.* London: HMSO, 1958.

5. **Registrar General.** *Decennial supplement England and Wales 1961. Occupational mortality tables.* London: HMSO, 1971.

6. **Registrar General.** *Decennial supplement England and Wales 1971. Series DS no 1.* London: HMSO, 1981.

7. **Coggon D, Inskip H, Winter P, Pannett B.** Lobar pneumonia: an occupational disease in welders. *Lancet* 1994;**344**:41–3.

8. **Palmer KT, Cullinan P, Rice S, Brown T, Coggon D.** Mortality from infectious pneumonia in metal workers: a comparison with deaths from asthma in occupations exposed to respiratory sensitisers. *Thorax* 2009;**64**:983–6.

9. **Beaumont JJ, Weiss NS.** Mortality of welders, shipfitters, and other metal trades workers in boilermakers Local No. 104, AFL-CIO. *Am J Epidemiol* 1980;**112**:775–86.

10. **Newhouse ML, Oakes D, Woolley AJ.** Mortality of welders and other craftsmen at a shipyard in NE England. *Br J Ind Med* 1985;**42**:406–10.

11. **Torén K, Qvarfordt I, Bergdahl IA, Järvholm B.** Increased mortality from infectious pneumonia after occupational exposure to inorganic dust, metal fumes and chemicals. *Thorax* 2011;**66**:992–6.

12. **McMillan GH, Pethybridge RJ.** The health of welders in naval dockyards: a proportional mortality study of welders and two control groups. *J Soc Occup Med* 1983;**33**:75–84.

13. **Palmer KT, Poole J, Ayres JG, Mann J, Burge PS, Coggon D.** Exposure to metal fume and infectious pneumonia. *Am J Epidemiol* 2003;**157**:227–33.

14. **Wong A, Marrie TJ, Garg S, Kellner JD, Tyrrell GJ; SPAT Group.** Welders are at increased risk for invasive pneumococcal disease. *Int J Infect Dis* 2010;**14**:e796–9.

15. **Wergeland E, Iversen BG.** Deaths from pneumonia after welding. *Scand J Work Environ Health* 2001;**27**:353.

16. **Cordes LG, Brink EW, Checko PJ,** *et al.* A cluster of Acinetobacter pneumonia in foundry workers. *Ann Intern Med* 1981;**95**:688–93.

17. **Avashia SB, Riggins WS, Lindley C,** *et al.* Fatal pneumonia among metalworkers due to inhalation exposure to *Bacillus cereus* containing *Bacillus anthracis* toxin genes. *Clin Infect Dis* 2007;**44**:414–6.

18. **Antonini JM, Roberts JR, Stone S, Chen BT, Schwegler-Berry D, Frazer DG.** Short-term inhalation exposure to mild steel welding fume had no effect on lung inflammation and injury but did alter defense responses to bacteria in rats. *Inhal Toxicol* 2009;**21**:182–92.

19. **Palmer K, Coggon D.** Does occupational exposure to iron promote infection? *Occup Environ Med* 1997;**54**:529–34.

20. **Flo TH, Smith KD, Sato S,** *et al.* Lipocalin-2 mediates an innate immune response to bacterial infection by sequestrating iron. *Nature* 2004;**432**:917–21.

21. **Bullen JJ.** The significance of iron in infection. *Rev of Infect Dis* 1981;**3**:1127–38.

22. **Kluger MJ.** Clinical and physiological aspects. In: Bullen JJ, Griffiths E (eds) *Iron and infection: molecular, physiological and clinical aspects.* Chichester: Wiley, 1987, pp. 243–82.

23. **Herbert V, Shaw S, Jayatilleke E, Stopler-Kasdan T.** Most free-radical injury is iron-related: it is promoted by iron, hemin, holoferritin and vitamin C, and inhibited by desferoxamine and apoferritin. *Stem Cells* 1994;**12**:289–303.

24. **Goyer RA.** Toxic effects of metals. In: Doull J, Klaassen CD, Amdur MO (eds) *Casarett and Doull's toxicology* (3rd edn). New York: Macmillan, 1986, pp. 582–635.

25. **Taylor MD, Roberts JR, Leonard SS, Shi X, Antonini JM.** Effects of welding fumes of differing composition and solubility on free radical production and acute lung injury and inflammation in rats. *Toxicol Sci* 2003;**75**:181–91.

26. **Palmer KT, McNeill Love RMC, Poole JR,** *et al.* Inflammatory responses to the occupational inhalation of metal fume, *Eur Respir J* 2006;**27**:366–73.

27. **van der Poll T, Opal SM.** Pathogenesis, treatment, and prevention of pneumococcal pneumonia. *Lancet* 2009;**374**:1543–56.

28. **Cundell DR, Gerard NP, Gerard C, Idanpaan-Heikkila I, Tuomanen EI.** Streptococcus pneumoniae anchor to activated human cells by the receptor for platelet-activating factor. *Nature* 1995;**377**:435–8.

29. **Rijneveld AW, Weijer S, Florquin S,** *et al.* Improved host defense against pneumococcal pneumonia in platelet-activating factor receptor-deficient mice. *J Infect Dis* 2004;**189**:711–6.

30. **Mushtaq N, Ezzati M, Hall L,** *et al.* Adhesion of *Streptococcus pneumoniae* to human airway epithelial cells exposed to urban particulate matter. *J Allergy Clin Immunol* 2011;**127**:1236–42.

31. **Suri R, Palmer K, Ross JAS, Coggon D, Grigg J.** Exposure to welding fume and adhesion of *Streptococcus pneumoniae* to A549 alveolar cells. *Thorax* 2012;**67** (Suppl 2): A51. doi:10.1136/thoraxjnl-2012-202678.109.

32. Department of Health. *Immunisation against infectious disease, 2006* (updated November 2011), Chapter 25 v2_0, p305. Available at: <http://www.dh.gov.uk/prod_consum_dh/groups/dh_digitalassets/documents/digitalasset/dh_131000.pdf> (accessed 24 January 2013).

33. Department of Health. *Immunisation against infectious disease, 2006* (updated March 2013), Chapter 25 v4_0, p306. Available at: <http://media.dh.gov.uk/network/211/files/2012/09/Green-Book-updated-140313.pdf> (accessed 26 April 2013). Top-level web page at <http://immunisation.dh.gov.uk/category/the-green-book/> (accessed 30 April 2013).

34. **Moberley SA, Holden J, Tatham DP, Andrews RM.** Vaccines for preventing pneumococcal infection in adults. *Cochrane Database Syst Rev* 2008;**1**:CD000422. doi: 10.1002/14651858.CD000422.pub2.

35. **Palmer KT, Cosgrove M.** Vaccinating welders against pneumonia. *Occup Med* 2012;**62**:325–30.

36. **Sen D, Chen Y.** Vaccinating welders against pneumonia (letter). *Occup Med* 2012;**62**:665–6. Authors' reply: 666–7.

Chapter 5

Retinal detachment and occupational lifting: rediscovering lost knowledge

Stefano Mattioli, Stefania Curti, Andrea Farioli, and Francesco S. Violante

Introduction

Some years ago, a female colleague of ours, an occupational physician, had an eye injury, an occupational injury caused by part of an overhead projector after a lecture, and a consequent retinal detachment (RD). Back at work, she told us that ophthalmologists had warned her to avoid lifting heavy objects, even shopping bags, because such actions could lead to re-detachment of the retina.

We therefore talked to another colleague, an ophthalmologist experienced in ergonomics, and discovered that there was an oral tradition concerning a supposed link between heavy lifting and RD. Searching the literature at that time, we failed to find clear evidence supporting this theory.

Retinal detachment: definition and epidemiology

RD is the separation of the neurosensory retina from the underlying retinal pigment epithelium.[1] RD is often preceded by posterior vitreous detachment—the separation of the posterior vitreous from the retina as a result of vitreous degeneration and shrinkage[2]—which gives rise to the sudden appearance of floaters and flashes. Late symptoms of RD may include visual field defects (shadows, curtains) or even blindness. The success rate of RD surgery has been reported to be over 90%;[3] however, a loss of visual acuity is frequently reported by patients, particularly if the macula is involved.[4] Since the natural history of RD can be influenced by early diagnosis, patients experiencing symptoms of posterior vitreous detachment are advised to undergo an ophthalmic examination.[5]

Epidemiology and individual risk factors for retinal detachment

Studies of the incidence of RD give estimates ranging from 6.3 to 17.9 cases per 100 000 person-years.[6] It has not been established whether this variability reflects real geographical differences or whether it is a consequence of methodological heterogeneity. Age is a well-known risk factor for RD. In most studies the peak incidence was recorded among subjects in their seventh decade of life. A secondary peak at a younger age (20–30 years) has been identified in large population studies and was attributed to RD among highly myopic patients.[6] Indeed, depending on the severity, myopia is associated with a four- to ten-fold increase in risk of RD.[7] The cumulative incidence of RD is six to eight times higher in the sixth year after cataract surgery and an increased risk has been reported to be still present after 20 years. Unsurprisingly, blunt trauma to the eye or the head is a direct cause of RD. Remarkably, traumatic RD (0.6–2 cases per 100 000 person-years) accounts for only a small proportion of the overall incidence of RD. The risk of RD is reported to be higher in males than in females, with relative risks, for males, ranging from 1.2 to 2.2. Gender imbalances in the distributions of myopia and traumatic RD may contribute to this difference. However, it has been hypothesized that other unknown gender-related risk factors may also be involved.[6,8]

Is retinal detachment a preventable disease?

While secondary prevention of RD is current practice, no effective primary prevention strategy is available at present. The idea is widespread among practitioners that RD is not preventable, probably the consequence of our historically poor understanding of the aetiology of RD. For instance, on the website of the Mayo Clinic—one of the top-ranked hospitals for ophthalmology in the US—it is possible to read that 'There's no way to prevent retinal detachment'.[9]

A recent study suggests that the short-term use of oral fluoroquinolones may be a strong risk factor for RD.[10] In addition, a case-control study of RD highlighted a possible association between obesity and risk of RD.[11] These surprising findings on personal risk factors for RD shed new light on the preventability of this disease. A question now arises: are there occupational risk factors for RD?

Literature review on occupational lifting and RD

The story seems to begin in the past, considering that in 1921 Edridge-Green stated in *The Lancet* that 'Any occupation which involves heavy lifting is not suitable for a myopic' and reported the case of a farmer who 'had to exert his strength to the upmost; he ruptured himself, became myopic to a low degree and blind in one eye through detachment of the retina'.[12]

The major textbook *Fitness for Work: The Medical Aspects*, in all its five editions (1988, 1995, 2000, 2007, 2012),[13–17] dedicated a chapter to vision, eye disorders, and occupation. All versions of this chapter included text on myopia and/or RD and occupation, although without citing references.

The authors of the chapters in each edition state that myopia of a high degree is associated with an increased risk of RD. In the first edition, Cross and Diamond added that myopics are unsuitable for heavy exertion, such as in digging or carrying heavy weights, and that after RD surgery patients should avoid the heaviest manual work.[13] In the second and third editions, Diamond and Munton appear to agree only with the latter statement, writing that 'Patients whose retina reattaches should subsequently avoid the heaviest ['heavy' in the third edition] manual work and some sports such as boxing or squash' and no longer discussing the issue of severe myopics performing heavy lifting.[14,15] In the fourth edition, Johnston and Pitts noted only that 'Myopia is associated with degeneration of the vitreous and peripheral retina, and an increased risk of RD' and did not discuss fitness for heavy work in cases of severe myopia or subjects treated surgically for RD.[16] In the fifth edition, Pitts and Mitchell propose a longer return to work interval after surgery in manual workers (2 months) than in sedentary workers (2 weeks), but make no proposal in relation to occupational lifting.[17]

We performed a search using PubMed to identify papers concerning the putative association of RD with occupational lifting. We used the 'more sensitive' search string we proposed in 2010 to study the occupational determinants of diseases,[18] adding the text words 'lifting' and 'physical exertion' within the search strategy. We obtained 165 citations: 95 related to eye injuries, three were papers on heavy lifting we ourselves had published in the last few years,[11,19,20] and a further six provided at least some indication of a relationship between heavy lifting and RD.[21–26]

In the 1970s, there was a debate in the Central and Eastern European literature about the possibility that RD, particularly in myopic subjects, could be due to lifting heavy weights. In a Latvian study of myopia complications, it was concluded that RD could be more frequent in myopics performing heavy physical work or exposed to occupational visual strain.[21] In Germany, hypotheses were discussed that RD in a severe myopic eye may be caused by hyperaemia of the choroid[22,23] or by a severe ciliary spasm[24] that had presumably occurred during heavy physical work. In Russia, Pivovarov and colleagues (1977) measured intraocular pressure in healthy subjects performing static physical efforts associated with various simulated lifting manoeuvres (with or without sudden holding of the breath). They found that lifting of weights over 15–20 kg was generally accompanied by an abrupt rise (~25 mmHg) and fall in intraocular pressure, particularly when the exertion was accompanied by sudden holding of the breath. They concluded that indirect trauma, in particular physical exertion, by causing peaks of intraocular pressure, could be considered among the determinants of RD. Moreover, in their opinion, severe myopics and patients treated surgically for RD should avoid lifting weights of more than 15 kg.[25] And at the end of the description of a Czech case-series, the authors suggested that RD could be prevented by advising severe myopic adolescents to carry out non-physically demanding work activities.[26]

Some years later, in a 1993 hospital-based case-control study in the US which explored putative risk factors for idiopathic rhegmatogenous RD—the study was restricted to subjects without any history of serious trauma, intraocular surgery, or pathologic myopia—no significant association emerged for 'vigorous physical activity', 'subjective impression of physical activity', or 'indoor/outdoor place of work'.[7] Unfortunately, the authors did not provide quantitative information regarding these factors and RD. Moreover, they did not define what they classed as 'physical activity': running and cycling are physical activities which may be vigorous, but no one has suggested that they are risk factors for RD.

Among studies concerning return to work after RD surgery, the most informative is probably a trial conducted in 1984 in the US to assess whether limiting physical activity after RD surgery is effective in limiting reoperation. Six months after surgery the rates of reoperation and final reattachment percentages in the active and inactive groups showed no statistically significant differences. The authors also provided a review of the literature regarding surgically treated RD and return to work.[27]

Finally, it should be noted that, unlike other blue-collar workers, farmers may be exposed not only to eye injuries and heavy lifting but also to fungicides, which Kamel and colleagues found to be associated with retinal degeneration, hence indirectly with RD.[28]

Physiopathological hypothesis

The most frequent form of RD, rhegmatogenous RD (RRD), is caused by the passage of liquefied vitreous through a retinal break, kept open by tractional forces generated by vitreous shrinkage.[1] It can therefore be hypothesized that external exposures associated with one of these three factors (retinal tear, liquefied vitreous, or tractional forces) may increase the risk of developing RRD.

Intraocular pressure—the fluid pressure inside the eye—is influenced by physical activity. Dynamic exercise causes an acute reduction in intraocular pressure, whereas physical fitness is associated with a lower baseline value.[29] Conversely, a sudden rise in intraocular pressure has been reported during the Valsalva manoeuvre.[30–32] In particular, Vieira and colleagues reported an important increase in intraocular pressure while lifting at 80% of the one-repetition maximum.[33]

Occupational physical activity may therefore cause both short- and long-term variations in intraocular pressure. On the one hand, physically demanding jobs may contribute to decreased baseline levels by increasing physical fitness but, on the other hand, lifting tasks may cause an important acute increase in pressure. Moreover, the eye of a manual worker who performs repeated lifting tasks involving the Valsalva manoeuvre may undergo several dramatic changes in intraocular pressure within a single working shift.

Recurring fluctuations of intraocular pressure might increase the risk of RRD through several pathways. They might:

1. induce tractional forces acting on the retina, which might cause the opening of a pre-existing retinal break
2. increase the risk of developing a retinal tear by increasing vitreous shrinkage
3. alter the physical state of the vitreous gel, speeding up vitreous liquefaction and causing an imbalance, with vitreoretinal adhesion, which is itself thought to be associated with complicated posterior vitreous detachment and therefore with RRD.[2]

Retinal detachment, myopia, and manual material handling: a case-control study

A case-control study was carried out to test the hypothesis that repeated lifting tasks involving the Valsalva manoeuvre could be a risk factor for RD.[11] Cases were enrolled from patients treated surgically for RD in a large urban hospital while controls were drawn from outpatients attending an eye clinic within the same catchment area. Due to the study design, all controls were near-sighted; therefore, to avoid confounding, the main analysis was restricted to myopic patients. Three categories of exposure to lifting were identified based on lifelong cumulative exposure, calculated as the product of the typically handled load (kg), frequency (number of lifting manoeuvres per week), and number of years of lifting. Since the authors hypothesized that the association between lifting and RD was mediated by the Valsalva manoeuvre, only information regarding loads heavier than 10 kg was used to estimate cumulative exposure. Odds ratios (OR) of RD and associated 95% confidence intervals (95% CI) were estimated through a multivariate logistic regression model (Table 5.1). Findings from the study supported the a priori hypothesis that heavy lifting was a strong risk factor for RD (OR 4.4, 95% CI 1.6–13). Intriguingly, body mass index (BMI) also showed a clear association with RD (top quartile: OR 6.8, 95% CI 1.6–29). Finally, degree of myopia, ocular surgery,

Table 5.1 Associations with retinal detachment

	Cases	Controls	OR (95% CI)	
			Univariate	Multivariate[a]
BMI (kg/m²)				
<21.0	9	23	1.9 (0.5–6.6)	1.2 (0.3–6.1)
21.0–22.9	5	24	1.0	1.0
23.0–25.4	14	26	2.6 (0.8–8.5)	2.2 (0.5–10)
≥25.5	33	26	6.1 (1.9–20)	6.8 (1.6–29)
Cumulative lifting (kg × freq × y)				
No manual lifting	25	67	1.0	1.0
≤8000	13	21	1.7 (0.7–3.8)	1.1 (0.4–3.0)
>8000	22	11	5.4 (2.1–13)	4.4 (1.5–13)
Myopia				
−0.5 to −5.75 dioptres	43	81	1.0	1.0
−6 to −9.75 dioptres	6	14	0.8 (0.3–2.3)	0.4 (0.1–1.5)
−10 dioptres or worse	12	4	5.7 (1.6–19)	4.2 (1.0–17)
Eye surgery (including cataract)				
No	39	93	1.0	1.0
Yes	22	6	8.7 (3.0–25)	7.1 (2.3–22)
Eye or head trauma				
No	38	88	1.0	1.0
Yes	23	11	4.8 (2.0–11.4)	5.0 (1.8–14)

[a] Adjusted for age and sex

Adapted with permission from Mattioli S, De Fazio R, Buiatti E, et al., Physical exertion (lifting) and retinal detachment among people with myopia, *Epidemiology*, Volume **19**, Issue 6, pp. 868–71, Copyright © 2008 Lippincott Williams & Wilkins

and ocular/head trauma were confirmed as important risk factors for RD. Based on their findings, the authors concluded that heavy occupational lifting (involving the Valsalva manoeuvre) may be a relevant risk factor for RD in myopics.

One important limitation of this study concerned the generalizability of the findings to non-myopic subjects. Because non-myopic cases were available, a case-case analysis was conducted to explore whether the risk of RD in workers performing lifting tasks is modified by the presence and the degree of myopia.[19] In that analysis, a constant effect of lifting was observed among four myopia strata (i.e. up to −0.5 dioptres, −0.5 to −4.75, −5 to −9.75, greater than −10). Hence, the authors concluded that heavy lifting may increase the risk of RD regardless of myopia. This hypothesis was indirectly confirmed in an extended case-control analysis in which both myopic and non-myopic cases were compared to myopic controls.[20]

Retinal detachment and manual work: a population-based study

A large population-based study carried out in Tuscany showed that surgically treated idiopathic RRD was almost twice as common among manual workers as non-manual workers.[34] This observation reinforces the evidence that work-related factors are relevant to RD onset.[11]

Interpretation of this finding must allow for the possibility that various factors, such as the prevalence of myopia and of severe myopia, occupational exposure, and BMI, could all be associated with the broad socio-occupational category of manual workers. Given that the prevalence of myopia of all degrees is strongly associated with both a higher level of education and higher socioeconomic status,[35,36] it seems unlikely that the higher rates of RRD recorded for manual workers could be explained in terms of a greater burden of severe myopia among this occupational category. Moreover, in the EPIC-Norfolk Eye Study, refractive error was associated with educational level but not with occupational class classified as manual/non-manual workers,[37] supporting the view that the association between lifting and RD is not substantially confounded by myopia. On the other hand, the finding appears consistent with the hypothesis that a relevant risk factor for idiopathic RRD may be heavy manual lifting requiring the Valsalva manoeuvre.[11,19] As a broad category, manual workers can be expected to perform such tasks much more frequently than non-manual workers, who will encounter this exposure mainly outside working hours (i.e. when engaging in sports or other hobbies, or performing domestic tasks).

High BMI is associated with surgically treated RD[11,19] but, even though people of lower socioeconomic status are more likely to be overweight or obese, its prevalence in Tuscany is very low.[38] Hence, it seems unlikely that the association with manual work in this study was substantially confounded by BMI.

Our findings from Tuscany appear to contrast with those from a study in Scotland,[39,40] where the incidence of RRD was associated with increasing affluence, as measured by the Scottish Index of Multiple Deprivation.[41] This apparent discrepancy could be related to major differences in the measures of interest (i.e. using a complex deprivation score rather than manual/non-manual work), and to different case definitions (diagnosed RRD cases instead of surgically treated cases of idiopathic RRD). Mitry and colleagues concluded that 'RRD cases from more deprived datazones frequently present with a more extensive area of detachment',[40] suggesting that case definition could be important.

This work indicates that the higher rates of RRD recorded among manual workers are consistent with the hypothesis that heavy lifting is an important risk factor. It underlines the importance of prevention and the identification of both occupational and non-occupational risk factors.

Prevention and research gaps

At present, only general guidance on prevention of RD can be given. We hypothesize that the Valsalva manoeuvre performed during lifting might increase the risk of RD. However, little is known about the changes in intraocular pressure during lifting. Experimental studies should be carried out to study the dose-response relationship between the lifted weight and the increase in intraocular pressure, also taking into account personal factors (e.g. gender, body shape) and working conditions (e.g. frequency of lifting, posture). There is also no firm epidemiological evidence about the exposure-response relationship between lifting tasks and the risk of RD. Future studies should investigate the time window between the exposure and occurrence of the disease. In addition, it will be important to investigate whether the elevation of risk is reversible following cessation of exposure.

If confirmed, the association between lifting and RD would open up new scenarios for prevention. Training on breathing techniques might be effective in reducing the number of Valsalva manoeuvres performed during a work shift. In the occupational health assessment of manual material handlers in relation to their exposure to biomechanical risk factors, eye examinations might be considered for workers with multiple risk factors to encourage early diagnosis of RD or its precursors. Finally, retinal diseases and their risk factors should be added to the criteria for the evaluation of fitness to work for jobs involving manual material handling.

Acknowledgements

We thank Professor David Coggon for his support for our efforts in rediscovering the occupational aetiology of retinal detachment. We are also grateful to Robin M.T. Cooke for his collaboration.

References

1. Ghazi NG, Green WR. Pathology and pathogenesis of retinal detachment. *Eye* 2002;**16**:411–21.

2. Johnson MW. Posterior vitreous detachment: evolution and complications of its early stages. *Am J Ophthalmol* 2010;**149**:371–82.

3. Kreissig I. Surgical techniques for repair of primary retinal detachment: Part II. Comparison of present techniques in relation to morbidity. *Folia Med* 2010;**52**:5–11.

4. Pastor JC, Fernández I, Rodríguez de la Rúa E, *et al*. Surgical outcomes for primary rhegmatogenous retinal detachments in phakic and pseudophakic patients: the Retina 1 Project—report 2. *Br J Ophthalmol* 2008;**92**:378–82.

5. **Byer NE.** Natural history of posterior vitreous detachment with early management as the premier line of defense against retinal detachment. *Ophthalmology* 1994;**101**:1503–13.

6. **Mitry D, Charteris DG, Fleck BW, Campbell H, Singh J.** The epidemiology of rhegmatogenous retinal detachment: geographical variation and clinical associations. *Br J Ophthalmol* 2010;**94**:678–84.

7. **The Eye Disease Case-Control Study Group.** Risk factors for idiopathic rhegmatogenous retinal detachment. *Am J Epidemiol* 1993;**137**:749–57.

8. **Wong TY, Tielsch JM, Schein OD.** Racial difference in the incidence of retinal detachment in Singapore. *Arch Ophthalmol* 1999;**117**:379–83.

9. **Mayo Clinic staff.** *Retinal detachment: prevention.* Available at: <http://www.mayoclinic.com/health/retinal-detachment/DS00254/DSECTION=prevention> (accessed 18 January 2013).

10. **Etminan M, Forooghian F, Brophy JM, Bird ST, Maberley D.** Oral fluoroquinolones and the risk of retinal detachment. *JAMA* 2012;**307**:1414–9.

11. **Mattioli S, De Fazio R, Buiatti E, et al.** Physical exertion (lifting) and retinal detachment among people with myopia. *Epidemiology* 2008;**19**:868–71.

12. **Edridge-Green FW.** The Arris and Gale Lecture on the cause and prevention of myopia. *Lancet* 1921;**197**:469–71.

13. **Cross AG, Diamond PAM.** Vision and eye disorders. In: Edwards FC, McCallum RI, Taylor PJ (eds) *Fitness for work: the medical aspects.* Oxford: Oxford University Press, 1988, pp. 101–13.

14. **Diamond PAM, Munton CGF.** Visual and ocular disorders. In: Cox RAF, Edwards F, McCallum RI (eds) *Fitness for work: the medical aspects* (2nd edn). Oxford: Oxford University Press, 1995, pp. 88–101.

15. **Diamond PAM, Munton G.** Vision and eye disorders. In: Cox RAF, Edwards FC, Palmer K (eds) *Fitness for work: the medical aspects* (3rd edn). Oxford: Oxford University Press, 2000, pp. 167–81.

16. **Johnston RV, Pitts J.** Vision and eye disorders. In: Palmer KT, Cox RAF, Brown I (eds) *Fitness for work: the medical aspects* (4th edn). Oxford: Oxford University Press, 2007, pp. 189–210.

17. **Pitts J, Mitchell SJ.** Vision and eye disorders. In: Palmer KT, Brown I, Hobson J (eds) *Fitness for work: the medical aspects* (5th edn). Oxford: Oxford University Press, 2012, pp. 174–95.

18. **Mattioli S, Zanardi F, Baldasseroni A, et al.** Search strings for the study of putative occupational determinants of disease. *Occup Environ Med* 2010;**67**:436–43. (Correction in *Occup Environ Med* 2010;**67**:799.)

19. **Mattioli S, Curti S, De Fazio R, et al.** Risk factors for retinal detachment (letter). *Epidemiology* 2009;**20**:465–6.

20. **Mattioli S, Curti S, De Fazio R, et al.** Occupational lifting tasks and retinal detachment in non-myopics and myopics: extended analysis of a case-control study. *Saf Health Work* 2012;**3**:52–7.

21. **Dambite GR, Flik LP.** Vliianie razlichnykh vidov truda na vozniknovenie tiazhelykh oslozhnenii pri blizorukosti. [Effect of different types of work on the development of severe complications in myopia.] *Oftalmol Zh* 1973;**28**:375–8.

22. **Scheerer R.** Netzhautablösung nach ungewohnter körperlicher Uberanstrengung. Augenärztliches Obergutachten zur Zusammenhangsfrage. [Retinal detachment following unaccustomed physical exertion. Ophthalmological senior expert testimony on the problem of causality.] *Klin Monbl Augenheilkd* 1974;**165**:670–2.

23. **Gärtner J.** Netzhautablosung durch Aderhautstauung? Zur Frage der Entstehung einer Amotio retinae nach ungewohnter koperlicher Anstrengung. [Retinal detachment, caused by hyperaemia of the choroid? Remarks on the supposed relationship between retinal detachment and 'indirect trauma'.] *Klin Monbl Augenheilkd* 1975;**166**:559–63.

24. **Schwab B, Gärtner J.** Kann das Heben schwerer Lasten einen zur Netzhautabhebung disponierenden Ziliarmuskelspasmus hervorrufen? Echographische Untersuchungen. [Can the lifting of heavy weights provoke a spasm of ciliary muscles conducive in turn to retinal detachment?] *Mod Probl Ophthalmol* 1977;**18**:64–7.

25. **Pivovarov NN, Malakhova LA, Bagdasarova TA, Chetvertukhin AP.** Rol' podniatiia tiazhesti v vozniknovenii otsloiki setchatki. [Role of weight lifting in the development of retinal detachment.] *Vestn Oftalmol* 1977;**6**:50–3.

26. **Synek S, Vlková E.** Pracovni zarazeni u nemocnych po operaci odchlipene sitnice. [Work capacity evaluation in patients after surgery for detached retina.] *Cesk Oftalmol* 1989;**45**:187–91.

27. **Bovino JA, Marcus DF.** Physical activity after retinal detachment surgery. *Am J Ophthalmol* 1984;**98**:171–9.

28. **Kamel F, Boyes WK, Gladen BC, et al.** Retinal degeneration in licensed pesticide applicators. *Am J Ind Med* 2000;**37**:618–28.

29. **Risner D, Ehrlich R, Kheradiya NS, Siesky B, McCranor L, Harris A.** Effects of exercise on intraocular pressure and ocular blood flow: a review. *J Glaucoma* 2009;**18**:429–36.

30. **Aykan U, Erdurmus M, Yilmaz B, Bilge AH.** Intraocular pressure and ocular pulse amplitude variations during the Valsalva maneuver. *Graefes Arch Clin Exp Ophthalmol* 2010;**248**:1183–6.

31. **Brody S, Erb C, Veit R, Rau H.** Intraocular pressure changes: the influence of psychological stress and the Valsalva maneuver. *Biol Psychol* 1999;**51**:43–57.

32. **Rafuse PE, Mills DW, Hooper PL, Chang TS, Wolf R.** Effects of Valsalva's manoeuvre on intraocular pressure. *Can J Ophthalmol* 1994;**29**:73–6.

33. **Vieira GM, Oliveira HB, de Andrade DT, Bottaro M, Ritch R.** Intraocular pressure variation during weight lifting. *Arch Ophthalmol* 2006;**124**:1251–4.

34. **Curti S, Mattioli S, Baldasseroni A, et al.** Incidence rates of surgically treated rhegmatogenous retinal detachment among manual workers, non-manual workers and housewives in Tuscany, Italy. *Occup Environ Med* 2011;**68**(Suppl 1):A55.

35. **Bar Dayan Y, Levin A, Morad Y, et al.** The changing prevalence of myopia in young adults: a 13-year series of population-based prevalence surveys. *Invest Ophthalmol Vis Sci* 2005;**46**:2760–5.

36. **Saw SM, Katz J, Schein OD, Chew SJ, Chan TK.** Epidemiology of myopia. *Epidemiol Rev* 1996;**18**:175–87.

37. **Foster PJ, Broadway DC, Hayat S, et al.** Refractive error, axial length and anterior chamber depth of the eye in British adults: the EPIC-Norfolk Eye Study. *Br J Ophthalmol* 2010;**94**:827–30.

38. **Istituto Nazionale di Statistica (Istat).** Indagine multiscopo sulle famiglie. Condizioni di salute e ricorso ai servizi sanitari 1999–2000. Roma: Istat, 2003. Available at: <http://www3.istat.it/dati/catalogo/20020313_01/> (accessed 18 January 2013).

39. **Saidkasimova S, Mitry D, Singh J, Yorston D, Charteris DG.** Retinal detachment in Scotland is associated with affluence. *Br J Ophthalmol* 2009;**93**:1591–4.

40. **Mitry D, Charteris DG, Yorston D,** *et al.* The epidemiology and socioeconomic associations of retinal detachment in Scotland: a two-year prospective population-based study. *Invest Ophthalmol Vis Sci* 2010;**51**:4963–8.

41. **The Scottish Government.** *Scottish Index of Multiple Deprivation. 2009 general report.* Edinburgh: The Scottish Government, 2009. Available at: <http://www.scotland.gov.uk/ Resource/Doc/289599/0088642.pdf> (accessed 18 January 2013.)

Part 2

Studying new populations

Chapter 6

What is the impact on mental health and well-being of military service in general and deployment in particular? A UK perspective

Nicola T. Fear, Josefin Sundin, and Simon Wessely

Why is studying mental health important, particularly in an occupational setting?

The role of 'work' has become prominent in the political arena as a possible determinant of health and well-being. The current coalition government of the UK has launched its 'No Health Without Mental Health' strategy, which outlines how employers, schools, local councils, housing organizations, voluntary groups, and health care bodies can promote good mental health.[1] 'Work stress' has been linked to behavioural problems, such as absenteeism from work; mental health problems, such as depression; and physical problems, including coronary heart disease.[2,3] Stress has also been linked to increased alcohol consumption which can have an impact on social and occupational functioning.[3] The profession of arms is one particular occupation in which one might expect to encounter 'work stress'. Our own centre, the King's Centre for Military Health Research (KCMHR), has been created to study the health of the UK Armed Forces including, but not restricted to, mental health.

Why is studying the military important?

Most modern military organizations are highly selected groups. In the UK, national service ended in 1963[4] and since then the UK military has been an all-volunteer force. Personnel choose to join, and then undergo various physical and technical training and they are required to have regular physical examinations throughout several stages of service, together with operational training for deployment.

It has long been known that war is associated with physical and psychological injury. Some uninformed commentators sometimes claim that the introduction of the diagnosis of post-traumatic stress disorder (PTSD) into the third edition of the Diagnostic and Statistical Manual,[5] the 'bible' of classification produced by the American Psychiatric Association, represented the first time that the psychological costs of conflict had been recognized, but this is a misreading of history.[6,7]

Several studies have shown that all modern conflicts have been associated with post-deployment syndromes characterized by unexplained medical symptoms.[8] In brief, these syndromes have included the following:

1. Debility syndrome, which was the most prevalent post-combat disorder in the nineteenth and early twentieth centuries amongst veterans of the late Victorian campaigns and the Boer Wars. Soldiers commonly presented with symptoms including general fatigue, rheumatic pains, and weakness for which physicians of the time were unable to find an explanation.[9]

2. Shell shock, which is associated with the First World War (1914–18) when soldiers in the trenches experienced unrelenting artillery bombardment. Symptoms included tiredness, irritability, giddiness, lack of concentration, and headaches.[10]

3. Gulf War syndrome, which emerged after the 1991 Gulf conflict, was defined as a collection of largely unexplained and often vague illnesses that affected the well-being of a minority of personnel who deployed to Iraq in 1991.[11–14]

Newer forms of psychological injury are likely to be less predictable, less well understood, harder to manage,[15] and compounded by external influences such as cultural factors[8] and media coverage of military health issues.[16]

There are many reports in the media which speculate about the consequences of military service, particularly deployment (for example,[17–19]). It is thus important to ensure that robust research is undertaken to either support or refute the claims made.

What was the approach of KCMHR?

The UK Ministry of Defence did not expect, and was unprepared for, the criticism that arose some years after the 1991 Gulf conflict in respect to their monitoring and handling of 'Gulf War syndrome'. In order to have early warning of any similar problem arising from the 2003 Iraq conflict, and to be in a position to respond appropriately, KCMHR were commissioned to develop and undertake a study of the health and well-being of UK military personnel deployed to the 2003 Iraq conflict and a comparable group of non-deployed service personnel to determine the health impact of deployment[20] and to monitor for the emergence of an 'Iraq War syndrome'.[21]

Phase 1 of the KCMHR cohort study compared a range of health outcomes between two randomly selected groups.[20] The first group consisted of approximately 10% of the fighting force that deployed during the war fighting phase of the 2003 Iraq conflict (codename Operation TELIC 1). The TELIC sample comprised individuals deployed between 18 January 2003 and 28 April 2003 (n = 7695). The second group comprised of individuals who were in the military at the same time but were not deployed on Operation TELIC 1 (termed Era) (n = 10 003). The sample included those who had left the military, those employed under a regular engagement (in full-time military employment), and those employed under a reservist engagement (individuals paid by the military only when they are carrying out military duties; reservists typically have civilian jobs when not working for the military) (Figure 6.1). Reservists were over-sampled at a ratio of 2:1 and the non-deployed group (Era) was increased by 10% because we anticipated that many individuals within this group would deploy

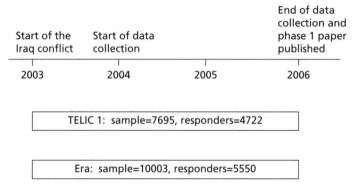

Figure 6.1 Timeline and sample for phase 1 of the KCMHR cohort study.[20]
Source: data from *The Lancet*, Volume **367**, Hotopf M et al., The health of UK military personnel who deployed to the 2003 Iraq war: a cohort study, pp. 1731–41, Copyright © 2006 Elsevier.

on later military operations to Iraq, and to take account of the fact that a number of non-deployed personnel would have had medical limitations placed on their ability to deploy. These individuals were randomly selected from UK Ministry of Defence databases (held by Defence Analytical Services and Advice (DASA)) and sampled to represent the order of battle for the war fighting phase of the Iraq conflict (TELIC 1). Contact details of eligible potential participants were provided by DASA to the researchers at KCMHR.

KCMHR developed a comprehensive self-report questionnaire which was sent to individuals, or individuals were visited by the research team at their military base. Over 50 base visits took place throughout the data collection period (2004–06). Overall, 10 272 personnel completed our phase 1 questionnaire (4722 from the TELIC sample and 5550 from the Era sample), resulting in a 59% response rate (with less than 1% actively refusing to participate).[20] Investigation of our responders and non-responders led us to conclude that there was no evidence of response bias from a health perspective[22] and that non-response was mainly due to the mobility of the study population.[23] The key results from phase 1 were published in 2006.[20,21]

The conflict in Iraq continued and UK Armed Forces experienced an increase in hostilities in the south of the country. At the same time, the campaign in Afghanistan intensified with UK Armed Forces deployed in large numbers to Helmand Province in southern Afghanistan, close to the Pakistan border. Fighting was intense and casualties were frequent, often resulting from improvised explosive devices causing trauma to those injured and those who observed them. So, in 2006, KCMHR was commissioned by the UK Ministry of Defence to undertake a further phase of the cohort study, to explore the longer-term impact of deployment to Iraq but also to explore the impact of deployment to Afghanistan.[24] In order to achieve this, we re-assessed the mental health of those who participated in phase 1 (who had given us consent for follow-up) as well as including two additional groups in order to represent the military structure (those who had joined the military since 2003; additional sample 1, the replenishment sample) and operational deployments (those deployed to Afghanistan between

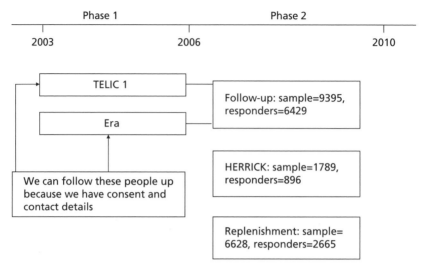

Figure 6.2 Timeline and sample for phase 2 of the KCMHR cohort study.[24]
Source: data from *The Lancet*, Volume **375**, Fear NT et al., What are the consequences of deployment to Iraq and Afghanistan on the mental health of the UK armed forces? A cohort study, pp. 1783–97, Copyright © 2010 Elsevier.

April 2006 and April 2007; additional sample 2, the HERRICK sample. Operation HERRICK is the UK military codename for the current military operations in Afghanistan) (Figure 6.2).

Of the 10 272 follow-up participants, 914 could not be followed-up because they had not given consent to be contacted again, had died, or could not be contacted because of insufficient address information. Thirty-seven participants who had returned completed questionnaires after phase 1 data collection had ended were included in the follow-up sample at phase 2. In total, 9395 participants were entered into the data collection for phase 2; 7884 were regular personnel and 1511 were reservists.

Additional sample 1, the 'replenishment sample', was randomly drawn from personnel who joined the military and were trained between the end of April 2003 and April 2007. For regulars, a sample fraction of approximately 7% was used. For reservists to be eligible they had to have received a bounty payment in 2007 and 2008 (bounty payments are made for attending a minimum number of training sessions the previous year). Reservists were oversampled at a ratio of 3:1. Overall, 7438 individuals were selected. Of these, 810 were ineligible because they had been incorrectly sampled, had died before we were able to contact them, or insufficient address information was supplied. The final size of the replenishment sample was 6628, of which 5128 were regular personnel and 1500 were reservists.

Additional sample 2, the 'HERRICK sample' was a random sample of military personnel who had deployed to Afghanistan between April 2006 and April 2007 (the period spanning Operations HERRICK 4 and 5). Approximately 10% of regular personnel and 90% of reservists who had served on Operations HERRICK 4 and 5 were sampled (1491 and 334 respectively). Thirty-six individuals originally sampled were not eligible and the final HERRICK sample contained 1789 individuals (1455 regulars and 334 reservists).

The characteristics of our overall sample were compared to the composition of the UK military at April 2007.[25,26] The distribution of age, sex, rank, and engagement type was similar, the only exception being service. Our sample had proportionally more Army personnel (67%) than in the UK military in 2007 (56%); this is because our sample reflected those likely to be deployed on operations.

As for phase 1, data were collected using an extensive self-report questionnaire. Data were collected between 2007 and 2009. The overall numbers who responded were: 6429 from the follow-up sample, 896 HERRICK sample, and 2665 from the replenishment sample, resulting in a 56% response rate.

The non-responders were more likely to be young males who hold lower ranks.[20,23,24] We were also able to use the data that we had already collected on all of those who took part in phase 1 to see if mental health at phase 1 influenced response at phase 2. Using that data, we found no evidence to suggest that response was associated with mental health status.[24] The key paper from phase 2 was published in 2010.[24]

Our response rate is comparable with that achieved by other large population-based studies, especially of mobile populations dominated by young men. The only other military study which collects longitudinal data on identified individuals (the US-based Millennium cohort study) has a response rate of 36%[27] and another US study, the RAND study, has a response rate of approximately 5%.[28]

Key measures used

Both phases collected data using self-report questionnaires.[20,21] These questionnaires used identical health measures so that changes over time could be accurately examined. The PTSD checklist (PCL) was used, a 17-item measure, with a score of 50 or more being used to define probable PTSD.[29] Symptoms of common mental disorder were assessed using the General Health Questionnaire, a 12-item measure, and a score of 4 or more was used to define 'caseness'.[30] Alcohol misuse was defined as scoring 16 or more on the Alcohol Use Disorders Identification Test questionnaire.[31]

What is the impact of deployment to the recent conflicts in Iraq and Afghanistan?

Phase 1 of our study showed that, for regulars, there was no impact of deployment on prevalence rates of probable PTSD, or of symptoms of common mental disorders (Table 6.1).[20] A small difference in prevalence was seen for alcohol misuse, with those in the deployment group more likely to report alcohol misuse than those in the non-deployed group. For reservists, we showed that there was an impact of being deployed on both probable PTSD and symptoms of common mental disorders. It is worth noting that although the rate of probable PTSD was highest in deployed reservists this rate, at 6%, was still low.

The finding for reservists led the UK Ministry of Defence to make changes to the way reservists were mobilized, demobilized, and the support they received post-deployment.

Table 6.1 Prevalence (%) of mental health outcomes among phase 1 participants, by regular and reserve status and deployment status[20]

	Regulars		Reservists	
	Not deployed to Iraq (Era)	**Deployed to Iraq (TELIC)**	**Not deployed to Iraq (Era)**	**Deployed to Iraq (TELIC)**
Probable PTSD	4	4	3	6
Symptoms of common mental disorders	19	20	16	26
Alcohol misuse	14	18	8	10

Source: data from *The Lancet*, Volume **367**, Hotopf M et al., The health of UK military personnel who deployed to the 2003 Iraq war: a cohort study, pp. 1731–41, Copyright © 2006 Elsevier

In-service mental health care was extended to reservists demobilized since January 2003 following overseas operational deployment and the Army introduced the 'one-Army' concept which integrated reservists with their regular counterparts prior, during, and post-deployment.

One of the key early objectives of the study was to see if there had been a repeat of the 'Gulf War syndrome' saga.[11–14] We, therefore, looked at the reporting of 53 symptoms among the TELIC and Era samples to see if there was any evidence of an 'Iraq War syndrome'. Perhaps surprisingly, there was no evidence of differential reporting in symptoms between the two groups.[21] Many of the factors that had been implicated in the media and popular imagination in the genesis of 'Gulf War syndrome', such as exposure to depleted uranium, use of pesticides, anthrax vaccination, and the use of pyridostigmine bromide as a protection against nerve gas agents, were present during both the 1991 Gulf War and the 2003 invasion of Iraq. The lack of a similar multi-symptom syndrome after the 2003 invasion suggests that these exposures were perhaps not responsible for the observed increase in multi-symptom illness seen in the aftermath of the 1991 conflict.

Returning to the most recent Iraq War, as is now well known, but had not been anticipated, the conflict did not resemble the brief campaign of 1991, but instead turned into a prolonged counter-insurgency campaign. Furthermore, in 2006 the UK commitment to Afghanistan intensified. One consequence was that the Ministry of Defence now decided to extend our study to cover these developments. Phase 2 gave us the opportunity to examine the longer-term impact of deployment to Iraq; to see if the changes to the way reservists were deployed and their post-service health care access had led to any changes in their mental health, and to explore the impact of multiple deployments.[24]

Phase 2 showed that the impact of deployment among regulars was again limited to alcohol misuse, with no impact on probable PTSD or on symptoms of common mental disorders (Table 6.2). These data also indicate that the mental health of the UK Armed Forces had not changed between phase 1 and 2 of our study. This finding, whilst reassuring, was surprising given the duration of the Iraq conflict and the escalation of the UK commitment to Afghanistan, where fighting was intense.

Table 6.2 Prevalence (%) of mental health outcomes among phase 2 participants, by regular and reserve status and deployment status[24]

	Regulars		Reservists	
	Not deployed to Iraq or Afghanistan	Deployed to Iraq or Afghanistan	Not deployed to Iraq or Afghanistan	Deployed to Iraq or Afghanistan
Probable PTSD	4	4	2	5
Symptoms of common mental disorders	20	20	19	19
Alcohol misuse	10	16	8	9

Adapted from *Lancet*, Volume **375**, Fear NT et al., What are the consequences of deployment to Iraq and Afghanistan on the mental health of the UK armed forces? A cohort study, pp. 1783–97, Copyright © 2010, with permission from Elsevier

Table 6.3 Prevalence (%) of mental health outcomes among phase 2 participants who were deployed, by deployment role[24]

	Combat	Combat support	Combat service support
Probable PTSD	7	2	4
Symptoms of common mental disorders	21	18	20
Alcohol misuse	23	11	14

Adapted from *Lancet*, Volume **375**, Fear NT et al., What are the consequences of deployment to Iraq and Afghanistan on the mental health of the UK armed forces? A cohort study, pp. 1783–97, Copyright © 2010, with permission from Elsevier

We anticipated that changes made by the UK Ministry of Defence in the way in which reservists were mobilized and deployed, and the support available on their return, might have reduced the previously observed impact of deployment on mental health. Unfortunately, although we found no impact of deployment on the reporting of symptoms of common mental disorder, the prevalence of probable PTSD among deployed reservists was almost doubled.

We also explored the impact of combat among those deployed. As expected, we saw that those deployed in a combat role (compared to those deployed in a non-combat role) were more likely to report probable PTSD, and this group were also more likely to report alcohol misuse (Table 6.3). The higher prevalence noted for alcohol misuse was mainly accounted for by age and gender; those in combat roles are predominantly young men and young men drink more.[24,32]

We had anticipated that those who had experienced more deployments to Iraq and Afghanistan would report more mental health problems.[33,34] These analyses were restricted to regular Army personnel who were still in service at the time of questionnaire completion. Army personnel, in general, deploy for periods of 6 months while the pattern of deployments differs for the other services and for reservists. Examination of

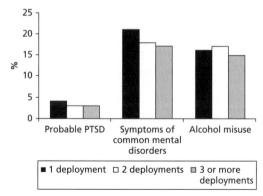

Figure 6.3 Total number of deployments (to 2010) among currently serving UK Army regulars and the prevalence rates (%) of mental health outcomes.[24]

Source: data from *The Lancet*, Volume **375**, Fear NT et al., What are the consequences of deployment to Iraq and Afghanistan on the mental health of the UK armed forces? A cohort study, pp. 1783–97, Copyright © 2010 Elsevier.

the prevalence rates of each disorder by number of deployments showed that there was no association with the reporting of mental health problems (Figure 6.3).[24] This lack of effect may be partially explained by selection, the 'healthy warrior effect', in which those who are unwell as a result of previous deployment have less chance of subsequent deployment,[35] whilst those who are more psychologically robust have more chance of deployment. Thus, rather than the counter-intuitive conclusion that deployment is 'good' for mental health, it is more likely that those with multiple deployments represent a more resilient group of individuals.

Comparisons with the UK general population

As the UK military are predominantly comprised of individuals from the UK general population (approximately 5% of the UK military are foreign nationals), it is useful to compare the military to the general population. It might be expected that, given the nature of the role of the Armed Forces, military personnel would be more likely than the general population to report mental health problems.

Initial comparisons with household-based surveys for symptoms of common mental disorders indicate that the rates are higher in the military than the general population. This may be the context in which these studies are administered;[36] they are often termed 'stress at work studies' which may lead to an over-reporting of symptoms and reflect dissatisfaction with the employer rather than overt mental health problems. When the military is compared to other occupational groups, similar rates of symptoms of common mental disorders are seen.

Our work has shown that compared to data collected as part of the Adult Psychiatric Morbidity Survey (data collected in 2007 from adults living in England) the rates of probable PTSD are comparable at approximately 4%.[37]

Comparisons with regards to alcohol misuse are not so favourable. Here, using a cut-off of 16 or more on the Alcohol Use Disorders Identification Test, the prevalence of misuse is 6% in the general population versus 13% in the UK military.[24,32,38] There are obvious demographic differences between the general population and the military, with the military being dominated by young men. But by making age- and gender-matched comparisons, we see that military men and women across all ages are more likely to report alcohol misuse than the general population (Figure 6.4).[32]

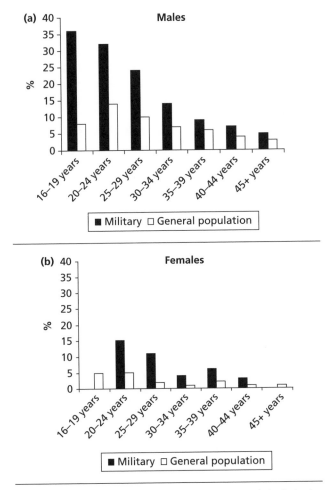

Figure 6.4 Comparison of prevalence rates (%) by age group of alcohol misuse between the UK military and the general population (based on data from the Adult Psychiatric Morbidity Survey) for males (a) and females (b).[37]

Source: data from McManus S et al., *Adult psychiatric morbidity in England, 2007: results of a household survey*, NHS Information Centre, Copyright © 2009, The Health & Social Care Information Centre, Social Care Statistics. Available at: <http://www.ic.nhs.uk/pubs/psychiatricmorbidity07>.

Comparisons with the US military

We might hypothesize that the health consequences of deployment would be similar between the US and UK militaries given that both have been fighting the same conflicts in the same environments for the last decade. However, the prevalence of PTSD is higher in the US military than the UK for those deployed (Figure 6.5).[24,39] Also, the prevalence rate of PTSD is higher post-deployment in the US military for both regulars and reservists. This is a further difference between the two nations. The expected trajectory of PTSD-related symptoms is a peak in reporting immediately after the trauma (in this case deployment) and the usual picture would be that these rates decrease as time since the trauma (i.e. deployment) increases.[40] This is not seen in the US, where rates of PTSD increase as time since deployment increases.[24,41] The same was anticipated to occur in the UK and a 'tidal wave' of probable PTSD had been predicted.[42] Our research shows that this is not the case.[24] We did find a modest increase in the prevalence of reported probable PTSD with time since return from deployment[24] but not to the extent expected by some. This increase represents more of a 'ripple' than the tidal wave predicted.

Why do we see these differences? As we are fighting the same enemy, on the same terrain, facing similar risks, using similar tactics, the reason for these differences is unlikely to lie in what is going in the operational location. We have identified a number of possible factors that may account for the differences observed:[24,41]

1. Sociodemographic differences. The US military is comprised of more reservists, non-officers, and young personnel, these are all factors associated with probable PTSD.[43]

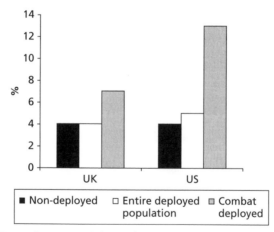

Figure 6.5 PTSD prevalence rates (%) stratified by country (US and UK).[24,39]
Source: data from Fear NT et al., What are the consequences of deployment to Iraq and Afghanistan on the mental health of the UK armed forces? A cohort study, *The Lancet*, Volume **375**, pp. 1783–97, Copyright © 2010 Elsevier and Kok BC et al., Posttraumatic stress disorder associated with combat service in Iraq or Afghanistan: reconciling prevalence differences between studies, *The Journal of Nervous and Mental Disease*, Volume **200**, pp. 444–50, Copyright © 2012 Lippincott Williams & Wilkins, Inc.

2. Deployment length differences. The US military deploy for approximately 12–15 months while the usual deployment length for the UK military is 6 months. This implies that US troops have twice the amount of time in a conflict zone and thus a higher chance of exposure to a traumatic experience.

3. Deployment locations. At the initial stages of the Iraq conflict, the US military were deployed to more hostile locations and they experienced more fatalities and casualties. This may have accounted for the differences observed originally between the two nations. However, once the UK commitment to Afghanistan increased, the patterns of fatalities and casualties changed.

4. Access to post-deployment health care. In the UK, serving military personnel have access to in-service health care and ex-service personnel fall under the remit of the National Health Service. In the US, since January 2008 military personnel, including reservists, have access to 5 years of Veterans Affairs health care after leaving service, for conditions that are determined by their Veterans Affairs doctor to be related to service in a combat area.[44] Prior to January 2008, the entitlement was for 2 rather than 5 years. Given that most people leave the military when they are still comparatively young, and well before they might be expected to develop age-related disease, even 5 years guaranteed access to health care will for the most part not provide much reassurance that future health needs will be taken care of.

Ex-service personnel

The media perception of ex-service personnel is that they are homeless, in prison, or have a mental health problem as a result of their military service (for example,[45–47]). It is not surprising that this perception is shared by the UK public. However, there is a growing body of evidence to show that these images are incorrect.[48]

Compared to serving personnel, those who left the military are more likely to report probable PTSD and symptoms of common mental disorders but they are no more likely to report alcohol misuse. We have also been able to look at Early Service Leavers (those that leave the military before they have completed the minimum term of service, in general this is 4 years).[49] Early Service Leavers compared to those who served for longer are more likely to report all mental health outcomes and alcohol misuse

Table 6.4 Prevalence (%) of mental health outcomes among Early Service Leavers compared to non-Early Service Leavers (based on phase 1 of the KCMHR cohort study)[49]

	Early Service Leavers	Non-Early Service Leavers
Probable PTSD	20	7
Symptoms of common mental disorders	46	27
Alcohol misuse	31	15

Source: data from Buckman JEJ et al., Early Service leavers: a study of the factors associated with premature separation from the UK Armed Forces and the mental health of those that leave early. *European Journal of Public Health*, 25 April 2012 [Epub ahead of print], Copyright © The Author 2012. Published by Oxford University Press on behalf of the European Public Health Association. All rights reserved. doi:10.1093/eurpub/cks042

(Table 6.4). However, it is not known if this increase is due to military experiences or to pre-service vulnerability. Our work shows that Early Service Leavers report higher levels of pre-enlistment vulnerability factors which are likely to be associated with their leaving and with the development of mental health problems. Using data from the 2007 Adult Psychiatric Morbidity Survey, which for the first time asked individuals if they had ever served in the military and if so for how long, we have been able to compare Early and non-Early Service Leavers.[50] Early Service Leavers report more money problems, alcohol misuse, and suicidal ideation. Other colleagues have looked at suicide rates within ex-service personnel and these data suggest that those who leave within 4 years of joining the military are more likely than their general population counterparts to commit suicide.[51]

There have been various estimates of the proportion of the prison population that are ex-service personnel; these range from 3.5%[52] to 9%.[53] The DASA statistics[52] are likely to represent a more robust estimate because DASA linked their service leavers' database (which includes details of name and date of birth) to the prisoner records supplied by the Ministry of Justice. Other estimates have relied on asking prisoners if they had ever served in the military and we know that recall bias may result in unreliable estimates. DASA were also able to compare the reasons for being in prison between ex-service personnel and the general prison population. What the DASA data showed was that, although ex-service personnel were less likely to be in prison than their general population counterparts, they were more likely to be in prison for sexual and violent offences.[52]

Conclusions

In summary, serving in the military does not necessarily mean that one will end up 'bad, sad, or mad'. PTSD is not the biggest problem seen among serving and ex-service personnel. Alcohol misuse is more prevalent and it is likely to have long-term implications for health, well-being, and functioning. There are, however, groups of individuals who are at increased risk of mental health problems which KCMHR has helped to identify. These include: reservists, Early Service Leavers, and those deployed in a combat role.

While the UK (and our NATO allies) remain in Afghanistan it is vital that we continue to monitor the health and well-being of our military. This need will not stop once the UK withdraws from Afghanistan; as we have learnt from experience, post-deployment syndromes may take many years to surface.

References

1. **Her Majesty's Government and The Department of Health.** *No health without mental health. A cross-government mental health outcomes strategy for people of all ages.* London: The Stationery Office, 2011. Available at: <http://www.dh.gov.uk/prod_consum_dh/groups/dh_digitalassets/documents/digitalasset/dh_124058.pdf> (accessed 5 February 2013).
2. **Kerr R, McHugh M, McCrory M.** HSE management standards and stress-related work outcomes. *Occup Med* 2009;**59**:574–9.

3. **Head J, Martikainen P, Kumari M, Kuper H, Marmot M.** *Work environment, alcohol consumption and ill-health. The Whitehall II Study.* Health and Safety Executive contract research report 422/2002. Norwich: Her Majesty's Stationery Office, 2002. Available at: <http://www.hse.gov.uk/research/crr_pdf/2002/crr02422.pdf> (accessed 5 February, 2013).

4. **Baynes J.** Recruiting the professional army 1960–90. In: Strachan H (ed.) *The British Army, manpower and society into the twenty-first century.* London: Frank Cass Publishers, 2000, pp 49–60.

5. **American Psychiatric Association.** *DSM-III: Diagnostic and statistical manual of mental disorders (3rd edn).* Washington DC: American Psychiatric Association, 1980.

6. **Jones E, Wessely S.** *Maudsley Monographs 47. Shell shock to PTSD: military psychiatry from 1900 to the Gulf War.* New York: Psychology Press, 2005.

7. **Jones E, Wessely S.** A paradigm shift in the conceptualization of psychological trauma in the 20th century. *J Anxiety Disord* 2007;**21**:164–75.

8. **Jones E, Hodgins-Vermaas R, McCartney H,** *et al.* Post-combat syndromes from the Boer war to the Gulf war: a cluster analysis of their nature and attribution. *BMJ* 2002;**324**:321–4. (Correction in *BMJ* 2002;**324**:397.)

9. **Jones E, Wessely S.** Case of chronic fatigue syndrome after Crimean war and Indian mutiny. *BMJ* 1999;**319**:1645–7.

10. **Jones E, Wessely S.** Hearts, guts and minds: somatisation in the military from 1900. *J Psychosom Res* 2004;**56**:425–9.

11. **Cherry N, Creed F, Silman A,** *et al.* Health and exposures of United Kingdom Gulf war veterans. Part I: the pattern and extent of ill health. *Occup Environ Med* 2001;**58**:291–8.

12. **Cherry N, Creed F, Silman A,** *et al.* Health and exposures of United Kingdom Gulf war veterans. Part II: the relation of health to exposure. *Occup Environ Med* 2001;**58**:299–306.

13. **Everitt B, Ismail K, David AS, Wessely S.** Searching for a Gulf War syndrome using cluster analysis. *Psychol Med* 2002;**32**:1371–8.

14. **Simmons R, Maconochie N, Doyle P.** Self-reported ill health in male UK Gulf War veterans: a retrospective cohort study. *BMC Public Health* 2004;**4**:27.

15. **Wessely S.** Risk, psychiatry and the military. *Br J Psychiatry* 2005;**186**:459–66.

16. **Paris M.** *Warrior nation: images of war in British popular culture, 1850–2000.* London: Reaktion, 2000.

17. **Collins T.** *Tsunami of post-traumatic stress haunts our heroes. The Sun,* 22 April, 2011. Available at: <http://www.thesun.co.uk/sol/homepage/news/campaigns/our_boys/3540966/Army-chiefs-on-how-to-help-Our-Boys.html> (accessed 5 February 2013).

18. **Elias M.** Many Iraq veterans fighting an enemy within. *USA Today,* 30 June, 2004. Available at: <http://usatoday30.usatoday.com/news/health/2004-06-30-vets-mental_x.htm> (accessed 5 February 2013).

19. **Daily Mail Reporter.** Army suicides among active-duty soldiers more than DOUBLED in July to reach record high. *Mail Online,* 17 August 2012. Available at: <http://www.dailymail.co.uk/news/article-2189656/Army-suicides-active-duty-soldiers-DOUBLED-July-month-reach-record-number.html#ixzz2FgeiTmEB> (accessed 5 February 2013).

20. **Hotopf M, Hull L, Fear NT,** *et al.* The health of UK military personnel who deployed to the 2003 Iraq war: a cohort study. *Lancet* 2006;**367**:1731–41.

21. **Horn O, Hull L, Jones M,** *et al.* Is there an Iraq war syndrome? Comparison of the health of UK service personnel after the Gulf and Iraq wars. *Lancet* 2006;**367**:1742–6.

22. Tate AR, Jones M, Hull L, *et al*. How many mailouts? Could attempts to increase the response rate in the Iraq war cohort study be counterproductive? *BMC Med Res Methodol* 2007;**7**:51.

23. Iversen A, Liddell K, Fear N, Hotopf M, Wessely S. Consent, confidentiality, and the Data Protection Act. *BMJ* 2006;**332**:165–9.

24. Fear NT, Jones M, Murphy D, *et al*. What are the consequences of deployment to Iraq and Afghanistan on the mental health of the UK armed forces? A cohort study. *Lancet* 2010;**375**:1783–97.

25. Defence Analytical Services and Advice. *UK defence statistics 2009*. Available at: <http://www.dasa.mod.uk/modintranet/UKDS/UKDS2009/ukds.html?PublishTime=09:30:00> (accessed 5 February 2013).

26. Defence Analytical Services and Advice. *Tri-Service Publication 7—UK reserves and cadets strengths at 1 April 2009*. Available at: <http://www.dasa.mod.uk/applications/newWeb/www/index.php?page=48&pubType=1&thiscontent=70&PublishTime=09:30:00&date=2009-11-23&disText=01%20Apr%202009&from=listing&topDate=2009-11-23> (accessed 5 February 2013).

27. Smith TC, Ryan MAK, Wingard DL, Slymen DJ, Sallis JF, Kritz-Silverstein D for the Millennium Cohort Study Team. New onset and persistent symptoms of post-traumatic stress disorder self reported after deployment and combat exposures: prospective population based US military cohort study. *BMJ* 2008;**336**:366–71.

28. Schell TL, Marshall GN. Survey of individuals previously deployed for OEF/OIF. In: Tanielian T, Jaycox LH (eds) *Invisible wounds of war: psychological and cognitive injuries, their consequences, and services to assist recovery*. Santa Monica, CA: RAND Corporation, 2008, pp. 87–115. Available at: <http://www.rand.org/content/dam/rand/pubs/monographs/2008/RAND_MG720.pdf> (accessed 5 February 2013).

29. National Center for PTSD. *PTSD checklist (PCL)*. US Department of Veterans Affairs, 1993. Available at: <http://www.ptsd.va.gov/professional/pages/assessments/ptsd-checklist.asp> (accessed 5 February 2013).

30. Goldberg DP, Gater R, Sartorius N, *et al*. The validity of two versions of the GHQ in the WHO study of mental illness in general health care. *Psychol Med* 1997;**27**:191–7.

31. Babor TF, Higgins-Biddle JC, Saunders JB, Monteiro MG. *AUDIT. The alcohol use disorders identification test. Guidelines for use in primary care* (2nd edn). Geneva: Department of Mental Health and Substance Dependence, World Health Organization, 2001. Available at: <http://whqlibdoc.who.int/hq/2001/who_msd_msb_01.6a.pdf> (accessed 5 February 2013).

32. Fear NT, Iversen A, Meltzer H, *et al*. Patterns of drinking in the UK Armed Forces. *Addiction* 2007;**102**:1749–59.

33. Reger MA, Gahm GA, Swanson RD, Duma SJ. Association between number of deployments to Iraq and mental health screening outcomes in US Army soldiers. *J Clin Psychiatry* 2009;**70**:1266–72.

34. Office of the Command Surgeon, US Forces Afghanistan (USFOR-A), and Office of The Surgeon General, United States Army Medical Command. *Mental Health Advisory Team (MHAT) 6. Operation Enduring Freedom 2009 Afghanistan*. US Army Medical Department Report, 6 November 2009. Available at: <http://www.armymedicine.army.mil/reports/mhat/mhat_vi/MHAT_VI-OEF_Redacted.pdf> (accessed 5 February 2013).

35. Wilson J, Jones M, Fear NT, *et al*. Is previous psychological health associated with the likelihood of Iraq War deployment? An investigation of the 'healthy warrior effect'. *Am J Epidemiol* 2009;**169**:1362–9.

36. Tversky A, Kahneman D. The framing of decisions and the psychology of choice. *Science* 1981;**211**:453–8.

37. McManus S, Meltzer H, Brugha T, Bebbington P, Jenkins R. *Adult psychiatric morbidity in England, 2007: results of a household survey*. NHS Information Centre, January, 2009. Available at: <http://www.ic.nhs.uk/pubs/psychiatricmorbidity07> (accessed 5 February 2013)

38. Coulthard M, Farrell M, Singleton N, Meltzer H. *Tobacco, alcohol and drug use and mental health*. London: The Stationery Office, 2002. Available at: <http://www.ons.gov.uk/ons/rel/psychiatric-morbidity/tobacco – alcohol-and-drug-use-and-mental-health/2000/index.html> (accessed 5 February 2013).

39. Kok BC, Herrell RK, Thomas JL, Hoge CW. Posttraumatic stress disorder associated with combat service in Iraq or Afghanistan: reconciling prevalence differences between studies. *J Nerv Ment Dis* 2012;**200**:444–50.

40. Kessler RC, Sonnega A, Bromet E, Hughes M, Nelson CB. Posttraumatic stress disorder in the National Comorbidity Survey. *Arch Gen Psychiatry* 1995;**52**:1048–60.

41. Sundin J, Fear NT, Iversen A, Rona RJ, Wessely S. PTSD after deployment to Iraq: conflicting rates, conflicting claims. *Psychol Med* 2010;**40**:367–82.

42. Harding T. Medical journal warns of 'tidal wave' of mental trauma among servicemen. *The Telegraph*, 13 May, 2010. Available at: <http://www.telegraph.co.uk/news/uknews/defence/7716014/Medical-journal-warns-of-tidal-wave-of-mental-trauma-among-servicemen.html#> (accessed 5 February 2013).

43. Iversen AC, Fear NT, Ehlers A, *et al*. Risk factors for post-traumatic stress disorder among UK Armed Forces personnel. *Psychol Med* 2008;**38**:511–22.

44. US Department of Veterans Affairs. *Federal benefits for veterans, dependents and survivors (2012 Online Edition)*. Available at: <http://www1.va.gov/opa/publications/benefits_book.asp> (accessed 5 February 2013).

45. Nestel ML. Thousands of veterans living on the streets. *The Daily*, 29 October, 2011. Available at: <http://www.thedaily.com/page/2011/10/29/102911-news-homeless-vets/> (accessed 5 February 2013).

46. Travis A. Revealed: the hidden army in UK prisons. *The Guardian*, 24 September 2009. Available at: <http://www.guardian.co.uk/uk/2009/sep/24/jailed-veteran-servicemen-outnumber-troops> (accessed 5 February 2013).

47. Gaber H. 'Souls being lost' after service in military—but there's help. *Arizona Daily Star*, 20 December, 2012. Available at: <http://azstarnet.com/news/local/souls-being-lost-after-service-in-military – -but/article_673ab423–72c1–5079–91e0–003bd147f1a5.html> (accessed 5 February 2013).

48. Iversen AC, Greenberg N. Mental health of regular and reserve military veterans. *Adv Psychiatr Treat* 2009;**15**:100–6.

49. Buckman JEJ, Forbes HJ, Clayton T, *et al*. Early Service leavers: a study of the factors associated with premature separation from the UK Armed Forces and the mental health of those that leave early. *Eur J Public Health* 2012. 25 April. [Epub ahead of print.] doi:10.1093/eurpub/cks042.

50. **Woodhead C, Rona RJ, Iversen AC,** *et al.* Mental health and health service use among post-national service veterans: results from the 2007 Adult Psychiatric Morbidity Survey of England. *Psychol Med* 2011;**41**:363–72.

51. **Kapur N, While D, Blatchley N, Bray I, Harrison K.** Suicide after leaving the UK armed forces—a cohort study. *PLoS Med* 2009;**6**:e26. doi:10.1371/journal.pmed.1000026.

52. **Defence Analytical Services and Advice.** *Estimating the proportion of prisoners in England and Wales who are ex-Armed Forces—updated estimate and further analysis.* 2010. Available at: <http://www.dasa.mod.uk/applications/newWeb/www/index.php?page=48&pubTyp e=3&thiscontent=550&PublishTime=13:00:00&date=2010–09–15&disText=Single%20 Report&from=listing&topDate=2010–09–15> (accessed 5 February 2013).

53. **NAPO.** *Ex-armed forces personnel and the criminal justice system.* August 2008. Available at: <http://www.napo.org.uk/about/veteransincjs.cfm> (accessed 5 February 2013).

Chapter 7

Methodological considerations in the epidemiology of work-related health problems in migrants

Elena Ronda, Emily Felt, Marc Schenker, and Fernando G. Benavides

The relevance of migration to occupational health

Human migration has always been an important global phenomenon. Several major motivations for migration include asylum seeking, environmental change, and family reunification but, overall, searching for work has been the largest driver of migratory flows in the last century. Immigration can be the key to improving one's quality of life and can increase opportunities for personal development, but it can also increase vulnerability and pose increased risks to health.

There are major difficulties in estimating flows of foreign labour, in part because there is a multiplicity of data sources, which are frequently partial in coverage, and because there are various definitions of what constitutes a migrant. There are also problems recording seasonal and other short-term workers.[1,2] Nevertheless, the International Organization for Migration estimates that there are about 214 million international migrants worldwide (3.1% of the world's population). One out of every 33 persons in the world today is a transnational migrant. This number does not include the much larger total of internal migrants, estimated to be as high as 750 million.[3]

The migrants we concern ourselves with here are those who fill the jobs characterized by low skill requirements, low wages, and working conditions that are often unacceptable for native workers. This chapter aims to shed light on work-related health issues for those migrants who may be under-represented in current research.[4]

Table 7.1 presents the principal sectors of employment for the native-born and foreign-born population in Europe.[5] Agriculture, manufacturing, construction, and domestic service, as well as unskilled jobs in general, are important sources of employment for migrants.[3] Foreign-born workers are under-represented in the public services and administration sectors, which are typically characterized by relatively more secure terms of employment and better working conditions. Migrant men are typically employed in construction and manufacturing, whereas migrant women are concentrated also in services, including health and education.[1]

The economic crisis of 2008 in developed countries has changed the dynamics of labour demand in many countries. In the US, Ireland, and Spain, migrant workers

Table 7.1 Percentage of native-born and foreign-born workers aged 25–54 in the total corresponding population of the principal sectors of employment, by gender, in 27 European countries[5]

	Male		Female	
	Native-born	**Foreign-born**	**Native-born**	**Foreign-born**
Manufacturing	22	22	17	16
Construction	13	19	15	13
Wholesale and retail trade, repair of motor vehicles and motorcycles	13	12	12	11
Accommodation and food service activities	2	8	4	10
Transportation and storage	8	8	1	10
Administrative and support service activities	3	5	4	8
Human health and social work activities	4	4	12	7
Professional, scientific, and technical activities	5	4	5	4
Information and communication	4	3	3	4
Public administration and defence; compulsory social security	8	3	8	4

Source: data from Awad I, *The global economic crisis and migrant workers: Impact and response*, Geneva, Copyright © International Labour Organization, 2009. Available at: <http://www.ilo.org/public/english/protection/migrant/download/global_crisis.pdf>

faced a decline in demand for labour in construction. But in some cases (e.g. US, Ireland) a number of sectors (e.g. health care, domestic service, and education) witnessed growth in employment and increased opportunities for migrants.[5]

In the first part of this chapter, we present an overview of general considerations for conducting epidemiological research with migrant workers; the second part reviews work-related health problems of migrant workers, as evidenced by recent research. In the third part we suggest considerations for researchers and policymakers.

General considerations for occupational epidemiological research on migrant workers

The epidemiology of work-related health problems in migrants raises methodological challenges, some of which are distinct from those of classical occupational epidemiology. The patterns of health status and risk factors tend to be different in migrant groups and the common absence of traditional sampling frames and tracking systems

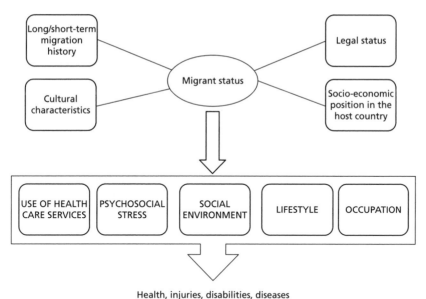

Figure 7.1 Conceptual framework showing the interaction between migrant status and health.

creates additional challenges.[6] There are many issues that arise when researchers wish to study the state of migrants' health and to explain the differences that may be found within and between groups (Figure 7.1).[7]

It is important to note some practical conceptual differences between studies on migrant health and classical occupational epidemiology: defining migrant workers, how researchers engage with migrant populations, how samples are selected and participants recruited, and how comparable the data may, or may not, be with data from the native-born population.

Definition of 'migrant'

An essential requirement for epidemiological research with migrants involves the definition of terms. Who do we refer to when we say 'migrant'? Despite considerable debate, there is still no consensus on this issue and there are complex conceptual, methodological, and technical challenges involved[2] with important implications for research.[8]

Migrant status may be indicated in several ways: by country of birth, citizenship, or by nationality. Migrant status is often conflated with membership in an ethnic or religious minority group. However, none of these definitions are equivalent, and the use of different concepts and non-standardized or poorly-defined indicators poses a particular problem for consistency in scientific research. Moreover, the definitions of 'migrant' commonly do not distinguish between categories, such as asylum seekers, trafficked persons, official labour migrants, irregular labour migrants, students, senior executives and skilled professionals, refugees, and others.[2] The International

Organization for Migration has attempted to improve the uniformity of terms.[9] In general, the term 'migrant' is understood to cover cases where the decision to migrate was taken freely by an individual for reasons of personal convenience; it therefore applies to persons and family members moving to another country or region to better their material or social conditions. A 'migrant worker' is a person who is to be engaged, is engaged, or has been engaged in a remunerated activity in a country of which he or she is not a national. A 'long-term migrant' is a person who moves to a country other than that of his or her usual residence for a period of at least a year, so that the country of destination effectively becomes his or her new country of usual residence.[9]

Heterogeneous groups of migrants are often analysed together despite wide divergences in their characteristics (socioeconomic, cultural, language, and migration experiences, among others). Researchers should be explicit as to whether their study population consists of migrants or of broader ethnic categories. Most of the research, certainly in Western Europe, pertains to the migrant (foreign-born) population as compared to the native (i.e. non-migrant) population. This differs from research in the US where ethnic groups, such as African Americans or Hispanics, are compared with the white ethnic population.[10]

Official data sources

Research is often based on routinely collected data from official registry statistics or surveys based on representative samples of the population. Most of these secondary data sources do not record migrant status and, if solicited, it is sometimes incorrectly reported.[11,12] In addition migrants may work in informal work arrangements or for labour intermediaries, or move between jobs, and so are often excluded inadvertently by these sources. For example, occupational injuries suffered by informal workers may not be covered by national social security or workers compensation systems and are therefore not recorded.

In surveys, one limitation commonly found is the small number of migrants in the sample. For instance, the Fourth European Working Conditions Survey (2005) included around 3% of migrants while Eurostat estimated in the same year that migrants make up 7% of the European workforce.[13] This fact might be due to the relatively small size of migrant communities in many geographic areas, but also to low response rates among migrants. Low response rates may be related to language problems, distrust in government institutions in the host country, or not being officially registered at a local address.[2,6,11] Undocumented migrants seldom figure in national surveys because of the difficulty of locating them and their fear of arrest and deportation. Oversampling is often required in surveys to yield statistically relevant information on small subgroups. Estimates may be biased if the fraction of the migrant population which is not included has a distinct sociodemographic or health profile. Another limitation of the small number of migrants included in official surveys is that it precludes the possibility of carrying out analyses by world region of origin (making it impossible to distinguish between migrants from countries with different levels of human development).

Primary research

The hidden nature of migrant populations makes it difficult to describe the underlying population of interest with complete accuracy, and very often prevents the use of random probability sampling. These problems are exacerbated in the case of undocumented migrants—an often difficult to access population, of unknown size, and for whom language, cultural barriers, and fear of reprisal complicate the process of conducting quality research.[11] Quota sampling methodology is therefore common in original research on migrants and this may affect the potential to extrapolate findings to a larger population, i.e. external validity.

Common biases

Selection bias, of unpredictable direction, may affect the results in the association between outcomes and exposure because migrant workers do not have the same probability of being included in the sample. An example of this bias was noted in a population-based study of Ecuadorian migrants in Spain compared to native-born Spaniards.[14] Contact was made by post; the proportion with an invalid postal address was higher among migrants because of their higher mobility. Although the selection was probabilistic, in order to be eligible, a person had to be registered in the municipal registry. Legal residence is not a prerequisite for registration in Spain, but those with higher mobility may have been under-represented.

The 'healthy migrant effect' is a well-documented bias by which migrants, especially recent arrivals, have better health on average than their host country peers, despite socioeconomic disadvantages and often less access to health services.[15] Those who migrate tend to be among the youngest and most fit in their countries and, in contrast, those who are less healthy have a lower propensity to emigrate. However, with increased time of residence in the host country this advantage disappears or is even reversed. One example is the 'Hispanic reproductive health paradox', in which Latina immigrants to the US have worsening pregnancy outcomes the longer they live in the US.[16]

Information bias may be important, if cultural differences affect migrants' responses to questionnaires. Standardized questionnaires and tests should, therefore, be valid cross-culturally. A survey on migrant and native-born workers in Spain compared self-perceived exposure to occupational risks.[17] Foreign-born male manual workers reported less exposure than their Spanish counterparts for most of the selected risks. This result contrasted with the increased risk of workplace injuries observed in migrant workers in construction, agriculture, and some other Spanish industries. In this example, a lower level of training and knowledge about occupational health may mean that foreign workers fail to recognize some job risks. A low level of information has been described in Hispanic immigrants recently arrived in the US.[18] More development and standardization of measurement instruments is needed in this area.

Confounding

Migrant workers may be disadvantaged if they live and work in poor conditions and have limited access to health care provision and social security benefits in the host country.[19] It is important to include these variables so they can be evaluated as potential confounders. Public health issues affecting migrants include many non-occupational factors such as education, housing, nutrition, health-related behaviours, and medical care delivery. It is advisable to study migrants in as many precise and meaningful categories as possible, and to examine the impact of gender, age, and socioeconomic status.[20]

Occupational epidemiology of migrants

Migrant status is an important epidemiological variable to explain variation in most working and employment exposures and in work-related health problems. The distinctive characteristics of migrants have been reviewed and documented elsewhere.[6,21–23] Some relevant conclusions include the following:

- There is an overall increased risk of occupational fatalities among migrants compared to native-born workers.[24–26] This is present within specific sectors such as agriculture[27] and construction.[28] Several possible explanations have been put forth, including worse employment and working conditions, a high incidence of temporary work and rotation between jobs, greater risk taking and reluctance to complain about hazardous conditions, and that many migrants perform different occupations from those they performed in their country of origin.

- Although the risk of non-fatal occupational injuries is, in general, higher for migrants, the findings are less consistent,[29] including in studies focused on specific occupations.[30,31] Migrants are more likely to be allocated to less desirable jobs, and such jobs may be more likely to be characterized by poor working conditions as is seen in the Fourth Survey of European working Conditions (Table 7.2).[13]

- Presenteeism (workers attending work whilst ill) may be common in some migrant groups because keeping their job is a high priority which takes precedence over concerns about health.[32,33]

- Self-reported health among migrants may be worse than among native-born populations, although there are differences according to country of origin, legal status, occupational, and socioeconomic factors.[34,35] The uncertainties involved in the migration process, coupled with poor employment and working conditions, may be factors that help to explain the high rates of depression, stress, somatic illnesses, anxiety disorders, and insomnia described in some studies.

Considerations for epidemiologists and implications for policymakers

The occupational epidemiology of migrant workers is an area that is currently understudied, in part due to methodological problems.[23] However, despite the challenges, informative research has the potential to greatly improve the health of these populations. Researchers are advised to seek out ways to overcome the challenges associated with mobile groups and consider that research may have little impact if it does not influence the policymaking process and the public discourse. These challenges should inform the development of new tools by epidemiologists.

Table 7.2 Prevalence (%) of self-reported exposure to poor working conditions in migrants and non-migrants in Europe by type of economic activity[13]

	Non-service[a]		Service	
	Non-migrant	**Migrant**	**Non-migrant**	**Migrant**
Vibrations from hand tools, machinery	32	44	8	12
Noise so loud that you have to raise your voice to talk to people	24	43	12	13
High temperature which makes you perspire	27	33	10	16
Low temperatures indoors or outdoors	22	23	9	8
Breathing fumes, dust, or powders	27	28	7	8
Tiring or painful position	40	34	18	19
Carrying or moving heavy loads	34	45	15	22
Standing or walking	59	65	55	69
Repetitive hand or arm movement	53	57	37	48
Shift work	16	15	18	25

[a] Manufacturing, agriculture, and construction

Source: data from Fourth European Working Conditions Survey, Office for Official Publications of the European Communities, Luxembourg, Copyright © European Foundation for the Improvement of Living and Working Conditions, 2007

Research findings show contradictory health outcomes for different migrant populations. The 'healthy migrant effect' in which migrants are often healthier than the host population, especially during their first years after arrival, offers opportunities to strengthen this health capital and conserve it. Because occupational risks to migrants may contribute to the decline in their health over time, intervention to improve working conditions and terms of employment of migrants may contribute to improved population health and potential long-term cost savings for health services.

Community-based participatory research, action-oriented research, and the use of cultural mediators are strategies which may offer opportunities for occupational epidemiology. Cultural mediators can be effective in bringing researchers and the study community together. Research has shown that certain groups are more likely to be active participants when they are involved in the design of the study and have the potential to see the benefits of its desired outcomes. Researchers, in gaining interaction with groups to which they normally have no access, gain the opportunity to explore contextual issues surrounding migrant livelihoods and to better interpret research findings.

To build an evidence base, reliable sources of information are needed. All routine health and labour surveys should capture indicators used for determining migrant status, e.g. country of birth, nationality, and time living in the host country. Standardized data collection instruments would be helpful for assessing occupational exposures and health outcomes and will improve comparisons between groups. Cross-country studies may always face difficulties when cultural differences do not permit easy comparison.

Despite the fact that such studies have significant costs, there is a need for large-scale research, such as cohort studies. The type of information offered by these more intensive research studies is invaluable. It is also likely that researchers will need to work directly with policymakers (or intermediaries with policy knowledge) to ensure that research questions are relevant to current policy questions and that research results inform policy changes.

The ITSAL (Inmigración, Trabajo y Salud) project is an example of a multi-method study that explores the occupational health conditions of foreign-born residents (documented and undocumented) working in Spain.[36] After qualitative studies including focus groups and interviews, a survey was carried out in 2006 with 2434 migrants and with comparable native-born workers selected from the same neighbourhoods (to minimize confounding by social class). Migrant workers were resurveyed in 2011. The ITSAL multi-method approach allows for the resolution of some of the problems related to studying migrant populations; for example, by including undocumented workers and sufficient numbers of migrants. The MICASA (Mexican Immigration to California Agricultural Safety Acculturation) study is an example of a long-term follow-up study concerning migrant populations.[37] This study relies on close cooperation with the community and interviewers who are familiar with and accepted by the community. More studies of this type are needed to understand determinants of health and disease among migrant populations.

References

1. **Salt J.** Trends in Europe´s international migration. In: Rechel B, Mladovsky P, Devillé W, Rijks B, Petrova-Benedict R, McKee M (eds) *Migration and health in the European Union.* Maidenhead: McGraw-Hill, 2011, pp. 17–36.

2. **Rechel B, Mladovsky P, Devillé W.** Monitoring the health of migrants. In: Rechel B, Mladovsky P, Devillé W, Rijks B, Petrova-Benedict R, McKee M (eds) *Migration and health in the European Union.* Maidenhead: McGraw-Hill, 2011, pp. 81–100.

3. **International Organization for Migration.** *Facts & figures.* Available at: <http://www.iom.int/cms/en/sites/iom/home/about-migration/facts – figures-1.html> (accessed 15 February 2013).

4. **Benach J, Muntaner C, Chung H, Benavides FG.** Immigration, employment relations, and health: developing a research agenda. *Am J Ind Med* 2010;**53**:338–43.

5. **Awad I.** *The global economic crisis and migrant workers: impact and response.* Geneva: International Labour Organization, 2009. Available at: <http://www.ilo.org/public/english/protection/migrant/download/global_crisis.pdf> (accessed 15 February 2013).

6. **Schenker MB.** A global perspective of migration and occupational health. *Am J Ind Med* 2010;**53**:329–37

7. **Ingleby D, Chimienti M, Hatziprokopiou P, Ormond M, De Freitas C.** The role of health in integration. In: Fonseca M, Malheiros J (eds) *Social integration and mobility: education, housing and health. IMISCOE Cluster B5 State of the Art Report.* Lisbon: Centro de Estudos Geográficos, Universidade de Lisboa, 2005. Available at: <http://mighealth.net/nl/images/c/ce/Cluster_B5.pdf> (accessed 15 February 2013).

8. **Bhopal R.** Glossary of terms relating to ethnicity and race: for reflection and debate. *J Epidemiol Community Health* 2004;**58**:441–5.

9. **Perruchoud R, Redpath-Cross J.** *International Migration Law No 25. Glossary on migration* (2nd edn). Geneva: International Organization for Migration, 2011. Available at: <http://publications.iom.int/bookstore/free/Glossary%202nd%20ed%20web.pdf> (accessed 15 February 2013).

10. **Foets M.** Improving the quality of research into the health of migrant and ethnic groups. *Int J Public Health* 2011;**56**:455–6.

11. **Levecque K, Benavides F, Ronda E, Van Rossen R.** Using existing health information systems for migrant health research in Europe: challenges and opportunities. In: Ingleby D, Krasnik A, Lorant V, Razum O (eds) *Health inequalities and risk factors among migrants and ethnic minorities. COST series on health and diversity. Volume 1.* Antwerp-Apeldoorn: Garant Publishers, 2012, pp. 53–68.

12. **Johnson M.** Problems and barriers in the collection of ethnicity and migration related data. In: Ingleby D, Krasnik A, Lorant V, Razum O (eds) *Health inequalities and risk factors among migrants and ethnic minorities. COST series on health and diversity. Volume 1.* Antwerp-Apeldoorn: Garant Publishers, 2012, pp. 39–52.

13. **Parent-Thirion A, Fernández Macías E, Hurley J, Vermeylen G.** *Fourth European Working Conditions Survey.* Dublin: European Foundation for the Improvement of Living and Working Conditions, 2005. Available at: <http://www.eurofound.europa.eu/publications/htmlfiles/ef0698.htm> (accessed 15 February 2013).

14. **Del Amo J, Jarrín I, García-Fulgueiras A,** *et al.* Mental health in Ecuadorian migrants from a population-based survey: the importance of social determinants and gender roles. *Soc Psychiatry Psychiatr Epidemiol* 2011;**46**:1143–52.

15. **Newbold KB.** Self-rated health within the Canadian immigrant population: risk and the healthy immigrant effect. *Soc Sci Med* 2005;**60**:1359–70.

16. **Hoggatt KJ, Flores M, Solorio R, Wilhelm M, Ritz B.** The 'Latina epidemiologic paradox' revisited: the role of birthplace and acculturation in predicting infant low birth weight for Latinas in Los Angeles, CA. *J Immigr Minor Health* 2012;**14**:875–84.

17. **Ronda E, Agudelo-Suárez AA, García AM, López-Jacob MJ, Ruiz-Frutos C, Benavides FG.** Differences in exposure to occupational health risks in Spanish and foreign-born workers in Spain (ITSAL project). *J Immigr Minor Health* 2013;**15**:164–71.

18. **Orrenius PM, Zavodny M.** Do immigrants work in riskier jobs? *Demography* 2009;**46**:535–51.

19. **Benach J, Muntaner C, Delclos C, Menéndez M, Ronquillo C.** Migration and 'low-skilled' workers in destination countries. *PLoS Med* 2011;**8**:e1001043. doi: 10.1371/journal.pmed.1001043.

20. **Norredam M, Kastrup M, Helweg-Larsen K.** Register-based studies on migration, ethnicity, and health. *Scand J Public Health* 2011;**39**(7 Suppl):201–5.

21. **González ER, Irastorza X** (eds). *Literature study on migrant workers.* Bilbao: European Agency for Safety and Health at Work, 2007. Available at: <https://osha.europa.eu/en/publications/literature_reviews/migrant_workers> (accessed 15 February 2013).

22. **Agudelo-Suárez AA, Ronda-Pérez E, Benavides FG.** Occupational health. In: Rechel B, Mladovsky P, Devillé W, Rijks B, Petrova-Benedict R, McKee M (eds) *Migration and health in the European Union.* Maidenhead: McGraw-Hill, 2011, pp. 155–68.

23. **Ahonen EQ, Benavides FG, Benach J.** Immigrant populations, work and health—a systematic literature review. *Scand J Work Environ Health* 2007;**33**:96–104.

24. López-Jacob MJ, Ahonen E, García AM, Gil A, Benavides FG. [Occupational injury in foreign workers by economic activity and autonomous community (Spain 2005)]. [Article in Spanish, English abstract.] *Rev Esp Salud Publica* 2008;**82**:179–87.

25. Richardson DB, Loomis D, Bena J, Bailer AJ. Fatal occupational injury rates in southern and non-southern States, by race and Hispanic ethnicity. *Am J Public Health* 2004;**94**:1756–61.

26. Corvalan CF, Driscoll TR, Harrison JE. Role of migrant factors in work-related fatalities in Australia. *Scand J Work Environ Health* 1994;**20**:364–70.

27. Hard DL, Myers JR, Gerberich SG. Traumatic injuries in agriculture. *J Agric Saf Health* 2002;**8**:51–65.

28. Dong X, Platner JW. Occupational fatalities of Hispanic construction workers from 1992 to 2000. *Am J Ind Med* 2004;**45**:45–54.

29. Strong LL, Zimmerman FJ. Occupational injury and absence from work among African American, Hispanic, and non-Hispanic White workers in the national longitudinal survey of youth. *Am J Public Health* 2005;**95**:1226–32.

30. Salminen S, Vartia M, Giorgiani T. Occupational injuries of immigrant and Finnish bus drivers. *J Safety Res* 2009;**40**:203–5.

31. Döös M, Laflamme L, Backström T. Immigrants and occupational accidents: A comparative study of the frequency and types of accidents encountered by foreign and Swedish citizens at an engineering plant in Sweden. *Saf Sci* 1994;**18**:15–32.

32. Gomes Carneiro I, Ortega A, Borg V, Høgh A. Health and sickness absence in Denmark: a study of elderly-care immigrant workers. *J Immigr Minor Health* 2010;**12**:43–52.

33. Agudelo-Suárez AA, Benavides FG, Felt E, Ronda-Pérez E, Vives-Cases C, García AM. Sickness presenteeism in Spanish-born and immigrant workers in Spain. *BMC Public Health* 2010;**10**:791. doi: 10.1186/1471-2458-10-791.

34. Sousa E, Agudelo-Suárez A, Benavides FG, *et al.* Immigration, work and health in Spain: the influence of legal status and employment contract on reported health indicators. *Int J Public Health* 2010;**55**:443–51.

35. Akhavan S, Bildt CO, Franzén EC, Wamala S. Health in relation to unemployment and sick leave among immigrants in Sweden from a gender perspective. *J Immigr Health* 2004;**6**:103–18.

36. Delclos CE, Benavides FG, García AM, López-Jacob MJ, Ronda E. From questionnaire to database: field work experience in the 'Immigration, work and health survey' (ITSAL Project). *Gac Sanit* 2011;**25**:419–22.

37. Stoecklin-Marois MT, Hennessy-Burt TE, Schenker MB. Engaging a hard-to-reach population in research: sampling and recruitment of hired farm workers in the MICASA study. *J Agric Saf Health* 2011;**17**:291–302.

Chapter 8

Epidemiological studies of older workers: research questions and methodological challenges

Harry S. Shannon

Introduction

Increasing attention is being paid to the ageing of the population worldwide. The proportion of the world's population over 60 is forecast to double from 11.6% in 2012 to 21.8% in 2050.[1]

One reason for the change is declining mortality rates, especially at older ages. Thus in the Organisation for Economic Co-operation and Development (OECD) countries overall, life expectancy at age 65 increased from 1960 to 2009 by 4.4 years for men and 5.6 for women.[2] A second reason is that fertility rates have also fallen; the OECD average is 1.74,[3] well below 2.1, the level needed for population replacement. Of particular relevance for work, the proportion of people between 15 and 64, the traditional working years, has fallen in Western countries, and will continue to do so.[3]

The United Nations Population Fund report on ageing was subtitled 'A celebration and a challenge', the 'celebration' due to the 'triumph of development', with lives extended through better nutrition, education, health programmes, etc.[1] Yet the way we respond to the challenge posed will determine if we reap what has been called the 'longevity dividend'—increased prosperity from 'a healthier, long-lived population'.[4] Among the concerns is the ability of economies to sustain social programmes, including health care and pensions. Policy options include: (1) lowering the standard of living for pensioners, (2) older retirement ages, (3) increasing contributions while working, and (4) increasing total transfers from workers to pensioners.[5] In Western countries, various governmental approaches have focused on option 2. For example, the European Union has adopted a policy to increase the proportion of 55–64-year-olds who are working to 50%; while Canada, *inter alia*, has announced an increase over time in the eligibility age for state pensions and other benefits,[6] whose indirect aim is presumably to extend working lives.

Griffiths posed two resultant questions: what will persuade older workers to stay in employment? How to ensure they remain healthy and productive?[7] For many workers, especially in poorer countries, the first question is somewhat moot—the International Labour Organization notes that, worldwide, just 40% of the working age population has legal pension coverage, and only 26% of the working population is effectively covered by old-age pension schemes. Without (and even with) help from their families, older workers must continue working until late in life. Indeed, in less developed regions, labour force participation in those over 65 is much higher than in more developed regions.[8] While this chapter focuses on the health and safety issues in Griffiths' second question, they are not unrelated to the first. Provided workers have a choice (e.g. financial provisions for retirement), workplace conditions, including the physical and psychosocial aspects of their work, must be attractive enough for workers to want to stay.

There is no consensus definition of who is an older worker,[9] and it is not required for this chapter. Rather, many functions and capabilities decline with age (albeit at highly variable rates between people) and occupational epidemiologists can study these processes in relation to occupational health and safety. I here outline possible research questions open to epidemiological approaches, before discussing methodological challenges in answering those questions.

Before doing so, I note that the changing nature of work creates a good deal of uncertainty about what jobs will look like over time. Western literature has emphasized the shift from manufacturing jobs to service work, but manufacturing jobs still exist. Globalization has moved them to other parts of the world—often with far poorer working conditions than before. We cannot ignore the effect on the health and safety of ageing workers doing those jobs, yet virtually all the literature to date on health and safety implications for the ageing workforce comes from Europe and North America.

Possible research questions

My list of possible research questions is of course not comprehensive. For ease of reading I have grouped the questions into categories, but recognize that there is considerable overlap. Some questions might apply to work at all ages, but I have concentrated on topics for which there may be special or unique problems for older workers.

Work exposures

The impact of 'common and potentially harmful worksite exposures' on older workers should be studied, especially their relationship with the normal processes of ageing.[10] Longer working lives increase cumulative exposures, as well as increasing the time since exposure—important when there is a long latency period between exposure and resultant disease. Further, some exposures may have a greater effect when they occur to older workers, e.g. carcinogens that are promoters rather than initiators.

Health promotion and chronic diseases

Older workers tend to have more chronic health conditions. We should understand how these conditions, and any medications taken for them, interact with workplace exposures, both during and after employment.[10] Prevention of chronic diseases in the first place would remove the need for such research, and a comprehensive research agenda was recently developed.[11] Will the increasing levels of obesity in many populations create particular problems as workers age?

Continuing employment and retirement

If workers are to remain in the workforce until later in life, Griffiths' two overarching questions noted earlier must be addressed. From them spring more specific questions. How does any age discrimination affect the health and well-being of older workers? What factors make older workers more vulnerable, or more resilient, to health effects of work? What components of work particularly influence the health of older workers, both positively and negatively? How does long- or short-term unemployment affect the ability of older workers to reintegrate safely into employment, and affect well-being and health at older ages? Given changing contexts, will current studies still be relevant in the future?[12]

The nature of work exposures has changed. As already noted, many manufacturing jobs have moved from higher- to lower-income countries. These trends, along with volatile economic conditions which can force people to continue working until late in life, mean that research questions should be carefully specified and try to anticipate trends, not simply assume constancy in the world of work.

We must also learn about transitions to retirement. If society wants (and needs) people to work longer, it has an obligation to ensure people do not work for *too* long. Exactly when is continuing to work harmful to workers' health and their ability to enjoy healthy retirement? For highly demanding jobs, when should retraining begin so those workers are ready to undertake less demanding work before their health is badly damaged? Conversely, there are occupations where reduced capacity to do the job properly can harm others—e.g. a surgeon who loses dexterity, or a firefighter who cannot rescue people. What is the optimal time for someone to stop work or move to lighter work—potentially based on a complex mix of factors including the physical and mental demands of the job, the individual worker's health status and level of job satisfaction, and social benefits available for retirees? Better still, how can workplaces examine their job structures and engage workers in redesigning jobs to accommodate the changing needs and abilities of older workers?

Work organization

The structure of work is important. For example, secure, full-time jobs with regular hours are increasingly disappearing, and employees are forced to accept irregular schedules demanded by the employer. Yet the greater sleep problems experienced with ageing mean that shift work poses potential problems. Folkard[13] hypothesized that older workers might be at higher risk of injury on night shifts, and called for epidemiological studies. While Costa[14] suggested research-based recommendations for managing older shift workers, Bohle and colleagues[15] noted that there was insufficient rigorous literature to be sure the proposals would have the desired impact. A similar complaint could be made about lack of evidence on ways to manage many other aspects of work organization and their effect on older workers.

Could work be distributed differently over a lifetime, with shorter work weeks but longer working lives? Christensen and colleagues reported preliminary evidence that this could increase life expectancy and health,[16] and more research is warranted. This question can be generalized—what flexible arrangements can allow older workers to continue employment while maintaining health (and productivity)? A Cochrane review tentatively concluded that there was a health benefit when the flexibility gave the worker some control, though not when it was for the employer's benefit, but the evidence was weak and better intervention studies were recommended.[17]

Workers' compensation and return to work after illness or injury

Older workers have fewer injuries, but take longer to recover. Wegman and McGee[10] recommended a full costing of illnesses and injuries in older workers. Burdorf[18] raises issues of sustained employability—of special importance in older workers. His questions include: when does work trigger an episode of disease, when does the episode cause work absence, and when do chronic diseases and repeated work absences limit the capacity to continue working? We might also ask what role workers' compensation systems (and other policies) play in rehabilitation and return to work in older workers. We also need to understand workplace adaptations and other prognostic factors that predict whether workers developing chronic conditions continue to work; an example for early osteoarthritis was recently reported.[19]

Special populations

Over the past few decades, women in Western societies have increased their participation in the paid workforce, and the proportion working at older ages has increased. That some of these women are also doing non-traditional jobs raises research questions. Payne and Doyal[20] note that women are more susceptible than men to conditions such as arthritis, women metabolize chemicals differently than men, and little is known about how health at work interacts with menopausal status.

Low-skilled migrants are especially vulnerable. Those admitted temporarily to a country are likely to be relatively young, but those who settle in the host country may have to continue working at demanding jobs until later in life, if they have had less time to accumulate pension rights. Moreover, they are typically less able to stand up for their rights in dangerous jobs.

As noted earlier, almost all relevant literature is from Europe and North America. While some may be generalizable to lower-income countries, it is unreasonable to assume this, and effort is needed to understand the health and safety implications of substantial continuing employment among older workers in lower-income countries. A research agenda for ageing listed poverty among older people in sub-Saharan Africa and Latin America as a priority area.[21] To ensure they are healthy enough to work and support themselves, the occupational health of older workers in these countries must be addressed.

Interventions

It is likely that various programmes for managing older workers will be developed and implemented. Grosch and Pransky[22] list target areas and corresponding possible interventions aimed at the workplace, workers, health care system, and benefits system. These and other interventions should be evaluated. At least at the individual level, randomized controlled trials should be done, such as that by Hughes and colleagues.[23] While interventions at the workplace level or jurisdictional level are much more difficult to assess as rigorously, this should not become an excuse not to do the evaluations.

Epidemiological/methodological challenges

Comprehensively addressing the questions listed in the previous section requires multidisciplinary approaches—for example, understanding the basic biological mechanisms of cell ageing, or developing psychological and sociological theories. Integrating these (and results from, e.g. qualitative research) with epidemiological methods is itself a challenge, but there are sufficient challenges in the epidemiological methods for me to focus only on those. I do not discuss general issues applicable to studies of workers of all ages unless there are special concerns related to older workers; they include identifying the sample, determining valid and reliable exposure measures over time (especially historical), measuring outcomes, and conducting appropriate analyses.

Conceptual models

All research is underpinned by explicit or implicit assumptions which influence the conduct of the research. This field is no different. Jex and colleagues summarize three perspectives on ageing:[24] (1) rate-of-living theory, arguing that people have a finite supply of energy and resources to use; (2) homeostasis, proposing that older adults subjected to a stressor have reduced ability to return to their pre-stressor state; and (3) life course perspective, in which events over one's life affect how one ages. Epidemiology focuses on the last approach, but different designs or analyses might be done if the other theories are used.

Study design

The single best improvement to epidemiological research on ageing workers is to conduct longitudinal studies, including follow-up of workers into retirement. Cross-sectional designs almost certainly incur the healthy survivor effect, since unhealthy workers may retire early.[25] Some long-running cohorts are available already especially in Scandinavia. Several newer prospective studies of ageing are under way (for example,[26,27]), although they have not been designed as occupational studies so that relatively little information has been collected about work and the workplace. As well, long-term effects will take many years to arise, and it will require considerable effort to retain participants in the studies.

Longitudinal studies pose distinctive challenges for lower-income countries. The United Nations Programme on Ageing lists as a key methodological issue the '[d]evelopment of multidimensional longitudinal study methods for use in developing countries, with special attention paid to cohort and multigenerational dimensions of longitudinal studies'.[21]

It will be worth exploring whether historical cohorts can be developed (perhaps from earlier cross-sectional studies) with enough reliable information to answer important questions in the short term. Using these existing samples depends on information already available, which varies across studies. Efforts to harmonize data collected in different ways[28] may allow more pooling of information, ideally via meta-analyses, to increase power. In addition, adding more detailed occupational information to current cohorts or regular ongoing surveys might answer many questions efficiently.

Measurement

We should not assume that work exposures of older workers are the same as those of younger ones, even when they have the same job title. Rael, for example, used detailed data to show that older construction workers had moved into supervisory roles, and did much lighter work than their younger co-workers.[29]

Studying ageing requires some extra measures, notably whether an older worker can still do his/her job. (Here I concentrate on whether workers remain sufficiently healthy, rather than consider the broader concept of employability, which includes whether a worker has the necessary knowledge and skills, competence, and adaptability to be able to find work.)

The term Work Ability was introduced in groundbreaking work in Finland in the 1980s, and represents the worker's current and near future state, and ability to do the job, regarding work demands, health, and mental resources.[30] Ilmarinen and colleagues also developed the Work Ability Index (WAI) based on scores relative to the individual's particular job. For such a simple and general measure, the WAI has proven to have very good predictive validity, yet its sensitivity and specificity for disability or retirement on disability pension for an individual is far from perfect, for example.[31] Ideally, the WAI would be further refined, perhaps becoming more specific to particular occupations, and additional assessment of translations and cross-cultural validations should be conducted.

For some 'knowledge workers', like physicians, even a relatively minor cognitive decline, which would not be likely to be detected by the WAI, might compromise their competence. It would be useful to develop a measure that can identify if/when they might pose a danger to their patients. Similar measures might be produced for other professionals, like lawyers, whose mistakes can have severe impacts on clients, albeit typically not life-and-death consequences.

Analysis

Most past studies have treated age as merely a confounding variable and rarely, if ever, have considered it an effect modifier. One exception is McCarthy and colleagues[32] who found that older workers may be more vulnerable to job strain. Jex and colleagues[24] argue that conceptually we should treat age as the variable of interest so that other variables are viewed as moderating the impact of age.

Burdorf[18] calls for new approaches to analysing workers' dynamic health paths, adopting a life course perspective and using trajectory analysis and multi-state models. These methods can be applied to existing long-term cohorts. Expanding on his ideas, there would be tremendous benefit to early identification of downward health (and work ability, etc.) trajectories, with a view to intervention. Regular regression analyses will have to be modified—Nuñez[33] recently used non-linear regression on British

Labour Force Survey data aiming to find inflection points at which the 'effect' of age accentuates occupational health problems. (Such analyses must account for selection bias; given the steady decline Nuñez found in the prevalence of chest and breathing problems from age 16–25 to 46–54, the bias was likely present in these survey data.) Provided possible selection problems can be dealt with, analyses of successive waves of regular surveys could mimic longitudinal studies by comparing members of birth cohorts over time as they age.

Various birth cohorts have been raised in different social, economic, and cultural times and, while there is no doubt wide variability within the cohorts, they may have different views of what life will (or even should) bring them. Further, age-specific disease prevalences differ by birth cohort. Reynolds and colleagues found that cardiovascular disease and arthritis were less common in later-born cohorts, but rates of other musculoskeletal conditions were higher.[34] Researchers should consider the possibility of such patterns in older workers.

Analyses should distinguish ageing *per se*, genetic factors, work exposures, and lifestyle in order to understand their relative and combined effects on health. Since few occupational studies have been done of older women, particular attention should be paid to any differences between the sexes. Multilevel approaches need to account for the nesting of workers within the workplace and, more generally, sort out interrelationships of age with social, cultural, technological, and economic factors. While these analyses will be complex, the results could highlight optimal points of intervention to maintain health into old age.

Discussion

The ageing of populations will, barring major catastrophic events, lead to an increasing proportion of older people in our workforces. Societies will face testing times in dealing with this shift. Researchers in many disciplines can provide solid evidence on which policymakers, workplaces, and individuals can base their decisions on how to respond. Occupational epidemiologists can provide a major component of this research base that will be needed to ensure healthy ageing, provided the various tough methodological questions can be handled. I trust we are up to the challenge.

References

1. **UNFPA and HelpAge International.** *Ageing in the twenty-first century: a celebration and a challenge.* New York: United Nations Population Fund, 2012. Available at: <http://unfpa.org/ageingreport/> (accessed 14 February 2013).

2. **Organisation for Economic Co-operation and Development.** Life expectancy and healthy life expectancy at age 65. In: *Health at a glance 2011: OECD indicators.* OECD Publishing, 2011. Available at: <http://dx.doi.org/10.1787/health_glance-2011-66-en> (accessed 14 February 2013).

3. **Organisation for Economic Co-operation and Development.** *OECD factbook 2011–2012: economic, environmental and social statistics.* OECD Publishing, 2012. doi: 10.1787/factbook-2011-en. Available at: <http://www.oecd-ilibrary.org> (accessed 14 February 2013).

4. **Olshansky SJ, Perry D, Miller RA, Butler RN.** Pursuing the longevity dividend: scientific goals for an aging world. *Ann N Y Acad Sci* 2007;**1114**:11–3.

5. **Pensions Commission.** *Pensions: challenges and choices. the first report of the pensions commission.* Norwich: The Stationery Office, 2004.

6. **Service Canada.** *Questions and answers regarding the changes to the Old Age Security Act.* Government of Canada, 2012. Available at: <http://www.servicecanada.gc.ca/eng/isp/oas/changes/faq.shtml> (accessed 14 February 2013).

7. **Griffiths A.** Healthy work for older workers: work design and management factors. In: Loretto W, Vickerstaff S, White PJ (eds) *The future for older workers: new perspectives.* Bristol: Policy Press, 2009, pp. 125–41.

8. **International Labour Organization.** *World social security report 2010/11. Providing coverage in times of crisis and beyond.* Geneva: ILO, 2010.

9. **Canadian Centre for Occupational Health and Safety.** *Aging workers.* CCOHS, 2012. Available at: <http://www.ccohs.ca/oshanswers/psychosocial/aging_workers.html> (accessed 14 February 2013).

10. **Wegman DH, McGee JP** (eds) for National Research Council and Institute of Medicine of the National Academies. *The health and safety needs of older workers.* Washington, DC: National Academies Press, 2004.

11. **Sorensen G, Landsbergis P, Hammer L,** *et al.* Preventing chronic disease in the workplace: a workshop report and recommendations. *Am J Public Health* 2011;**101**(Suppl 1):S196–207.

12. **Schalk R, van Veldhoven M, de Lange AH,** *et al.* Moving European research on work and ageing forward: overview and agenda. *Eur J Work Organ Psychol* 2010;**19**:76–101.

13. **Folkard S.** Shiftwork, safety, and aging. *Chronobiol Int* 2008;**25**:183–98.

14. **Costa G.** Some considerations about aging, shift work and work ability. In: Costa G, Goedhard WJA, Ilmarinen J (eds) *Assessment and promotion of work ability, health and well-being of ageing workers: Proceedings of 2nd International Symposium on Work Ability, Verona, Italy, 18–20 October 2004.* Elsevier, International Congress Series 2005:**1280**:67–72. Available at: <http://www.sciencedirect.com/science/journal/05315131/1280> (accessed 14 February 2013).

15. **Bohle P, Pitts C, Quinlan M.** Time to call it quits? The safety and health of older workers. *Int J Health Serv* 2010;**40**:23–41.

16. **Christensen K, Doblhammer G, Rau R, Vaupel JW.** Ageing populations: the challenges ahead. *Lancet* 2009;**374**:1196–208.

17. **Joyce K, Pabayo R, Critchley JA, Bambra C.** Flexible working conditions and their effects on employee health and wellbeing. *Cochrane Database Syst Rev* 2010;**2**:CD008009. doi: 10.1002/14651858.CD008009.pub2.

18. **Burdorf A.** The need for novel strategies to analyze the dynamic pattern of worker's [sic] health over time and the consequences for sustained employability. *Scand J Work Environ Health* 2012;**38**:485–8.

19. **Bieleman HJ, Reneman MF, Drossaers-Bakker KW, Groothoff JW, Oosterveld FGJ.** Prognostic factors for sustained work participation in early osteoarthritis: a follow-up study in the cohort hip and cohort knee (CHECK). *J Occup Rehabil* 2013;**23**:74–81.

20. **Payne S, Doyal L.** Older women, work and health. *Occup Med* 2010;**60**:172–7.

21. **United Nations Programme on Ageing and the International Association of Gerontology and Geriatrics.** *Research agenda on ageing for the 21st century: 2007 update.* New York: UN Programme on Ageing, 2007. Available at: <http://www.un.org/ageing/documents/AgeingResearchAgenda-6.pdf> (accessed 14 February 2013).

22. **Grosch JW, Pransky GS.** Safety and health issues for an aging workforce. In: Czaja SJ, Sharit J (eds) *Aging and work: issues and implications in a changing landscape.* Baltimore, MD: Johns Hopkins University Press, 2009, pp. 334–58.

23. **Hughes SL, Seymour RB, Campbell RT, Shaw JW, Fabiyi C, Sokas R.** Comparison of two health-promotion programs for older workers. *Am J Public Health* 2011;**101**:883–90.

24. **Jex SM, Wang M, Zarubin A.** Aging and occupational health. In: Shultz KS, Adams GA (eds) *Aging and work in the 21st century.* Applied Psychology Series. Murphy KR, Cleveland JN (series eds). Mahwah, NJ: Lawrence Erlbaum Associates, 2007, pp. 199–223.

25. **Park J.** Retirement, health and employment among those 55 plus. *Perspect Labour Income* 2011;**23**:1–12. Ottawa: Statistics Canada, Catalogue no. 75–001-X. Available at: <http://www.statcan.gc.ca/pub/75–001-x/2011001/pdf/11402-eng.pdf> (accessed 14 February 2013).

26. **Börsch-Supan A, Hank K, Jürges H.** A new comprehensive and international view on ageing: introducing the 'Survey of Health, Ageing and Retirement in Europe'. *Eur J Ageing* 2005;**2**:245–53.

27. **Raina PS, Wolfson C, Kirkland SA,** *et al.* The Canadian Longitudinal Study on Aging (CLSA). *Can J Aging* 2009;**28**:221–9.

28. **Fortier I, Doiron D, Little J,** *et al.* Is rigorous retrospective harmonization possible? Application of the DataSHaPER approach across 53 large studies. *Int J Epidemiol* 2011;**40**:1314–28.

29. **Rael EGS.** *An epidemiological study of the incidence and duration of compensated lost time occupational injury for construction workmen, Ontario, 1989: an assessment and application of Workers' Compensation Board and labour force data.* Master's thesis, University of Toronto, 1992.

30. **Ilmarinen J, Tuomi K.** Work ability of aging workers. *Scand J Work Environ Health* 1992;**18**(Suppl 2):8–10.

31. **Ilmarinen J, Rantanen J.** Promotion of work ability during ageing. *Am J Ind Med* 1999;**36**(Suppl 1):21–3.

32. **McCarthy VJ, Perry IJ, Greiner BA.** Age, job characteristics and coronary health. *Occup Med* 2012;**62**:613–9.

33. **Nuñez I.** The effects of age on health problems that affect the capacity to work: an analysis of United Kingdom labour-force data. *Ageing Soc* 2010;**30**:491–510.

34. **Reynolds SL, Crimmins EM, Saito Y.** Cohort differences in disability and disease presence. *Gerontologist* 1998;**38**:578–90.

Part 3

Applying epidemiology to sick leave, unemployment, disability, and work

Chapter 9

Who returns to work after sick leave and why? Implications for the effectiveness of interventions for musculoskeletal disorders

Alex Burdorf

Musculoskeletal disorders and return to work

Musculoskeletal disorders have long been recognized as an important source of morbidity and disability in many occupational populations.[1,2] Most musculoskeletal disorders, for most people, are characterized by recurrent episodes of pain that vary in severity and in their consequences for work. Most episodes subside uneventfully within days or weeks, often without any intervention, though about half of people continue to experience some pain and functional limitations after 12 months.[3,4]

In working populations, musculoskeletal disorders may lead to a spell of sickness absence. Sickness absence is increasingly used as a health parameter of interest when studying the consequences of functional limitations due to disease in occupational groups. Since duration of sickness absence contributes substantially to the indirect costs of illness, interventions increasingly address return to work (RTW).[5]

Predicting RTW for low back pain

Given the increased interest in RTW issues, it may come as a surprise that few studies have documented RTW across all workers on sick leave. Usually, studies select a group of workers on prolonged sick leave, typically 4–8 weeks, and report on the probability that a worker will return in full capacity. Although of great value, these studies do not provide insights into the natural course of RTW because most workers return to work after only a few days of sickness absence.

The Clinical Standards Advisory Group in the United Kingdom reported RTW within 2 weeks for 75% of all low back pain (LBP) absence episodes and suggested that approximately 50% of all work days lost due to back pain in the working population are from the 85% of people who are off work for less than 7 days.[6] In studies on the duration of compensation claims for lost time due to back injury in Canadian provinces, complete RTW patterns have been documented (see Figure 9.1). The fastest RTW curve after a spell of sickness absence due to LBP pain showed a 30% RTW after 1 week, 59% after 2 weeks, 93% after 3 months, and 96% after almost 6 months.[7] The

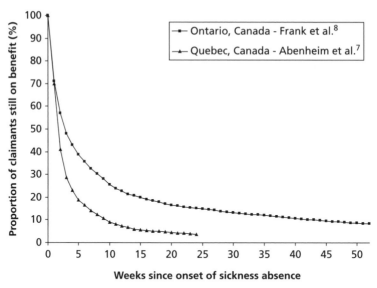

Figure 9.1 Observed return to work curves after a compensation claim for lost time due to sick leave for low back pain in occupational populations.

Adapted with permission from Abenhaim L et al., The prognostic consequences in the making of the initial medical diagnosis of work-related back injuries, *Spine*, Volume **20**, pp. 791–5, Copyright ©1995 Lippincott-Raven Publishers; and Frank JW et al., Disability resulting from occupational low back pain. Part II: What do we know about secondary prevention? A review of the scientific evidence on prevention after disability begins, *Spine*, Volume **21**, pp. 2918–29, Copyright ©1996 Lippincott-Raven Publishers.

slowest RTW curve showed a 29% RTW after 1 week, 43% after 2 weeks, 79% after 3 months, and 85% after 6 months.[8]

The difference between the two RTW curves is striking. Both jurisdictions have similar RTW patterns within the first week of sickness absence with approximately 30% of the workers returning to work. After the first week, the curves deviate markedly and RTW is much quicker in Quebec than in Ontario. For example, the difference in RTW is 15% after 2 weeks and 14% after 3 months. Whereas in Quebec about 93% of workers are back at work on full duties within 3 months, this takes more than a year in Ontario. The difference between the two RTW curves may stem from various sources, such as the definition of RTW, case criteria for workers with LBP, eligibility criteria for compensation, and the involvement of health care providers.

Several studies have summarized the prognostic factors for RTW among workers absent from work with LBP in order to understand the observed differences in RTW across observational and experimental studies. A systematic review on 18 publications identified 79 prognostic factors within eight categories. The most important predictors for prolonged absence from work were severity of LBP, older age, strenuous work such as physically demanding work, whole-body vibration, high job strain, female gender, social isolation, and higher compensation payments.[9] A second systematic review looked specifically for psychosocial predictors of delayed RTW in 24 studies. From these studies, moderate to strong evidence was inferred that lack of positive recovery expectation and fear avoidance beliefs contributed to slower RTW, and that anxiety, depression, job dissatisfaction, and perceived stress did not influence RTW.[10] Interestingly, the two reviews presented conflicting evidence with regard to factors such as depression, stress, and recovery expectation.

These contradictory findings strongly suggest that RTW depends on contextual factors and study populations. Individual studies also show the complexity of predicting who will return to work promptly and who will not. In a Dutch cohort of over 600 workers on sick leave for 3–6 weeks due to LBP, five factors contributed to the prediction model: job dissatisfaction, fear avoidance beliefs, pain intensity, duration of LBP at the start of sick leave, and female gender. However, the explained variance was low, 6% of the prediction model, and also the predictive power was low, with an area under the curve of 0.64.[11] In Quebec, over 1000 workers who consulted their general practitioner because of sickness absence for LBP were followed up for 2 years. The best prediction model included seven factors: patient's recovery expectations, radiating pain, previous back surgery, pain intensity, frequent change of position because of back pain, irritability and bad temper, and difficulty sleeping. Although the negative predictive value for prolonged RTW was good at 94%, the positive predictive value was only 31%, illustrating the problem of accurately identifying workers who need supportive health care and structured interventions.[12]

Effectiveness of interventions in musculoskeletal disorders

Several evaluation studies on RTW interventions have been conducted in recent years. A systematic review of ten workplace-based RTW interventions concluded that there was strong evidence that work disability duration is significantly reduced by work accommodation offers and by contact between health care provider and workplace, and moderate evidence that it is reduced by interventions which include early contact with worker by the workplace, ergonomic work site visits, and presence of a RTW coordinator. For these five intervention components, there was moderate evidence that they reduce costs associated with work disability duration. Employers, labour representatives, and occupational health service providers were identified as important stakeholders in successful interventions. Although this review presents useful guidance for occupational health professionals, the authors were 'struck by the limited details provided about the interventions offered' and intervention content seemed to have at best a modest fit with the identified prognostic factors for RTW.[13]

A recent thorough systematic review evaluated 42 studies on all possible RTW interventions. Interventions included exercise therapy, behavioural change techniques, workplace-based adaptations, and provision of additional services. The overall median relative risk (RR) for RTW was 1.21 with an interquartile range of 1.00–1.60. Table 9.1 summarizes the main findings for the most important categories of RTW interventions.[14]

Most interventions appeared beneficial with median RRs for RTW varying between 1.20 and 1.40 and interquartile ranges between 1.00 and 1.70, suggesting modest effects

Table 9.1 Effects of interventions on sickness absence due to musculoskeletal disorders, expressed as the relative risk of returning to work in the intervention group compared to the control group and of a reduced duration of sickness absence

	Number of studies	Relative risk		Number of studies	Sickness absence	
		Median	IQR[a]		Median	IQR[a]
Workplace interventions:						
all types	11	1.30	1.00–1.60	6	1.64	0.43–3.42
job modifications	4	1.12	1.00–1.60	1	1.29	0.54–1.73
Behavioural interventions:						
set graded tasks	11	1.40	1.16–1.90	5	1.67	1.11–3.30
provide instructions	18	1.20	1.00–1.60	14	1.11	0.33–2.64
Exercise therapy:						
physical therapy	4	1.25	1.10–1.70	1	0.32	N/A[b]
work simulation	11	1.20	1.00–1.60	4	0.69	0.10–1.22

[a] IQR = interquartile range, [b] N/A = not applicable

Adapted, with permission, from Palmer KT et al., Effectiveness of community- and workplace-based interventions to manage musculoskeletal-related sickness absence and job loss: a systematic review, *Rheumatology*, Volume **51**, pp. 230–42, Copyright ©2011, Oxford University Press

in favour of the intervention. The median reduction in sickness absence was 1.11 days per months, interquartile range 0.32–3.20. Additional analyses to determine the key features of the most successful interventions could not demonstrate particular interventions to be superior, although simple interventions (<12 hours) appeared more effective than effort-intensive interventions (>30 hours), interventions with graded tasks were slightly more effective, and interventions with workplace adaptations were more beneficial in reducing work days lost. The observation that time-intensive interventions were apparently less effective may give some support to the notion that structured interventions of a fixed duration sometimes delay timely return to work.[15] This systematic review also established that cost-benefit analyses did not show any statistically significant net economic benefits. Based on all this evidence, Palmer and colleagues prudently concluded that the benefits of RTW interventions were typically small and of doubtful cost-effectiveness.[14] Thus, simple, low-cost interventions are often to be preferred and expensive interventions should be implemented only with an accompanying rigorous cost-benefit evaluation.

Why do interventions show these contradictory findings?

The systematic reviews on interventions that promote a faster and more sustainable RTW show that RTW is a complex process. The probability of returning to work after sickness absence is not only determined by improvement in health, but also by several individual factors (i.e. sociodemographic and psychological characteristics) and environmental factors, such as workplace-based factors, occupational health care, and company policy. In addition, RTW is also influenced by national social security legislation and provisions for sickness benefits. When sickness absence is prolonged, the RTW becomes a complex process involving various stakeholders (e.g. worker, employer, health care provider, and insurer) who may have different perspectives on how to achieve a successful RTW.[16] Since these factors vary across all RTW interventions described in the scientific literature, it is difficult to extrapolate the results of individual studies and systematic reviews to a particular population in a specific context.

A crucial factor in understanding why interventions are effective or not is the timing of the enrolment of workers on sick leave into the intervention. The RTW pattern over time, as depicted in Figure 9.1, has important consequences for appropriate timing of the best window for effective clinical and occupational interventions. The evidence presented by Palmer and colleagues clearly suggests that a stepped care approach is required. In the first step of rapid RTW, most workers will return to work even without specific interventions. Simple, short interventions involving effective coordination and cooperation between primary health care and the workplace will be sufficient to help the majority of workers to achieve an early RTW. In the second step, more expensive, structured interventions are reserved for those who are having difficulties returning, typically between 4 weeks and 3 months. However, to date there is little evidence on the optimal timing of such interventions for workers on sick leave due to LBP.[14,15]

Modelling the timing of enrolment in the intervention

It might reasonably be anticipated that the specific combination of the sick leave pattern over time and the effectiveness of the intervention will largely determine the optimum time for structured interventions for workers still off work. In evidence-based medicine, the strategy would be to provide guidance for the optimum enrolment of absent workers into RTW interventions, relying on separate evaluation studies that have used different enrolment criteria, or on a very large evaluation study that enables subgroup analysis according to time of enrolment into the intervention. The systematic reviews described in this chapter[13,14] suggest that such an approach is very costly and time-consuming. The meta-analytic approach by Palmer and colleagues was not able to distinguish clearly the interrelation between the content of the RTW intervention and the timing of enrolment of workers on the effectiveness of the intervention.

An alternative strategy relies on examining the theoretical effects of different timing of existing RTW interventions and on evaluating the consequences for costs and benefits of these interventions. This approach consists of three steps. In the first step, selected RTW curves are fitted to a mathematical function that best describes the RTW rate over time. In step 2, measures of effect of an intervention are incorporated in the mathematical function to calculate the theoretical effects on RTW rates of different start times for the intervention. In the third step, the theoretical effects are linked to the costs and benefits of the intervention in order to evaluate consequences for the cost-benefits of RTW interventions.[15]

Any RTW curve over time can be described with a mathematical Weibull function.[15] This Weibull function is characterized by a scale parameter λ and a shape parameter k.

The scale parameter λ is a function of different covariates that include the intervention effect, preferably expressed as hazard ratio (HR) between the intervention group and the reference group in a Cox's proportional hazards regression model. The shape parameter k reflects the relative increase or decrease in survival time, thus expressing how much the RTW rate will decrease with prolonged sick leave. Each of the RTW curves depicted in Figure 9.1 fits such a Weibull model very well. The slow RTW curve can be described by a scale parameter $\lambda = 5.4$ and a shape parameter $k = 0.42$, whereas the values for the fast RTW are $\lambda = 2.1$ and $k = 0.54$. The difference in shape parameter reflects a faster decline in the RTW rate over time for the slow RTW curve in Ontario, Canada, as compared with the fast RTW curve in Quebec, Canada.

Based on information from Table 9.1, a HR as measure of effect can be introduced as a covariate in the scale parameter λ in the Weibull model and the difference in areas under the curve between the intervention model and the basic model will give the improvement in sickness absence days due to the intervention. By introducing different times of starting the intervention among those workers still on sick leave, the impact of timing of enrolment can be evaluated. Subsequently, the estimated changes in total sickness absence days can be expressed in a benefit/cost ratio (BC ratio), where benefits are the costs saved due to a reduction in sickness absence and costs are the expenditures relating to the intervention.[15]

The impact of timing of enrolment on effectiveness of interventions

The modelling approach assumes a median effect of a RTW intervention to have RR = 1.21 and a large effect to have RR = 1.60.[14] Timing of enrolment was introduced into the model with increments of 2 weeks. Since it is reasonable to assume that some time will elapse between the start of the intervention and its effect on RTW, time lags of 2 and 4 weeks were also introduced.

Figure 9.2 presents the theoretical reductions in sickness absence days per worker enrolled in the intervention at different times in the sickness episode, under the assumption of an immediate effect, i.e. the intervention works from the first day of enrolment. The first observation is that the theoretical interventions were much more beneficial on the slow RTW curve than on the fast RTW curve. In fact, a powerful intervention (with HR = 1.60) among workers with a fast RTW had improvements on sickness absence days which were comparable to those of a considerably less powerful intervention (with HR = 1.21) among workers with a slow RTW. For the slow RTW curve, at the optimum effectiveness the intervention with HR = 1.60 resulted in almost 6 days of sickness absence less than the intervention with HR = 1.21. For the fast RTW curve, the maximum difference between the interventions was 3.6 days of sickness absence. The effect of different starting times for the interventions suggests that an intervention with a smaller effect should be delivered earlier in the RTW process (within 4 weeks) than an intervention with a larger effect, where the most appropriate time window is somewhere between 4 and 10 weeks.

Figure 9.3 describes the evaluation of the trade-off between benefits and costs (BC ratio), the actual starting time of the intervention, and the assumed delay in time

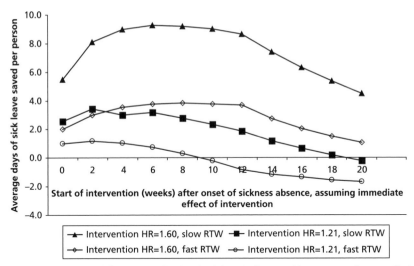

Figure 9.2 Estimated effects on reduction in sickness absence (days per worker enrolled in the intervention) of interventions starting at different points in the episode of absence, stratified by intervention effect (HR = 1.21 or 1.60), and by RTW curve (slow or fast).

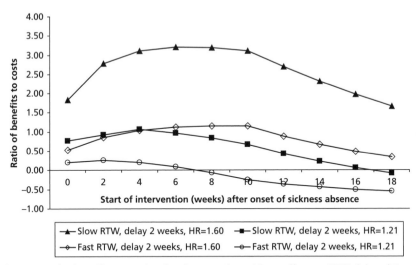

Figure 9.3 The benefit-cost ratio of an intervention with an effect on RTW delayed 2 weeks after enrolment in the intervention, stratified by intervention effect (HR = 1.21 or 1.60), and by RTW curve (slow or fast).

before the intervention will have its effect on RTW. This evaluation assumes interventions with effect sizes of HR = 1.60 and HR = 1.21, costs for the intervention of €500 per worker, and average employer-related costs of €200 for 1 day of sickness absence. The latter estimate is based on the median income of Dutch households in 2011 and on

Table 9.2 Results of the sensitivity analysis for changes in parameter values on the ratio of benefits to costs (BC ratio) of RTW interventions

Type of RTW curve	Size of intervention effect	Delay in the effect	Cost of intervention	Maximum BC ratio
Slow RTW	HR = 1.60	2 weeks	€250–€1000	1.60–7.20
		4 weeks	€250–€1000	1.39–5.54
	HR = 1.21	2 weeks	€250–€1000	0.53–2.14
		4 weeks	€250–€1000	0.41–1.62
Fast RTW	HR = 1.60	2 weeks	€250–€1000	0.58–2.30
		4 weeks	€250–€1000	0.44–1.76
	HR = 1.21	2 weeks	€250–€1000	0.13–0.50
		4 weeks	€250–€1000	0.06–0.22

social insurance premiums paid by Dutch employers. For the scenario where the RTW curve is fast, only interventions with a large effect (HR = 1.60) and a short time span of 2 weeks between delivery and effect will achieve a beneficial BC ratio of up to 1.15, when offered between 6 to 8 weeks after the onset of the episode of sickness absence. For an intervention with median effectiveness (HR = 1.21), the costs will always exceed the benefits. For scenarios with the slow RTW curve, an average intervention will quickly have a BC ratio below 1. The most 'profitable' scenario is an intervention with large effectiveness, and that works within 2 weeks, within a slow RTW setting. In this scenario, BC ratios are projected to vary from 1.7 to 3.2 with an optimum enrolment of workers at around 6–8 weeks into the episode of sickness absence.

In this modelling approach, five different parameters are amenable to change: type of RTW curve, size of the intervention effect, delay until the effect, cost of intervention, and cost of a day of sickness absence. Table 9.2 presents the sensitivity analysis for different combinations of parameter values. The anticipated effects of the intervention and the type of RTW curve have the largest impact on the estimated BC ratios. When keeping all other parameters constant, a change in effectiveness from HR = 1.21 to HR 1.60 introduces changes in BC ratios of 3- to 8-fold. The difference between a fast RTW curve and a slow RTW curve (i.e. the difference between Quebec and Ontario) is associated with differences in BC ratios of 2.8- to 6.8-fold. The sensitivity analysis also demonstrates that for many combinations it will be difficult to achieve sufficient cost savings to exceed the costs of the intervention (i.e. achieve BC ratio >1).

Implications for the effectiveness of RTW interventions

This study shows that the cost-benefits of a structured RTW intervention among workers on sick leave will be determined by the effectiveness of the intervention, the natural speed of RTW in the target population, the timing of the enrolment of workers into the intervention, and the costs of both the intervention and of a day of sickness absence. Since these factors are most likely interrelated and current studies do not provide clear guidance as to their relative importance, the most important question remains: when precisely should which intervention be implemented?

For workers absent from work due to musculoskeletal disorders, a stepped care approach is attractive. The steepness of RTW curves in the first weeks should ensure that most workers with musculoskeletal complaints will return to work rapidly, typically 50–70% in the first 2 weeks. With such a high RTW in the first few weeks, the only early interventions which are likely to be cost-beneficial are inexpensive work-focused enhancements to early routine care, such as simple accommodations in the workplace. The median reduction in sickness absence of 1.1 days per months across all RTW interventions, as reported by Palmer and colleagues,[14] indicates that these early interventions should not exceed €250 per worker. Structured interventions at this early stage are unlikely to have an additional impact on the already good prognosis and, thus, will not be cost-beneficial. The analysis of the timing for RTW interventions suggests that the optimum time window for an effective intervention is at approximately between 4 and 10 weeks. Interestingly, most randomized controlled trials of RTW interventions for workers with LBP have included workers 4–12 weeks into the episode of sick leave, often with enrolment starting after week 4.[15] It can be expected that RTW interventions initiated after about 12 weeks will have a low probability of success due to the decreased RTW rate at this time. After about 12 weeks on sickness absence, RTW will be complex and intensive interventions will be required that address social factors in addition to health care and workplace interventions.[17,18]

Traditionally, occupational health professionals have focused on measures of effectiveness in randomized controlled trials, such as effect size, RR, or HR. Conclusions about effectiveness of specific interventions often rely heavily on these measures. However, Figures 9.2 and 9.3 illustrate that even an intervention that is highly effective (HR = 1.60) in a target population with a naturally slow RTW will become cost-ineffective in a different target population with a much faster RTW. It has been noted before that differences in underlying RTW curves may partly explain the contradictory results of similar interventions in different occupational populations.[19]

The findings on the time delay before an intervention expresses its effects point at another pitfall hampering the effectiveness of interventions. Participation in an intervention for several weeks may obstruct the natural RTW and, hence, introduce a detrimental effect. The introduction of a delay in effect for several weeks strongly reduces the likelihood of a cost-beneficial intervention.[18] Thus, intervention at 8–12 weeks after onset of sickness absence with a required participation for more than 4 weeks should only be considered for an individual worker with a poor prognosis due to the presence of several prognostic predictors of a delayed RTW.

Recommendations

The cost-effectiveness of a RTW intervention will be determined by the effectiveness of the intervention, the costs of the intervention and of a day of sickness absence, the natural course of RTW in the target population, the timing of the enrolment of workers into the RTW intervention, and the time lag before the intervention takes effect. The latter three factors are seldom taken into consideration in systematic reviews and guidelines for management of RTW, although their impact may easily be as important as classical measures of effectiveness, such as effect size or HR. The following recomm-endations summarize the key issues:

1. The effectiveness of an RTW intervention is not a fixed trait, but highly depends on characteristics of the target population, workplace-based factors, occupational health care, company policy, and national social security legislation.

2. Studies on the effectiveness of an RTW intervention should publish details with respect to the RTW curve, distribution of time of enrolment into the intervention, and average duration of the intervention in relation to RTW.

3. Since generalizability of a specific RTW intervention to other populations in other countries is low, systematic reviews and guidelines should refrain from presenting conclusive evidence that a particular intervention warrants implementation above another intervention.

4. Before implementing an intervention, it should be verified whether the features of the RTW pattern in the target population, as well as the nature and timing of the intervention, are conducive to success.

References

1. **Dagenais S, Caro J, Haldeman S.** A systematic review of low back pain cost of illness studies in the United States and internationally. *Spine J* 2008;**8**:8–20.

2. **Virta L, Joranger P, Brox JI, Eriksson R.** Costs of shoulder pain and resource use in primary health care: a cost-of-illness study in Sweden. *BMC Musculoskelet Disord* 2012;**13**:17. doi: 10.1186/1471-2474-13-17.

3. **Elders LAM, Burdorf A.** Prevalence, incidence, and recurrence of low back pain in scaffolders during a 3-year follow-up study. *Spine* 2004;**29**:E101–6.

4. **Hestbaek L, Leboeuf-Yde C, Manniche C.** Low back pain: what is the long-term course? A review of studies of general patient populations. *Eur Spine J* 2003;**12**:149–65.

5. **Viikari-Juntura E, Burdorf A.** Return to work and job retention—increasingly important outcomes in occupational health research. *Scand J Work Environ Health* 2011;**37**:81–4.

6. **Great Britain Department of Health.** Clinical Standards Advisory Group. *Epidemiology review: the epidemiology and cost of back pain. The annex to the Clinical Standards Advisory Group's report on back pain.* London: Her Majesty's Stationery Office, 1994.

7. **Abenhaim L, Rossignol M, Gobeille D, Bonvalot Y, Fines P, Scott S.** The prognostic consequences in the making of the initial medical diagnosis of work-related back injuries. *Spine* 1995;**20**:791–5.

8. **Frank JW, Brooker AS, DeMaio SE,** *et al.* Disability resulting from occupational low back pain. Part II: what do we know about secondary prevention? A review of the scientific evidence on prevention after disability begins. *Spine* 1996;**21**:2918–29.

9. **Steenstra IA, Verbeek JH, Heymans MW, Bongers PM.** Prognostic factors for duration of sick leave in patients sick listed with acute low back pain: a systematic review of the literature. *Occup Environ Med* 2005;**62**:851–60.

10. **Iles RA, Davidson M, Taylor NF.** Psychosocial predictors of failure to return to work in non-chronic non-specific low back pain: a systematic review. *Occup Environ Med* 2008;**65**:507–17.

11. **Heymans MW, Anema JR, van Buuren S, Knol DL, van Mechelen W, de Vet HCW.** Return to work in a cohort of low back pain patients: development and validation of a clinical prediction rule. *J Occup Rehabil* 2009;**19**:155–65.

12. **Dionne CE, Bourbonnais R, Frémont P, Rossignol M, Stock SR, Larocque I.** A clinical return-to-work rule for patients with back pain. *CMAJ* 2005;**172**:1559–67.

13. **Franche R-L, Cullen K, Clarke J,** *et al.* Workplace-based return-to-work interventions: a systematic review of the quantitative literature. *J Occup Rehabil* 2005;**15**:607–31.

14. **Palmer KT, Harris EC, Linaker C,** *et al.* Effectiveness of community- and workplace-based interventions to manage musculoskeletal-related sickness absence and job loss: a systematic review. *Rheumatology* 2012;**51**:230–42.

15. **van Duijn M, Eijkemans MJ, Koes BW, Koopmanschap MA, Burton KA, Burdorf A.** The effects of timing on the cost-effectiveness of interventions for workers on sick leave due to low back pain. *Occup Environ Med* 2010;**67**:744–50.

16. **Aust B, Helverskov T, Nielsen MBD,** *et al.* The Danish national return-to-work program—aims, content, and design of the process and effect evaluation. *Scand J Work Environ Health* 2012;**38**:120–33.

17. **Waddell G, Burton AK, Kendall NAS,** for the Vocational Rehabilitation Task Group of the Industrial Injuries Advisory Council. *Vocational rehabilitation: what works, for whom, and when?* London: The Stationery Office, 2008. Available at: <http://www.dwp.gov.uk/docs/hwwb-vocational-rehabilitation.pdf> (accessed 7 February 2013).

18. **Waddell G, Burton AK.** *Concepts of rehabilitation for the management of common health problems.* London: The Stationery Office, 2004. Available at: <http://www.dwp.gov.uk/docs/hwwb-concepts-of-rehabilitation.pdf> (accessed 7 February 2013).

19. **Elders LAM, van der Beek AJ, Burdorf A.** Return to work after sickness absence due to back disorders—a systematic review on intervention strategies. *Int Arch Occup Environ Health* 2000;**73**:339–48.

Chapter 10

Unemployment at a young age and future unemployment, sickness absence, disability pension, and death in Sweden

Magnus Helgesson, Bo Johansson,
Ingvar Lundberg, and Eva Vingård

Introduction

Unemployment has, since the start of the economic crises in 2008, increased in most Western countries. Work is an important part of most people's lives, and the loss of employment can be detrimental, not only to the personal economy but also to health and well-being. Unemployed persons have, in general, worse health, both mentally and physically, than employed persons.[1,2] An economic 'scar' of lower income can be seen many years after the initial unemployment period.[3] Economic hardship can be one of the contributing factors to decreased well-being among the unemployed.[4] Whether unemployment leads to poor health or poor health leads to unemployment is an important and difficult question. Studies support both positions; today there is a consensus that the effect goes in both directions. A vicious circle can probably be started by either unemployment or poor health. Sweden had been relatively spared from unemployment since the 1930s but then entered a recession at the beginning of the 1990s which had similarities with the current crisis in Europe. The unemployment rate, especially among young people, increased substantially from a few per cent in 1990 to around 20% in 1993 (Figure 10.1).[5]

Periods of unemployment, especially longer spells, can make the entry, or re-entry, to the labour market problematic because unemployment may, from an employer's perspective, be interpreted as low productivity.[6] Ultimately unemployment can end up in social exclusion, especially for vulnerable groups such as individuals with low education, with functional disabilities, or immigrants.[7,8] Countries differ in their welfare and employment regulation. A study from the UK showed that, in the UK, the risk of dismissal from employment was similar throughout the follow-up period of 8 years while the risk in Sweden and Holland decreased with longer employment.[9] The structure of the labour market and the welfare regime, e.g. social insurances and government programmatic spending, will, in great part, be decisive factors in how stable the labour market is and in particular in how detrimental the consequences of unemployment will be.[9]

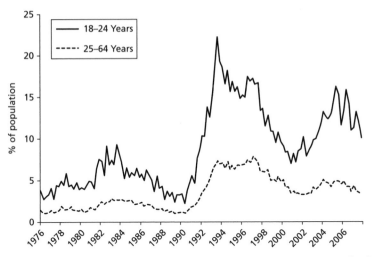

Figure 10.1 Unemployment rate in Sweden 1976–2007. Source: Statistics Sweden.[5]

Young adults are, in general, more affected by unemployment than are older workers.[10] Two longitudinal studies, one from Sweden and one from Norway, concluded that periods of unemployment early in working life increase the risk of future unemployment.[11,12] Young people generally have better initial health than older adults but possibly changes in those lifestyle factors (e.g. alcohol, drugs, eating habits) which are correlated with unemployment can influence health rapidly.[10,13,14] A meta-analysis on 20 million individuals indicated a hazard ratio of death from any cause of 1.63 for unemployed individuals compared to the employed.[15] A longitudinal study from Sweden concluded that unemployed individuals had a slightly elevated risk of premature death during the first 4 years of an 8-year follow-up period. However, adjustment for socioeconomic factors and previous sickness absence erased most of the effect.[16] There are many studies that conclude that unemployment leads to later ill health[1,2] and death[15] but, to our knowledge, very few studies examining unemployment and future sickness absence and disability pension, outcomes related to both health and work participation. An ecological study from Iceland found an increased incidence of disability pension due to mental and behavioural disorders 1 year after a peak in the unemployment rate.[17] In Finland, individuals who were unemployed in 1998, both short-term and long-term, had an elevated risk of disability pension due to depression 5 years later, in 2003.[18]

Sweden has, compared to many other countries, a relatively large immigrant population. In the 1950s and 1960s, immigration was mainly for economic reasons and almost all immigrants found work but after 1970 there was greater immigration of refugees and of family members seeking reunification. Today around 15% of the population was born outside Sweden.[19] Immigrants have had increasing difficulties succeeding in the Swedish labour market since the economic downturns in the 1970s. The research on work and health in the native compared to the immigrant population is fragmentary.[20–22] On the one hand, receipt of a disability pension is more common among immigrants in both Sweden and in Norway.[23,24] But, in a recent study from Sweden, most immigrant workers did not seem to have worse health, measured as hospitalization, than Swedish-born workers. Immigrants from other Nordic countries had, however, worse health than Swedish-born workers.[25] Time since immigration and arrival at a young age have been seen to be a decisive factor for future health status.[26]

The aim of this large study was to examine if exposure to unemployment during a recession period was associated with future unemployment, sickness absence, disability pension, or death for first-generation immigrant and native young men and women living in Sweden.

Methods

The study was a register-based prospective cohort study. The baseline year was 1992 and the cohort was followed from 1993 to 2008. The study group comprised all foreign-born individuals aged 20–24 who were living in Sweden in 1992 and had immigrated before 1990 (n=25 607). A random sample of native Swedes in the same age group (n=174 016) was also included (Table 10.1). 'Immigrant' refers, in this study, to a person born outside Sweden with two non-Swedish-born parents. A 'native Swede' was defined as a person born in Sweden with two Swedish-born parents. To be classified as unemployed the person must have been registered as unemployed at the National Labour Office. One hundred days of unemployment or more is an official measure of long-term unemployment among young individuals at the Swedish Public Employment Service and is the time point when individuals are entitled to extra support.

To form as healthy a cohort as possible, individuals who received unemployment benefit in 1990 and 1991, or who received a disability pension in 1990–92, or who were

Table 10.1 Distribution of unemployment in 1992 for the study population

		Total	**0 days**	**1–99 days**	**≥100 days**
Native Swedes	Women	83 406	59 397 (71.2%)	15 278 (18.3%)	8731 (10.5%)
	Men	90 610	60 042 (66.2%)	16 403 (18.1%)	14 165 (15.6%)
Immigrants	Women	13 544	8471 (62.5%)	2781 (20.5%)	2292 (16.9%)
	Men	12 063	6756 (56.0%)	2400 (19.9%)	2907 (24.1%)
	Total	199 623	134 666	36 862	28 095

Source: data from Magnus Helgesson et al., Unemployment at a young age and later sickness absence, disability pension and death in native Swedes and immigrants, *The European Journal of Public Health,* first published online August 28, 2012, Copyright © The Author 2012. Published by Oxford University Press on behalf of the European Public Health Association

hospitalized due to pulmonary, cardiovascular, musculoskeletal, or psychiatric diagnoses in 1990–92 were excluded. Also, approximately 17 000 persons, both immigrants and native Swedes, who emigrated temporarily or permanently from Sweden during the follow-up period were excluded because their time under risk of sickness absence and disability pension was uncertain and death in another country is not consistently reported in Sweden.

Odds and hazard ratios with 95% confidence intervals were analysed for the studied outcomes by logistic regression and Cox regression models methods using SAS version 9.2. Potential confounders included in the analyses were age, income in 1991, native country, place of residence in Sweden, educational background, and income from sickness absence in 1990 and 1991.

Data on social insurance up to 2008 were obtained from the Longitudinal Integration Database for Health Insurance and Labour Market Studies. Mortality data were collected from the Cause of Death Register. The National Patient Register provided data on hospitalization.

Results

Table 10.1 shows that baseline unemployment in 1992 in these young adults was related to gender and to immigrant status: men were more likely to be unemployed, as were immigrants. Amongst young immigrant men, 24.1% had been unemployed in 1992 for 100 days or more. Immigrants also had during the follow-up a higher risk of 100 days or more of unemployment compared to native Swedes (not in tables). However, there were no consistent risk differences between unemployed immigrants and unemployed native Swedes for any of the studied outcomes.

Young people who were unemployed in 1992, both for 1–99 days and for 100 days or more, had a higher risk of 100 or more days of unemployment during follow-up to 2008 (Table 10.2). The effect was seen in every time period, but declined over time. Those with 100 or more days of unemployment in 1992 were at a greater risk of future unemployment than those with 1–99 days, and men had a greater risk than women. Immigrant status did not appear to influence the risk of subsequent unemployment. During the first 5 years of follow-up, educational background was of importance to the results and those with lower educational attainment had a greater risk of subsequent unemployment (Table 10.3). Unemployment at baseline was also examined in finer detail and there was an increasing risk of future unemployment for every step of 50 days in 1992 until the maximum exposure to unemployment noted in this study (Table 10.4).

Table 10.5 displays the results of similar analyses for sickness absence. Individuals with long-term unemployment in 1992 had a higher probability of subsequent sickness absence than did individuals with no recorded unemployment; the elevated risk was rather similar across the three periods of follow-up. There was also a higher risk of receiving a disability pension during follow-up amongst the unemployed, especially the long-term unemployed (Table 10.6). And there was an increased risk of death during follow-up among the unemployed of every group except native Swedish women; the number who died was, however, very small (Table 10.6).

Table 10.2 Adjusted[a] odds ratio (OR) (95% confidence interval) for ≥100 days of future unemployment for individuals who were unemployed 1–99 or ≥ 100 days in 1992, compared with individuals with no unemployment in the same year

			1993–1997		1998–2002		2003–2007	
			N	OR	N	OR	N	OR
Native Swedes	Women	1–99 days	10 456	3.55 (3.41–3.69)	4633	1.63 (1.56–1.70)	2914	1.33 (1.26–1.40)
		≥100 days	7101	6.90 (6.51–7.31)	3677	2.54 (2.41–2.67)	2260	1.84 (1.74–1.94)
	Men	1–99 days	11 373	4.54 (4.37–4.72)	4337	1.82 (1.74–1.90)	2722	1.47 (1.40–1.55)
		≥100 days	11 282	7.92 (7.57–8.29)	4794	2.52 (2.41–2.63)	3000	1.92 (1.83–2.02)
Immigrants	Women	1–99 days	2245	3.97 (3.56–4.42)	1375	1.58 (1.44–1.74)	858	1.31 (1.18–1.44)
		≥100 days	2046	7.64 (6.63–8.82)	1360	2.25 (2.03–2.48)	835	1.59 (1.44–1.76)
	Men	1–99 days	1976	4.37 (3.87–4.94)	1187	1.81 (1.64–2.01)	747	1.30 (1.16–1.45)
		≥100 days	2583	7.78 (6.82–8.88)	1579	2.20 (1.99–2.42)	1049	1.63 (1.47–1.80)

[a] Adjusted for: age, education, income in 1991, residence in Sweden 1992, native country, and sickness absence in 1991–92

Source: data from Magnus Helgesson et al., Unemployment at a young age and later sickness absence, disability pension and death in native Swedes and immigrants, *The European Journal of Public Health*, first published online 28 August 2012, Copyright © The Author 2012. Published by Oxford University Press on behalf of the European Public Health Association

Table 10.3 Adjusted[a] odds ratio (OR) (95% confidence interval) for ≥100 days of future unemployment during the period 1993–97 for individuals who had different educational backgrounds and were unemployed 1–99 or ≥ 100 days in 1992, compared with individuals with no unemployment in the same year

		Elementary school		Upper secondary school		University	
		N	OR	N	OR	N	OR
Native Swedes	Women						
	1–99 days	1497	4.46 (3.88–5.14)	7767	3.82 (3.65–4.00)	1173	2.32 (2.11–2.56)
	≥100 days	1614	9.94 (8.27–11.94)	4853	7.40 (6.91–7.93)	610	3.92 (3.40–4.52)
	Men						
	1–99 days	1501	5.83 (5.12–6.63)	8480	4.92 (4.70–5.15)	1358	2.70 (2.46–2.97)
	≥100 days	2037	13.24 (11.39–15.39)	8203	8.60 (8.15–9.08)	1002	3.69 (3.30–4.13)
Immigrants	Women						
	1–99 days	731	5.41 (4.32–6.78)	1284	3.64 (3.17–4.19)	139	2.37 (1.69–3.30)
	≥100 days	741	9.84 (7.43–13.04)	1121	7.19 (5.96–8.67)	93	5.40 (3.29–8.88)
	Men						
	1–99 days	677	5.66 (4.39–7.30)	1107	4.46 (3.81–5.22)	98	2.28 (1.57–3.33)
	≥100 days	933	11.23 (8.46–14.90)	1390	7.76 (6.54–9.21)	115	3.29 (2.22–4.88)

[a] Adjusted for: age, income in 1991, residence in Sweden 1992, native country, and sickness absence in 1991–92

Source: data from Magnus Helgesson et al., Unemployment at a young age and later sickness absence, disability pension and death in native Swedes and immigrants, *The European Journal of Public Health*, first published online August 28, 2012, Copyright © The Author 2012. Published by Oxford University Press on behalf of the European Public Health Association

Table 10.4 Adjusted[a] odds ratio (OR) (95% confidence interval) for ≥ 100 days of future unemployment for individuals, both native Swedes and immigrants, exposed to different lengths of unemployment in 1992, compared with individuals with no unemployment in the same year

		1993–1997		1998–2002		2003–2007	
		N	OR	N	OR	N	OR
1–49 days	Native Swedes	10 916	3.58 (3.46–3.71)	4378	1.57 (1.51–1.64)	2763	1.29 (1.24–1.36)
	Immigrants	1982	3.65 (3.28–4.06)	1169	1.52 (1.39–1.67)	724	1.19 (1.08–1.31)
50–99 days	Native Swedes	10 913	4.66 (4.49–4.85)	4592	1.88 (1.81–1.96)	2873	1.49 (1.42–1.56)
	Immigrants	2239	4.73 (4.23–5.28)	1393	1.85 (1.69–2.02)	881	1.40 (1.28–1.54)
100–149 days	Native Swedes	7915	5.94 (5.66–6.23)	3443	2.16 (2.06–2.26)	2191	1.70 (1.62–1.79)
	Immigrants	1768	6.44 (5.61–7.40)	1069	1.93 (1.75–2.13)	707	1.55 (1.40–1.72)
150–199 days	Native Swedes	4718	7.88 (7.36–8.44)	2200	2.59 (2.44–2.74)	1331	1.85 (1.73–1.97)
	Immigrants	1141	6.95 (5.82–8.30)	736	2.26 (2.00–2.55)	447	1.50 (1.32–1.70)

(Continued)

Table 10.4 (Continued)

		1993–1997		1998–2002		2003–2007	
		N	OR	N	OR	N	OR
200–249 days	Native Swedes	3145	10.18 (9.29–11.15)	1512	2.96 (2.76–3.18)	898	2.00 (1.85–2.17)
	Immigrants	812	8.41 (6.71–10.54)	531	2.40 (2.08–2.77)	354	1.80 (1.56–2.07)
250–299 days	Native Swedes	1640	11.53 (10.10–13.17)	799	3.07 (2.79–3.38)	502	2.23 (2.01–2.48)
	Immigrants	500	11.94 (8.60–16.58)	329	2.68 (2.23–3.22)	208	1.75 (1.46–2.10)
≥ 300 days	Native Swedes	965	14.94 (12.32–18.12)	517	3.70 (3.27–4.20)	338	2.70 (2.36–3.09)
	Immigrants	408	17.82 (11.32–28.04)	274	2.78 (2.26–3.43)	168	1.68 (1.37–2.06)

[a] Adjusted for: sex, origin, age, income in 1991, residence in Sweden 1992, native country, and sickness absence in 1991-92

Source: data from Magnus Helgesson et al., Unemployment at a young age and later sickness absence, disability pension and death in native Swedes and immigrants, *The European Journal of Public Health*, first published online August 28, 2012, Copyright © The Author 2012. Published by Oxford University Press on behalf of the European Public Health Association

Table 10.5 Adjusted[a] odds ratio (OR) (95% confidence interval) for ≥60 days of sickness absence for individuals unemployed 1–99 or ≥100 days in 1992 compared with individuals with no unemployment in the same year. Within each group, zero days of unemployment is the reference category

			1993–1997		1998–2002		2003–2007	
			N	OR	N	OR	N	OR
Native Swedes	Women	1–99 days	1543	1.04 (0.97–1.11)	3163	1.10 (1.05–1.15)	3530	1.15 (1.10–1.20)
		≥100 days	1237	1.27 (1.19–1.37)	2243	1.30 (1.23–1.38)	2462	1.36 (1.29–1.44)
	Men	1–99 days	979	1.08 (1.00–1.17)	1396	1.23 (1.15–1.32)	1489	1.21 (1.13–1.29)
		≥100 days	1114	1.25 (1.15–1.34)	1580	1.49 (1.40–1.59)	1676	1.48 (1.39–1.58)
Immigrants	Women	1–99 days	305	1.02 (0.88–1.19)	707	1.11 (1.00–1.24)	841	1.34 (1.21–1.48)
		≥100 days	324	1.34 (1.16–1.55)	649	1.24 (1.11–1.38)	712	1.33 (1.20–1.48)
	Men	1–99 days	159	1.03 (0.84–1.26)	300	1.25 (1.08–1.46)	315	1.22 (1.06–1.42)
		≥100 days	231	1.10 (0.92–1.32)	393	1.28 (1.11–1.47)	460	1.45 (1.27–1.65)

[a] Adjusted for: age, income in 1991, education, residence in Sweden 1992, native country, and sickness absence in 1991–92

Source: data from Magnus Helgesson et al., Unemployment at a young age and later sickness absence, disability pension and death in native Swedes and immigrants, *The European Journal of Public Health*, first published online August 28, 2012, Copyright © The Author 2012. Published by Oxford University Press on behalf of the European Public Health Association

Table 10.6 Adjusted[a] hazard ratio (HR) (95% confidence interval) for disability pension and death over the whole follow-up period of 15 years; individuals unemployed 1–99 or ≥100 days in 1992 compared to individuals with no unemployment. Within each group, zero days of unemployment is the reference category

			Disability pension		Death	
			N	HR	N	HR
Native Swedes	Women	1–99 days	798	1.05 (0.96–1.14)	75	1.15 (0.88–1.50)
		≥100 days	801	1.53 (1.41–1.66)	43	1.02 (0.73–1.43)
	Men	1–99 days	451	1.23 (1.10–1.37)	142	1.18 (0.97–1.44)
		≥100 days	617	1.62 (1.46–1.79)	177	1.56 (1.30–1.87)
Immigrants	Women	1–99 days	248	0.98 (0.85–1.14)	26	1.59 (0.98–2.60)
		≥100 days	276	1.26 (1.09–1.45)	23	1.65 (0.99–2.75)
	Men	1–99 days	158	1.08 (0.89–1.32)	37	1.01 (0.68–1.51)
		≥100 days	250	1.38 (1.16–1.63)	53	1.15 (0.81–1.64)

[a] Adjusted for: age, income in 1991, education, residence in Sweden 1992, native country, and sickness absence in 1991–92

Source: data from Magnus Helgesson et al., Unemployment at a young age and later sickness absence, disability pension and death in native Swedes and immigrants, *The European Journal of Public Health*, first published online August 28, 2012, Copyright © The Author 2012. Published by Oxford University Press on behalf of the European Public Health Association

Discussion

Unemployment in early working life clearly affected the probability of future unemployment 15 years after exposure. This finding is similar to those of previous longitudinal studies in Scandinavia. In the Swedish study, individuals who became unemployed directly after compulsory school had more than a twofold risk of unemployment during the 5-year follow-up compared to individuals in work or in labour market programmes.[11] In the Norwegian study, previous unemployment increased the risk of future unemployment substantially, more than, for example, educational attainment and school dropout.[12] Our study showed a dose-response relationship between duration of unemployment in 1992 and future unemployment, with an increase in risk for every step of 50 days up to the maximum of 300 days or more. An English study had a similar outcome, with the longer the period of unemployment at age 16–23 the more months of unemployment at age 23–33 and 33–42.[27]

The relationship between unemployment and health is complex and the question about causation or selection to future unemployment, poor health, or death is debated. There are five groups of theories which provide plausible causal links between unemployment and poor health.[28] The economic deprivation models assume that unemployment means having less money and this affects the prerequisites for good health. The control models assume that the passive situation means low control over life which is a risk factor for ill health. The stress models focus on how individuals cope with the situation of unemployment, and the social support models assume that human contact means that individuals can handle stress in a better way. Finally, the models of latent functions assume that any work, almost without exception, has a profound effect on health so that when an individual loses a job those protective functions are lost; the best known theory of latent functions was developed by Jahoda in the 1930s.[29] The authors concluded that all models correlate fairly well to poor health, and support the causation theory.[28]

A Swedish study provided strong evidence for a selection effect; individuals on sick leave before assessment had an elevated risk of future unemployment.[16] Another study from Sweden, however, showed that poor mental health was associated with future unemployment even after adjustment for previous sickness absence, in particular with longer spells of unemployment.[30] A Finnish study showed a health selection effect when comparing unemployed individuals in a boom and in a recession. Unemployed individuals in a boom had poorer health than unemployed individuals in a recession. In prosperous times mostly those with poor health will remain unemployed, while in recessions also 'healthier' individuals become unemployed.[31] Other studies imply that predictors of future unemployment can be detected already in childhood and adolescence.[32,33]

Very few previous studies have, to our knowledge, studied exposure to unemployment and subsequent risk of sickness absence and disability pension as outcomes. We found an association between unemployment and both sickness absence and receipt of a disability pension. Some previous studies show an association between unemployment and poor well-being, a state that may be associated with disability,[1,2] and depression.[18] In Sweden, sickness benefit is payable for almost all forms of disease, so the severity and character of illness eligible for benefit can hence vary substantially.

This study showed a slight increase of death for unemployed individuals in all groups except native Swedish women. The elevated risk was highest in native Swedish men. One should bear in mind that our cohort is young with few deaths during follow-up, and so our conclusions relating to unemployment and risk of death must be tentative. Roelfs and co-workers showed a similar elevated odds ratio for death among unemployed individuals compared to employed, especially among young adults, in a meta-analysis of worldwide data. These findings were assumed to be related to the latent sickness hypothesis, health-related behaviours, or coping/stress hypothesis.[15] Lundin and co-workers found that the elevated risk of death among unemployed individuals compared to the employed essentially disappeared after adjustment for previous sickness absence.[16]

This study showed that immigrants had a higher baseline risk of unemployment than did native Swedes but unemployed immigrants followed the same pattern as native Swedes when exposed to unemployment. In other words, the absolute burden of unemployment was highest in immigrants, but immigrants were no more vulnerable to the subsequent adverse effects of unemployment than were native Swedes. The reasons for the higher baseline unemployment rate in immigrants to Sweden are not fully understood. Previous research has indicated that the mental health of young immigrants is worse than the mental health of young native Swedes[34] and that immigrants in all age groups lost jobs to a greater extent and had less access to new jobs in the economic crisis in the early 1990s.[35] Immigrants were, in many cases, newcomers to the Swedish social security system, but that is also true for young native Swedish individuals. Young native Swedes and immigrants seem to be equally affected by disqualification from receiving welfare benefits.[35] In this young cohort any differences between native Swedes and young immigrants may have become diluted because most immigrants came to Sweden in early or late childhood and had been brought up in the Swedish educational, health, and welfare systems. Arrival at young age and time since arrival is associated with better self-rated health as shown in previous studies.[26]

Conclusion

Unemployment among young adults was associated with an increased risk of unemployment, sickness absence, disability pension, and death as long as 15 years after exposure. This emphasizes the importance of making efforts to reduce unemployment among young individuals, in order to prevent individual suffering, preserve economic growth, and reduce future spending on health care and welfare systems. Young immigrants had a higher baseline rate of unemployment, both for short-term (1–99 days) and long-term unemployment (100 days or more), but they followed the pattern of native Swedes in relation to future unemployment and ill health. Education had a protective effect on future unemployment.

Acknowledgement

This chapter is based, with permission, on Magnus Helgesson, Bo Johansson, Tobias Nordqvist, Ingvar Lundberg, and Eva Vingård, Unemployment at a young age and later sickness absence, disability pension and death in native Swedes and immigrants,

The European Journal of Public Health first published online 28 August 2012 doi:10.1093/ eurpub/cks099, Copyright © The Author 2012, published by Oxford University Press on behalf of the European Public Health Association.

References

1. **Paul KI, Moser K.** Unemployment impairs mental health: Meta-analyses. *J Vocat Behav* 2009;**74**:264–82.

2. **McKee-Ryan F, Song Z, Wanberg CR, Kinicki AJ.** Psychological and physical well-being during unemployment: a meta-analytic study. *J Appl Psychol* 2005;**90**:53–76

3. **Strandh M, Nordlund M.** Active labour market policy and unemployment scarring: a ten-year Swedish panel study. *J Soc Policy* 2008;**37**:357–82.

4. **Janlert U, Hammarström A.** Alcohol consumption among unemployed youths: results from a prospective study. *Br J Addict* 1992;**87**:703–14.

5. **Statistics Sweden (SCB).** *Arbetskraftsundersökningarna (Workforce review).* 2010. Available at: <http://www.scb.se/Pages/ProductTables.aspx?id=23272> (accessed 6 February 2013).

6. **Lockwood B.** Information externalities in the labor-market and the duration of unemployment. *Rev Econ Stud* 1991;**58**:733–53.

7. **Hammer T (ed.).** *Youth unemployment and social exclusion in Europe: a comparative study.* Bristol: The Policy Press, University of Bristol, 2003.

8. **Kieselbach T.** Youth unemployment and health effects. *Int J Soc Psychiatry* 1988;**34**:83–96.

9. **Layte R, Levin H, Hendrickx, Bison I.** Unemployment and cumulative disadvantage in the labour market. In: Gallie D, Paugam S (eds) *Welfare regimes and the experience of unemployment in Europe.* Oxford: Oxford University Press, 2000, pp. 153–74.

10. **Reine I, Novo M, Hammarström A.** Does the association between ill health and unemployment differ between young people and adults? Results from a 14-year follow-up study with a focus on psychological health and smoking. *Public Health* 2004;**118**:337–45.

11. **Hammarström A, Janlert U.** Do early unemployment and health status among young men and women affect their chances of later employment? *Scand J Public Health* 2000;**28**:10–5.

12. **Hammer T.** History dependence in youth unemployment. *Eur Sociol Rev* 1997;**13**:17–33.

13. **Breslin F, Mustard C.** Factors influencing the impact of unemployment on mental health among young and older adults in a longitudinal, population-based survey. *Scand J Work Environ Health* 2003;**29**:5–14.

14. **Hammarström A.** Health consequences of youth unemployment—review from a gender perspective. *Soc Sci Med* 1994;**38**:699–709.

15. **Roelfs DJ, Shor E, Davidson KW, Schwartz JE.** Losing life and livelihood: a systematic review and meta-analysis of unemployment and all-cause mortality. *Soc Sci Med* 2011;**72**:840–54.

16. **Lundin A, Lundberg I, Hallsten L, Ottosson J, Hemmingsson T.** Unemployment and mortality—a longitudinal prospective study on selection and causation in 49321 Swedish middle-aged men. *J Epidemiol Community Health* 2010;**64**:22–8.

17. **Thorlacius S, Ólafsson S.** From unemployment to disability? Relationship between unemployment rate and new disability pensions in Iceland 1992–2007. *Eur J Public Health* 2010;**22**:96–101.

18. **Lamberg T, Virtanen P, Vahtera J, Luukkaala T, Koskenvuo M.** Unemployment, depressiveness and disability retirement: a follow-up study of the Finnish HeSSup population sample. *Soc Psychiatry Psychiatr Epidemiol* 2010;**45**:259–64.

19. **Statistics Sweden (SCB).** *Population statistics.* Available at: <http://www.scb.se/Pages/Product____25799.aspx> (accessed 6 February 2013).

20. **Ahonen EQ, Benavides FG, Benach J.** Immigrant populations, work and health – a systematic literature review. *Scand J Work Environ Health* 2007;**33**:96–104. (Correction in: *Scand J Work Environ Health* 2007;**33**:240.)

21. **European Agency for Safety and Health at Work.** *Literature study on migrant workers.* 2007. Available at: <https://osha.europa.eu/en/publications/literature_reviews/migrant_workers/view> (accessed 6 February 2013).

22. **Wren K, Boyle P.** *SALTSA programme report no 1:2001. Migration and work-related health in Europe–a literature review.* 2001. Available at: <http://www.ekhist.uu.se/Saltsa/publications.htm> (accessed 6 February 2013).

23. **Claussen B, Smeby L, Bruusgaard D.** Disability pension rates among immigrants in Norway. *J Immigr Minor Health* 2010;**14**:259–63.

24. **Osterberg T, Gustafsson B.** Disability pension among immigrants in Sweden. *Soc Sci Med* 2006;**63**:805–16.

25. **Johansson B, Helgesson M, Lundberg I,** *et al.* Work and health among immigrants and native Swedes 1990–2008: a register-based study on hospitalization for common potentially work-related disorders, disability pension and mortality. *BMC Public Health* 2012;**12**:845. doi: 10.1186/1471-2458-12-845.

26. **Leão TS, Sundquist J, Johansson SE, Sundquist K.** The influence of age at migration and length of residence on self-rated health among Swedish immigrants: a cross-sectional study. *Ethn Health* 2009;**14**:93–105.

27. **Gregg P, Tominey E.** The wage scar from male youth unemployment. *Labour Econ* 2005;**12**:487–509.

28. **Janlert U, Hammarström A.** Which theory is best? Explanatory models of the relationship between unemployment and health. *BMC Public Health* 2009;**9**:235. doi: 10.1186/1471-2458-9-235.

29. **Jahoda M.** Impact of unemployment in the 1930s and the 1970s. *Bull Br Psychol Soc* 1979;**32**:309–14.

30. **Backhans MC, Hemmingsson T.** Unemployment and mental health—who is (not) affected? *Eur J Public Health* 2011;**22**:429–33.

31. **Martikainen PT, Valkonen T.** Excess mortality of unemployed men and women during a period of rapidly increasing unemployment. *Lancet* 1996;**348**:909–12.

32. **Caspi A, Wright BRE, Moffitt TE, Silva PA.** Early failure in the labor market: Childhood and adolescent predictors of unemployment in the transition to adulthood. *Am Sociol Rev* 1998;**63**:424–51.

33. **Montgomery SM, Bartley MJ, Cook DG, Wadsworth ME.** Health and social precursors of unemployment in young men in Great Britain. *J Epidemiol Community Health* 1996;**50**:415–22.

34. **Malmberg-Heimonen I, Julkunen I.** Out of unemployment? A comparative analysis of the risks and opportunities longer-term unemployed immigrant youth face when entering the labour market. *J Youth Stud* 2006;**9**:575–92.

35. **Bergmark Å, Palme J.** Welfare and the unemployment crisis: Sweden in the 1990s. *Int J Soc Welf* 2003;**12**:108–22.

Part 4

Extending the epidemiological approach

What do surveillance schemes tell us about the epidemiology of occupational disease?

Raymond Agius, Malcolm R. Sim, and
Vincent Bonneterre

Introduction

In the public health setting, disease and injury surveillance has been an important tool in identifying trends over time, in assisting in the development of better targeting of prevention programmes, and in monitoring the effectiveness of interventions. Some examples from the public health arena include monitoring the impact of anti-smoking programmes on reducing the incidence of lung cancer by using data collected by cancer registries and the trends in traffic accidents by using surveillance data collected by road traffic authorities.[1]

In the occupational health context, datasets to allow effective surveillance of work-related disease and injury have historically been less advanced. One of the earliest diseases for which surveillance was established is mesothelioma, with several countries establishing mesothelioma surveillance either by using cancer registrations, as in Australia[2] and France,[3] or mortality data, as in the UK.[4] Mesothelioma has some advantages over most other occupational diseases in the ease of establishing reliable monitoring data because it is a rare tumour and its cause is limited to one particular hazard, asbestos, which is usually encountered only from occupational exposure. This contrasts with most other malignant and non-malignant work-related conditions, such as lung cancer, back pain, or dermatitis, which are common in the community and for which there are many work- and non-work-related contributing factors.

In the absence of reliable surveillance data systems for most occupational diseases, many countries have relied on workers' compensation data. However, for work-related diseases such data fall far short of providing a reliable estimate of their extent, because such conditions and their relationship with work are often not well recognized by treating doctors and there are many barriers which reduce the likelihood of success when a worker with an occupational disease makes a claim.[5] Therefore, relying on such data usually leads to a major underestimate of the true incidence of work-related diseases and this has prompted the need for specific surveillance programmes.[6] In the US, it has been estimated that up to 80% of work-related injury and disease is missed.[7]

Due to the limitations of compensation data systems, several countries have established specific work-related diseases surveillance systems. Two of the earliest surveillance programmes were established in Finland[8] and, starting in 1989, in the UK[9] for occupational respiratory disease. An analogous model, SENSOR (Sentinel Event Notification System for Occupational Risks), was developed at around the same time in the US.[10] Not all states participated and usually the main centres for reports were state health departments so capture may have been limited. SENSOR draws a distinction between new cases of occupational asthma and those where asthma is aggravated by work.[11] In more recent years, similar programmes have been established in many other countries, such as South Africa, France, Canada, and Australia. In the UK, The Health and Occupation Reporting network (THOR) has expanded to encompass a range of medically-certified sources including general practitioners (GPs) with special training.[12] Such surveillance programmes have been providing useful data on work-related disease trends for many years. However, the sustainability of these programmes can be uncertain and the information they are able to provide may vary.

Methodological issues

In order to obtain information of the highest quality and utility, surveillance schemes have to be designed, set up, and managed with the same methodological rigour as high-calibre prospective cohort studies. Whether surveillance schemes are voluntary or not, considerable effort has to be invested to ensure a satisfactory and sufficient denominator, the best numerator quality, and the most complete ascertainment. Although the force of statute is relied upon in some surveillance schemes, even in these the initial and continuing motivation of the reporters (usually physicians) is paramount.

Probably the first challenge is to establish a denominator base for surveillance and reporting which is either comprehensive and encompasses the whole population being studied or else constitutes a measurable and representative sample of the population. Thus, for example, in establishing surveillance schemes for occupational respiratory and skin disease in the UK the aim was to cover the entire country by including, as far as possible, all specialists in these disciplines.[13] This entailed eliciting the active support of the specialist societies and recognized authorities in the respective fields. Although many incident reports can be gleaned by appealing to the greater good this motive alone may not suffice to achieve the best data capture. In order to engage physicians, regular meetings, or participation in learned society meetings, newsletters (at least quarterly), and provision of educational material and other resources to satisfy continuing professional development have been found to be essential collective adjuncts. Rapid responses to individual queries for guidance or for summary abstracts of the data, and the involvement of the reporters in peer-reviewed publications from the surveillance centre, are also important motivators for the stakeholders. Nevertheless, a population coverage that falls short of the target remains a concern, although it is possible, in part, to address this by quantitative adjustments.[14]

In determining the numerator, some early surveillance schemes relied on the judgement of the reporters as to what constituted a case, although the current consensus is that valid criteria for reporting are essential and should be audited.[15] A comprehensive case definition for numerator cases should include not only the clinical criteria but also the threshold for occupational attribution. However, physicians have different criteria for determining occupational attribution, such as whether the occupational cause is deemed to be a necessary or sufficient cause, or whether attribution is based on the balance of probability.[16] Specific studies have been undertaken to determine the degree of agreement within and between groups of reporting physicians in making judgements on diagnoses and their occupational attribution, for example, in mental disorders[17] and in occupational asthma.[18] Although these studies show that there is interobserver variation in making judgements on numerator data, it is generally not of sufficient magnitude to negate the validity of the findings, provided their limitations are not ignored.

There is a surveillance 'pyramid' within which the patient's own perception is at the base, the GP is at a higher level, and the clinical specialist is close to the apex. The source of the surveillance reports affects the numerator because case severity and case mix differ according to the level in the pyramid.[19] Although incidence rate estimates may be expected to be lower at the higher levels in the surveillance pyramid this is not necessarily always the case. Self-referral and medical referral patterns may vary within and between countries. Although surveillance undertaken by physicians who specialize in the organ system concerned or in occupational disease (or in both aspects) may be considered to be the medical 'gold standard' it can suffer from a more limited patient catchment because of various referral filters. Surveillance by GPs will capture numerator cases as close to the base of the pyramid as possible, but may suffer from greater diagnostic variation than surveillance by specialists. Limiting recruitment to GPs with a special interest, and some training, in occupational medicine is a compromise between the two levels.[20]

When surveillance is part of a statutory or other compulsory scheme then incident case identification is a continuous and ongoing process. However, when surveillance is voluntary, for a research objective, it may be preferable to sample over shorter, randomly selected intervals, so as to reduce the demands associated with the data collection and 'reporting fatigue'. Evidence so far suggests that sampling over shorter time intervals results in higher incidence estimates than continuous sampling.[21]

There are several considerations in determining incidence from surveillance data. It is possible to calculate an incidence rate based on the general population, on the population of working age, or on the total working population,[19] since these denominator bases are generally readily available, but such rates are not the most useful in determining risk. Therefore, incidence rates are usually calculated in respect of specific occupations or industries.[22] Valid incidence rates are dependent on valid numerator and denominator data but some shortcomings in data quality can be circumvented. Thus, when coverage of the population of interest is unrepresentative, absolute incidence rates would be erroneously low. However, if this systematic shortcoming applies in an equal manner to all occupations being studied it is nevertheless possible to calculate rate ratios and thus compare risks (though not quantify risks absolutely).[23,24] Ideally, incidence rates should be expressed in relation to quantitative estimates of exposure but most surveillance schemes would require additional data collection as special exercises to achieve this aim.

The monitoring of temporal trends in incidence from surveillance schemes presents challenges which range from secular changes in the denominator through to reporting fatigue. Nevertheless, through the use of multilevel models it may be possible to demonstrate temporal trends in the incidence of occupational disease. Thus in the UK there was evidence of a modest reduction in reported incidence of both occupational asthma and contact dermatitis.[25] The methodology has also been used in other contexts, namely mental ill health and musculoskeletal ill health, where the findings suggested a reduction in reported incidence of work-related musculoskeletal ill health accompanied by an increased incidence of work-related mental ill health.[26] However such findings should be interpreted in context. For example, the explanation for this finding may lie in a shift in subjects who are distressed by their work from a primarily musculoskeletal label, notably back pain, to that of a mental disorder because the former cases are now more actively rehabilitated while the diagnosis of the latter is less stigmatized. Although reporting fatigue is an important consideration in tempering conclusions drawn from such multilevel models, it is possible to take account of this potential bias in various ways. For example, when evaluating interventions, temporal trends in outcomes resulting from other exposures can be used to control for fatigue.[23,24] The phenomenon of reporting fatigue may be characterized by an 'excess of zeroes' beyond what is expected of a Poisson distribution and this effect can be quantified.[27]

Therefore, provided certain assumptions are made, appropriate models used, or steps taken to address potential biases, it is possible to use surveillance data to study temporal trends in the incidence of work-related illness in a valid manner.

Ethical issues

Work-related disease and injury surveillance has some additional potential ethical problems on top of the usual ethical problems related to worker research. Because disease surveillance programmes involving physician notifications are undertaken in a clinical diagnosis and treatment environment, this can raise issues about privacy and about security of data transfer to ensure that individuals cannot be identified.[28] Because of concerns by workers about the possible impact on their employment, they may not agree to have their data included in a surveillance system. Participating physicians may be concerned about a potential conflict of interest between their clinical and research roles. The ethical requirement to ensure the de-identification of patient notifications can inhibit later follow-up studies which require contact with the patient or data linkage and this can be a barrier to the most effective use of surveillance data in research. Individual-level data, even when ostensibly anonymized, may have the potential to identify individuals because of unique demographic and employment combinations. When data are presented in a tabular form the convention is not to populate cells with fewer than five cases.

Exposure surveillance

Whereas quantification of the denominator population by industry or by job title is relatively easy, measuring exposure on a large scale is much more demanding. Thus, in order to evaluate interventions through occupational disease surveillance, surrogate measures such as implementation of legislation, exposure standards, or market availability have been used.[23,24,27] One of the criticisms of occupational disease surveillance is that, for diseases with longer latency, it takes too long to ascertain sufficient cases, with resulting delays in implementing prevention activities. Therefore, work exposure surveillance programmes have been developed to complement disease surveillance programmes in order to help identify earlier signals, based on exposure patterns, which can be used to better target programmes aimed at reducing workplace exposures and therefore disease. This method has been used effectively in Finland to document an overall reduction in the prevalence of, and level of exposure to, 41 chemical agents in workplaces from 1950 to 2008.[29] Another example is the CAREX (CARcinogen EXposure) database in the European Union, which provides selected exposure data, and also estimates of the number of exposed workers by country, carcinogen, and industry.[30] When used in combination with work-related disease surveillance data, this can be a powerful tool to monitor both exposure and disease and paint a more complete picture of the likely impact on the health of workers over time.

Examples of findings—associations between industry/job/exposure and ill health

Historically, surveillance programmes, especially those involving physician notifications, have started by surveillance of occupational respiratory disease, so data for these conditions are available for many countries. This provides the opportunity to compare countries and investigate the reasons for differences. Selected examples are used to illustrate this.

In respect of occupational asthma Table 11.1 shows that there is considerable variability in incidence rates between countries, although not all countries have estimated incidence. For those countries which have estimated incidence, the highest incidence was in Finland, where it was about four times greater than in the other countries. Such large differences are likely to be due to differences in definitions, reporting rates, and denominators, but also may reflect differences in industry and exposure patterns between the countries. This is supported by the data on the most commonly reported agents shown in Table 11.1, which also indicate variability in the pattern of commonly reported agents.

Musculoskeletal disorders are another example where surveillance data have helped to provide information on prevalence and incidence rates or trends in working populations in several countries or regions.[36] Besides describing the distribution by industrial sectors and jobs, these schemes have also contributed to the management of physical, organizational, and psychosocial work-related risk factors.[37]

Evaluation of interventions through the use of occupational disease surveillance

One of the main benefits of occupational disease surveillance is its capacity to monitor the effects of interventions at a national or international level. At the simplest level, earlier approaches involved counting incident numerator cases on a year-by-year basis and drawing conclusions from these data. Thus Figure 11.1 shows data on asthma

Table 11.1 Comparison of work-related asthma findings from notification surveillance programmes in different countries

Programme, country, publication year	Incidence of work-related asthma	Most commonly reported agents (%)
SWORD UK, 2005[9]	Respiratory physicians: 22/million workers Occupational physicians: 87/million workers	Respiratory physicians: Isocyanates 14% Flour/grain 9% Wood dust 6% Metals 4% Solder/colophony 4% Glutaraldehyde 3% Resins 3% Welding fume 3% Laboratory animals 3%
SHIELD West Midlands, UK, 2008[31]	42/million workers (95% CI 37–45)	Isocyanates 21% Metal working fluids 11% Adhesives 7% Chrome 7% Latex 6% Glutaraldehyde 6%
SORDSA South Africa, 2001[32]	13.1/million employed people	Latex 24% Isocyanates 20% Platinum salts 12% Flour/grain 12%, Glue/resin 5% Solder/colophony/welding fume 4% Vanadium 3%
SABRE Australia, 2004[33]	30.9/million workers (95% CI 26.8–35.5)	Wood dust 14% Non-specific dust 7% Isocyanates 6% Paint fumes 4% Potroom fume 4% Products of thermal combustion 4% Solvents 3% Welding fume 3% Latex 3%
Occupational disease system Finland, 2000[8]	174/million workers	Animal epithelia/hairs/ secretions 38% Flour/grain/fodder 22% Mites 5% Isocyanates 5% Welding fume 4% Wood dust 3% Moulds 3% Formaldehyde 2%

(Continued)

Table 11.1 *(Continued)*

Programme, country, publication year	Incidence of work-related asthma	Most commonly reported agents (%)
eWoRLD California, Michigan, New Jersey, Massachusetts, US, 2012[34]	3284 cases 1993–2006. No incidence estimated	Miscellaneous chemicals 20% Mineral/inorganic dusts 15% Pyrolysis products 12% Indoor air pollutants 10% Solvents 8% Moulds 6%
ONAP France, 2003[35]	24/million workers (27 for men, 19 for women)	Flour 20% Isocyanates 14% Latex 7% Aldehyde 6% Persulphate salts 6% Wood dust 4%

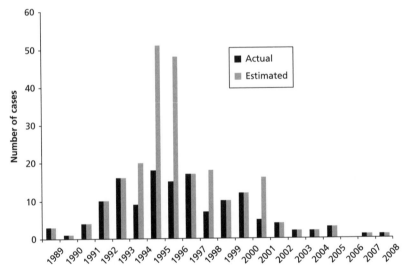

Figure 11.1 Temporal trends in reported cases of asthma attributed to occupational exposure to latex by respiratory physicians in the UK (1991–2010). The vertical bars indicate the number of incident cases of latex asthma reported per year both as actual cases and as estimated cases which takes into account the sampling fraction (since some physicians reported for only one randomly selected month per year).
Source: previously unpublished data from SWORD.

related to latex collected from respiratory physicians in the SWORD (Surveillance of Work-related and Occupational Respiratory Disease) scheme in the UK. As the figure shows, there was a progressive rise in annual reports of cases in the 1990s and, once steps were implemented to provide powderless antigen free latex gloves, there was a steady decline.

Methods of studying interventions through occupational disease surveillance have now developed considerably and, through investigating incidence rate ratios in a controlled approach, the incidence of occupational skin disease caused by latex can be shown to have fallen significantly.[23] At an international level, a European Union directive to control exposure to chromium VI (CrVI) has been evaluated using UK data from THOR and was shown to have been associated with a significant fall in incidence of CrVI dermatitis.[24] It is therefore encouraging both for researchers and for policymakers to note that occupational disease surveillance can provide useful answers to help quantify the health benefits of statutory interventions.

Occupational disease 'vigilance'

Surveillance usually follows trends in incidence of types of work-related ill health that are already recognized both as clinicopathological entities and in terms of specified causes. Even where surveillance has been initiated for the ostensible purpose of highlighting new work-related diseases or causes of disease, the methods used for 'alerts' or 'vigilance' tend to be unspecified or unsystematic. Therefore, it was recognized that other systems should be set up for this 'sentinel' purpose, in order to 'tackle the unforeseen'. This kind of system should not only be sensitive to potential new work-related diseases but also needs to be followed by appropriate investigation and other actions. To determine level of proof when quantitative data are limited, such a system would need to include a process involving expert knowledge. The last step is one of dissemination of information.

In France, an occupational diseases surveillance and prevention network has been set up entitled 'Réseau National de Vigilance et de Prévention des Pathologies Professionnelles' (RNV3P)[38] which is also part of a European Union network for Monitoring trends in Occupational Diseases and tracing new and Emerging Risks (MODERNET).[39] They have defined new diseases as: (1) disease related to a new agent (e.g. nanoparticles) or (2) agent not previously described as causing this disease (new disease-agent 'couplet'), or (3) disease whose association with an agent is already known, but is now reported in a new occupational setting (new disease-agent-occupational setting 'triplet').

There are several challenges for occupational disease 'vigilance'. Firstly, it is neither organ-specific nor agent-specific. Secondly, past and present exposures at work, often complex, are either not known, or not well characterized. Thirdly, physicians may not be familiar with causal hypotheses based on toxicology or other disciplines. Finally, interactions between non-occupational and occupational exposures, as well as individual susceptibility, make the assessment of work-relatedness more complex.

This approach draws from the experience of pharmacovigilance and of observational studies used in postmarketing surveillance in the pharmaceutical industry. Pharmacovigilance attempts to elicit early signals of new associations between drugs and diseases. One approach is primarily qualitative, relying on case reports identified, shared, and discussed by experts. Another approach is primarily quantitative and relies on mining existing databases. Both approaches are used by the MODERNET consortium in building a sentinel surveillance system and performing systematic data analysis of existing databases. At its simplest level, any sentinel surveillance system works on the assumption that a physician will highlight a case of a potentially new occupational disease. The association might be reported several times within a database without physicians being aware that their colleagues have reported the same association. Provided that some of these reports have used the same codes (for disease, agent, or occupational setting), systematic data-mining could highlight this 'hidden' information. These hypothesis generation methods have been tested on the French RNV3P network.[40,41]

Research on more complex methods derived from social networks is also in progress[38,41] and work on quantitative structure-activity relationships to predict sensitization risks, notably for asthma, has been undertaken and linked to THOR.[42]

Conclusion

Occupational disease surveillance schemes can provide a wealth of information on the incidence of occupational diseases and work-related ill health and on their distribution by industry, occupation, and causal agent. When undertaken well, such surveillance is an important method in observational epidemiology for providing between-country comparisons of the incidence of occupational disease. Occupational disease surveillance can also show not only secular trends over time but, more importantly, the effects of interventions. Information from occupational disease surveillance has been shown to be of value to policymakers in the UK[43] and around the world. The way ahead must continue to involve partnerships between epidemiologists, the public bodies that benefit from the information, and the physicians and other reporters who provide the data. In order to benefit the largest number of workers, further international collaboration is also essential.

References

1. Sivak M, Schoettle B. An analysis of U.S. road fatalities per population: changes by age from 1958 to 2008. *Traffic Inj Prev* 2011;**12**:438–42.

2. Leigh J, Driscoll T. Malignant mesothelioma in Australia, 1945–2002. *Int J Occup Environ Health* 2003;**9**:206–17.

3. Le Stang N, Belot A, Gilg Soit Ilg A, *et al.* Evolution of pleural cancers and malignant pleural mesothelioma incidence in France between 1980 and 2005. *Int J Cancer* 2010;**126**:232–8.

4. McElvenny DM, Darnton AJ, Price MJ, Hodgson JT. Mesothelioma mortality in Great Britain from 1968 to 2001. *Occup Med* 2005;**55**:79–87.

5. Biddle J, Roberts K, Rosenman KD, Welch EM. What percentage of workers with work-related illnesses receive workers' compensation benefits? *J Occup Environ Med* 1998;**40**:325–31.

6. Sim MR. The need for an occupational disease surveillance system in Australia. *J Occup Health Saf Aust NZ* 2007;**23**:557–62.

7. Wolfe D, Fairchild AL. The need for improved surveillance of occupational disease and injury. *JAMA* 2010;**303**:981–2.

8. Karjalainen A, Kurppa K, Virtanen S, Keskinen H, Nordman H. Incidence of occupational asthma by occupation and industry in Finland. *Am J Ind Med* 2000;**37**:451–8.

9. **McDonald JC, Chen Y, Zekveld C, Cherry NM.** Incidence by occupation and industry of acute work related respiratory diseases in the UK, 1992–2001. *Occup Environ Med* 2005;**62**:836–42.

10. **Baker EL.** Sentinel Event Notification System for Occupational Risks (SENSOR): the concept. *Am J Public Health* 1989;**79**(Suppl):18–20.

11. **Goe SK, Henneberger PK, Reilly MJ,** *et al.* A descriptive study of work aggravated asthma. *Occup Environ Med* 2004;**61**:512–7.

12. **Hussey L, Turner S, Thorley K, McNamee R, Agius R.** Work-related sickness absence as reported by UK General Practitioners. *Occup Med* 2012;**62**:105–11.

13. **Meredith SK, Taylor VM, McDonald JC.** Occupational respiratory disease in the United Kingdom 1989: a report to the British Thoracic Society and the Society of Occupational Medicine by the SWORD project group. *Br J Ind Med* 1991;**48**:292–8.

14. **Carder M, McNamee R, Turner S, Hussey L, Money A, Agius R.** Improving estimates of incidence of specialist-diagnosed, work-related respiratory and skin disease. *Occup Med* 2011;**61**:33–9.

15. **Spreeuwers D, de Boer AGEM, Verbeek JHAM, van Dijk FJH.** Evaluation of occupational disease surveillance in six EU countries. *Occup Med* 2010;**60**:509–16.

16. **Chen Y, Agius R, McNamee R,** *et al.* Physicians' beliefs in the assessment of work attribution when reporting musculoskeletal disorders. *Occup Med* 2005;**55**:298–307.

17. **O'Neill E, McNamee R, Agius R, Gittins M, Hussey L, Turner S.** The validity and reliability of diagnoses of work-related mental ill-health. *Occup Environ Med* 2008;**65**:726–31.

18. **Turner S, McNamee R, Roberts C,** *et al.* Agreement in diagnosing occupational asthma by occupational and respiratory physicians who report to surveillance schemes for work-related ill-health. *Occup Environ Med* 2010;**67**:471–8.

19. **Hussey L, Carder M, Money A, Turner S, Agius R.** Comparison of work-related ill-health data from different GB sources. *Occup Med* 2013;**63**:30–7.

20. **Hussey L, Turner S, Thorley K, McNamee R, Agius R.** Work-related ill health in general practice, as reported to a UK-wide surveillance scheme. *Br J Gen Pract* 2008;**58**:637–40.

21. **McNamee R, Chen Y, Hussey L, Agius R.** Time-sampled versus continuous-time reporting for measuring incidence. *Epidemiology* 2010;**21**:376–8.

22. **Turner S, Carder M, van Tongeren M,** *et al.* The incidence of occupational skin disease as reported to The Health and Occupation Reporting (THOR) network between 2002 and 2005. *Br J Dermatol* 2007;**157**:713–22.

23. **Turner S, McNamee R, Agius R, Wilkinson, SM, Carder M, Stocks SJ.** Evaluating interventions aimed at reducing occupational exposure to latex and rubber glove allergens. *Occup Environ Med* 2012;**69**:925–31.

24. **Stocks SJ, McNamee R, Turner S, Carder M, Agius RM.** Has European Union legislation to reduce exposure to chromate in cement been effective in reducing the incidence of allergic contact dermatitis attributed to chromate in the UK? *Occup Environ Med* 2012;**69**:150–2.

25. **McNamee R, Carder M, Chen Y, Agius R.** Measurement of trends in incidence of work-related skin and respiratory diseases, UK 1996–2005. *Occup Environ Med* 2008;**65**:808–14.

26. **Carder M, McNamee R, Turner S, Hodgson JT, Holland F, Agius RM.** Time trends in the incidence of work-related mental ill-health and musculoskeletal disorders in the UK. *Occup Environ Med* 2013;**70**:317–24.

27. **Paris C, Ngatchou-Wandji J, Luc A,** *et al.* Work-related asthma in France: recent trends for the period 2001–2009. *Occup Environ Med* 2012;**69**:391–7.

28. Pearce N, Dryson E, Feyer A-M, Gander P, McCracken S, Wagstaffe M. *Surveillance of occupational disease and injury in New Zealand: report to the Minister of Labour.* Wellington: NOHSAC, 2005. Available at: <http://www.dol.govt.nz/publications/nohsac/pdfs/surveillance-disease-injury-minister-rep.pdf> (accessed 21 February 2013).

29. Kauppinen T, Uuksulainen S, Saalo A, Mäkinen I. Trends of occupational exposure to chemical agents in Finland in 1950–2020. *Ann Occup Hyg* 2012. 10 December. [Epub ahead of print.] doi:10.1093/annhyg/mes090.

30. Kauppinen T, Toikkanen J, Pedersen D, *et al.* Occupational exposure to carcinogens in the European Union. *Occup Environ Med* 2000;**57**:10–8.

31. Bakerly ND, Moore VC, Vellore AD, Jaakkola MS, Robertson AS, Burge PS. Fifteen-year trends in occupational asthma: data from the Shield surveillance scheme. *Occup Med* 2008;**58**:169–74.

32. Hnizdo E, Esterhuizen TM, Rees D, Lalloo UG. Occupational asthma as identified by the Surveillance of Work-related and Occupational Respiratory Diseases programme in South Africa. *Clin Exp Allergy* 2001;**31**:32–9.

33. Elder D, Abramson M, Fish D, Johnson A, McKenzie D, Sim M. Surveillance of Australian workplace Based Respiratory Events (SABRE): notifications for the first 3.5 years and validation of occupational asthma cases. *Occup Med* 2004;**54**:395–9.

34. National Institute for Occupational Safety and Health. *Work-Related Lung Disease Surveillance System (eWoRLD). Work-related asthma: state-based surveillance.* Available at: <http://www2a.cdc.gov/drds/WorldReportData/SubsectionDetails.asp?ArchiveID=1&Subsectiontitleid=23> (accessed 23 February 2013).

35. Ameille J, Pauli G, Calastreng-Crinquand A, *et al.* Reported incidence of occupational asthma in France, 1996–99: the ONAP programme. *Occup Environ Med* 2003;**60**:136–41.

36. Ha C, Roquelaure Y, Leclerc A, Touranchet A, Goldberg M, Imbernon E. The French Musculoskeletal Disorders Surveillance Program: Pays de la Loire network. *Occup Environ Med* 2009;**66**:471–9.

37. Roquelaure Y, Ha C, Rouillon C, *et al.* Risk factors for upper-extremity musculoskeletal disorders in the working population. *Arthritis Rheum* 2009;**61**:1425–34.

38. Bonneterre V, Faisandier L, Bicout D, *et al.* Programmed health surveillance and detection of emerging diseases in occupational health: contribution of the French national occupational disease surveillance and prevention network (RNV3P). *Occup Environ Med* 2010;**67**:178–86.

39. COST MODERNET website. Available at: <http://www.costmodernet.org/> (accessed 25 February 2013).

40. Bonneterre V, Bicout DJ, de Gaudemaris R. Application of pharmacovigilance methods in occupational health surveillance: comparison of seven disproportionality metrics. *Saf Health Work* 2012;**3**:92–100.

41. Faisandier L, Bonneterre V, de Gaudemaris R, Bicout DJ. Occupational exposome: a network-based approach for characterizing occupational health problems. *J Biomed Inform* 2011;**44**:545–52.

42. Jarvis J, Seed MJ, Elton R, Sawyer L, Agius R. Relationship between chemical structure and the occupational asthma hazard of low molecular weight organic compounds. *Occup Environ Med* 2005;**62**:243–50.

43. Osman J, Benn T. Monitoring occupational disease: past, present and future. In: McCaig R, Harrington M (eds) *The changing nature of cccupational health.* Norwich: HMSO, 1998, pp. 89–117.

Chapter 12

Investigating outbreaks of occupational asthma

Katherine M. Venables

Introduction

This chapter covers the investigation of a possible epidemic of occupational asthma in a workplace, but the general approach can be adapted to other respiratory disorders, non-respiratory conditions, and to community outbreaks. Dealing with a possible outbreak of occupational asthma is a common experience for not only occupational epidemiologists but also practitioners in occupational health, public health, and respiratory medicine. Real outbreaks of occupational asthma are significant events: they are preventable, the exposures may be sufficient to cause severe and even life-threatening asthma, and they may cause employees to lose their jobs and businesses to close. The investigation should therefore be carried out thoughtfully and carefully. Firstly, it is important to understand how asthma is diagnosed and defined, and the ways in which asthma may behave in an epidemic form in community and occupational outbreaks.

Diagnosis and definition of asthma

Symptomatically, a person with asthma may notice wheeze, cough, breathlessness, or chest tightness. Clinical investigations may reveal bronchial hyper-responsiveness (which can be measured in relation to several non-specific stimuli) and airway narrowing. But none of these features is diagnostic—all may be seen in a range of respiratory and cardiac conditions. The defining feature of asthma is its variability, or episodic nature. Symptoms and clinical features are usually worse at night, in the early morning, on exercise, on breathing in irritants, after colds or flu, or after inhaling an allergen to which the person is sensitized. For most people, symptoms are mild, intermittent, and barely affect everyday life but, for a minority, asthma is a disabling chronic disease.

Asthma can be difficult to define because, so far, no single genetic or environmental cause has been identified and many believe that it is part of a spectrum of airway disorders characterized by chronic inflammation. Scadding's general definition is the most inclusive and widely accepted.[1] This states that asthma is 'wide variations in airflow limitation over short periods of time'. It can be operationalized for use in epidemiology in terms of variable symptoms, variable lung function, or non-specific bronchial hyper-responsiveness.

Epidemics and outbreaks

The terms 'epidemic' and 'outbreak' are used interchangeably in this chapter. An epidemic (from the Greek επί epi (upon), δήμος demos (people)) is defined as 'the occurrence in a community or region of cases of an illness, specific health-related behaviour, or other health-related events clearly in excess of normal expectancy'[2] and might be more relevant when a whole industrial sector is affected, as was the case when enzyme detergents were introduced or latex gloves became widely used in health care.[3,4] An outbreak is 'an epidemic limited to localised increase in the incidence of a disease e.g. in a village, town, or closed institution; upsurge is sometimes used as a euphemism for outbreak'.[2]

Lay perceptions of asthma epidemics

Asthma is often mentioned in media reports of community anxiety about possible sources of environmental contamination. For example, a typical recent piece in a regional newspaper in the UK about a plan to recover coal from an old colliery spoil heap highlighted an interview with a mother who was angry that she might not be able to safeguard her asthmatic children from a dust which she perceived as toxic.[5]

The global epidemic

Asthma occurrence varies over time and place. An increase in the prevalence of asthma in the second half of the twentieth century caused considerable professional and media interest. Because of the difficulties in defining asthma, data sources that use a consistent definition are especially valuable and some of the most convincing evidence came from Finland.[6] Figure 12.1 shows the steadily increasing prevalence of asthma noted in young men over time, using information from medical records relating to military conscription. At the same time, the prevalence of asthma in children was surveyed in many separate studies around the world using simple, but consistent, field epidemiology techniques; for example, prevalence in Australian primary school children more than doubled between 1982 and 1992.[7] What has received less attention in the media is that this epidemic may now have levelled off. The Finnish conscription data shows this[8] and, by 2002, the prevalence of asthma in Australian children had plateaued.[7]

Such marked variations in asthma occurrence over only a generation cannot have a genetic cause and must be related to major changes in external factors, such as those associated with economic development. An increase has been noted in several studies of migrants from less- to more-developed countries. One intriguing consequence of the reunification of Germany at the end of the Cold War was the discovery that the prevalence of asthma in children living in former East Germany was lower than in West Germany.[9] Many theories have been proposed to explain these variations including changes in exposure to allergens in the home (e.g. house dust mite[10]) or diet (e.g. cows' milk), parental smoking, childhood infections, access to health care, treatment for asthma, and variations in diagnostic behaviour and symptom labelling. It is likely that real changes in underlying causal factors and incidence are occurring, as well as changes in medical care.[11,12] Several countries noted an epidemic of asthma deaths—a

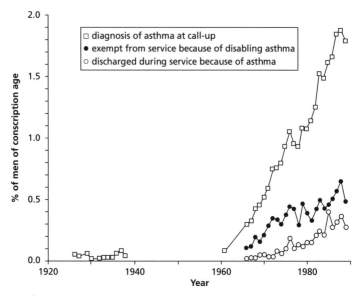

Figure 12.1 Increasing prevalence of asthma in young Finnish men in the twentieth century.[6]

Adapted by permission from BMJ Publishing Group Limited. *British Medical Journal*, Prevalence of asthma in Finnish young men, Haahtela T et al., Volume **301**, No. 6746 pp. 266–8, Copyright © 1990.

real increase in incidence—in the 1960s, mainly in the young, which was associated with sales and prescriptions of newer asthma preparations. A longer and more sustained increase occurred in the 1980s.[11] Variations in deaths from asthma illustrate some of the interesting issues of numbers versus rates, labelling, diagnostic transfer, and the effects of treatment.

Airborne pollutants, including aeroallergens

Compared with non-asthmatics, many asthma patients have increased broncho-constriction on inhaling cold dry air, or airway irritants such as sulphur dioxide. So it is not surprising that some patients may have clinically-relevant bronchoconstriction after, for example, heavy work in a cold, dusty workplace. At the level of large populations, air pollution influences respiratory mortality and morbidity in a way that is not yet fully understood.[13] Although small in size compared to clinical airway responses, these effects are of public health importance because of the large populations exposed.

Thunderstorms

Thunderstorms are perhaps the most dramatic and interesting cause of epidemics of asthma. The explanation is not entirely clear but one convincing suggestion is that storms disrupt ambient grass pollen grains, causing them to release large numbers of inhalable particles that deposit allergen in the respiratory tract.[14,15] Allergens are not usually regarded as an airborne pollutant, but it appears that the storms act as a kind of natural inhalation challenge test, affecting members of the population who are sensitized to pollen.

One of the first thunderstorm-associated asthma outbreaks to be reported occurred in Birmingham, UK, in July 1985.[16] In June 1994, a very large epidemic occurred affecting the whole of London and the South-East of the UK and estimated to have provoked about 1000 excess episodes of asthma over one night.[17] Figure 12.2 shows the time-course of attendances at accident and emergency departments in London and shows a striking peak—a fivefold increase—in attendances starting immediately after the rainfall associated with the storm, and attendances then falling off over the next 12 hours.[18] This was an extreme event and it is entirely plausible that similar smaller epidemics go unnoticed. Firstly, it overwhelmed the services available: in several accident and emergency departments off-duty staff were called in and emergency supplies of medication were requested. An important factor contributing to its subsequent investigation was the involvement of a London poisons unit (now part of the Health Protection Agency, <http://www.hpa.org.uk/>). The toxicologist on call realized that this was not a chemical incident, as originally suspected, and also initiated the data collection that was then used by the UK Department of Health to estimate the size of the epidemic. A multidisciplinary group was set up and subsequent follow-up confirmed a high prevalence of allergy to grass pollen in the affected cases. This outbreak raised public awareness of thunderstorm-related asthma and the Meteorological Office in the UK continues to provide health alerts for patients with asthma when a thunderstorm is predicted (<http://metoffice.gov.uk>).[19]

Soya beans and asthma in Barcelona

There have been some very prominent community epidemics of asthma related to air pollution by a potent allergen. The best investigated so far is the series of outbreaks in Barcelona related to soya bean unloading in the port. Like the 1994 UK thunderstorm-related outbreak, several serendipitous coincidences are believed to have contributed to the detection of the outbreaks and to the correct assignment of causation.

Soya beans started to be unloaded at the port of Barcelona in late 1979 and, in 1981, the first epidemic of asthma was noted. By 1983, doctors in Barcelona wrote of 'days where the attendance of patients with acute severe asthma was so severe that our emergency room and intensive care unit were overloaded'.[20] A collaborative group was formed in 1984, including epidemiologists. A prospective monitoring system for emergency respiratory hospital attendances was set up at the main hospitals. Cases appeared to cluster in place as well as time (Figure 12.3).[21] Attention was initially focussed on an industrial area as a possible source of air pollution but, in 1987, it was appreciated that the outbreaks coincided with times when cargo ships were unloading in the harbour. So the time series data collected were analysed in a case-control manner with the 'cases' being asthma epidemic days, defined rigorously and objectively using emergency attendance data, and 'controls' being non-epidemic days. The results clearly showed that soya bean unloading was linked with epidemic days.[22] A particular harbour silo was identified as the cause and unloading was stopped until appropriate filters had been installed. One of the forces driving multidisciplinary collaboration and practical control measures was that, coincidentally, Barcelona was to host the Olympic Games in 1992.

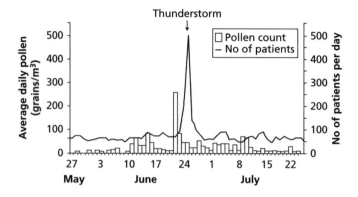

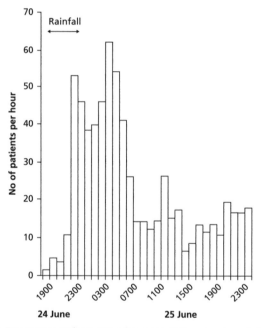

Figure 12.2 Emergency asthma attendances in 12 London hospitals in the thunderstorm-related asthma epidemic of 24/25 June 1994.[18] Upper panel shows daily attendances, lower panel hourly attendances.

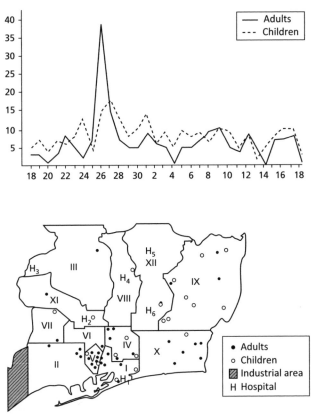

Figure 12.3 One of a series of epidemics of asthma in Barcelona. Emergency hospital attendances, November/December 1984. Distribution of adult and child cases in time (upper panel) and place (lower panel).[21]

Reprinted from *The Lancet*, Volume **327**, Antó JM, Sunyer J, Asthma Collaborative Group of Barcelona: A point-source asthma outbreak, pp. 900–3, Copyright © 1986, with permission from Elsevier.

A case-control study on epidemic asthma cases confirmed the association with allergic sensitization to soya.[23] Subsequent studies confirmed that soya bean could be identified in dust samples in the city air, that the particles contained soya allergen, that the levels of soya allergen varied according to port unloading activity, and that preventive measures did, indeed, prevent the epidemics. The outbreaks ceased when an adequate filter was installed.[24,25] In later years, outbreaks re-started when controls broke down and again ceased with engineering controls.[26] This investigation has had important practical public health consequences in the city of Barcelona, with cargo unloading protocols developed, and monitoring of air, emergency attendances, and a patient panel.

Other potent natural allergens: the example of castor bean

The Barcelona epidemics emphasized that 'natural' materials can be much more powerful causes of asthma epidemics than synthesized chemicals. Soya is not the only potent 'natural' allergen. Castor beans and their processing, for example, have been implicated in several large epidemics, including one causing deaths, and other smaller outbreaks. A good example of a community outbreak of asthma with over 200 cases caused by castor bean processing came from South Africa in 1952.[27] Another epidemic reported in 1952 came from São Paulo, Brazil, and caused 150 cases with nine deaths.[28] Castor allergens are such potent causes of allergy, including asthma, that their traces in felt made from recycled hessian sacks which had previously contained castor beans have caused small occupational outbreaks in the upholstery department of a furniture factory[29] and in a felt manufacturing factory.[30] Merchant seamen exposed to the beans in the hold of their cargo ship have also become sensitized.[31] Traces of castor allergen in the sacks containing green coffee bean have been implicated as a cause of occupational allergy and asthma in coffee workers.[32]

Occupational epidemics

Inhaled occupational allergens are potent causes of asthma. Several hundred are known, and the list is repeatedly updated as new chemicals come into industrial use, and as new manufacturing processes are developed.[33] Even common environmental allergens (such as insects, animals, plants, and moulds) are a much higher risk in the occupational setting, because occupational exposures are higher than in the general environment, and people are exposed across a whole working shift for a working week instead of only occasionally.

Most 'new causes' of occupational asthma are reported in the scientific literature as case reports which include a detailed clinical and immunological investigation of one or more index cases. But a close reading of these reports discloses that many are, in fact, of small outbreaks. Outbreaks of occupational asthma are, indeed, so common that I believe that most are not reported, either in the scientific literature or to regulatory agencies. As well as 'new causes', established allergens will cause an outbreak whenever engineering or other controls break down. An alertness to the presence of other cases in the same work area should be a key part of the routine workplace health surveillance after any case of occupational asthma is detected.

Outbreaks in a single factory

An outbreak of asthma in Wales in the 1970s illustrates some general principles.[34] Two index cases were detected in a plant which coated sheet steel with plastics. A cross-sectional survey detected further cases, in a prevalence of about 10%. The information collected about the date of onset of first symptoms pinpointed one particular year and scrutiny of the factory records showed that a known respiratory sensitizer—an isocyanate—had been introduced into a coating in that year. The index cases were studied in a clinical laboratory and had positive inhalation challenge tests to the isocyanate at a low exposure. After the isocyanate was removed from the process, 80% of the cases lost their symptoms or improved. As another and recent example, an outbreak of occupational asthma due to chromium and cobalt in metal-working fluids in a Birmingham engineering firm was reported in 2012.[35] Again, a cross-sectional survey of the workforce and a workplace assessment was carried out in parallel with

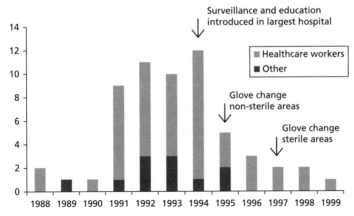

Figure 12.4 The epidemic of asthma due to latex. Workers' compensation claims in Ontario for asthma due to natural rubber latex.[4]
Adapted with permission from Liss GM, Tarlo SM, Natural rubber latex-related occupational asthma: association with interventions and glove changes over time, *American Journal of Industrial Medicine*; Volume 40, Issue 4, pp. 347–53, Copyright © 2001 Wiley-Liss, Inc.

detailed clinical investigations in order to characterize the outbreak and advise on control measures.

Industrial sector-wide epidemics

Whole industrial sectors may be affected by an epidemic of asthma. Latex allergy, including asthma, caused an important epidemic in health care workers in the late twentieth century with the increased use of latex gloves for infection control. Liss and Tarlo[4] made use of workers' compensation data to follow the epidemic in Ontario, Canada, over the 1980s and 1990s and evaluate the effects of interventions (Figure 12.4).

One of the better known examples of a sector-wide epidemic of occupational asthma is that due to the incorporation of protease enzymes derived from *Bacillus subtilis* into laundry detergents in the late 1960s. Many cases of asthma were reported from the UK[3] and elsewhere. Driven, no doubt, by concerns for consumer safety as much as occupational health, several cross-sectional surveys were carried out in the UK[36,37] and around the world and high prevalence rates were reported of respiratory symptoms and of positive skin prick tests against enzyme preparations. Although consumers were not thought to be affected, it was clear that engineering controls were needed to protect workers. The detergent industry cooperated amongst itself, and with regulators and academics, in devising dust control measures and health surveillance procedures and this was lauded in review articles and textbooks for many years as a successful example of a multimodal intervention to control a risk of occupational asthma and allergy. However, in 2000, two cross-sectional surveys were reported, from the UK[38] and Finland,[39] of occupational asthma and allergy prevalences in detergent workers that were similar to those described 30 years previously. This illustrates the importance of continued vigilance after control measures are adopted. It also illustrates why quality scoring systems for systematic reviews include the funding source; industry authors may be biased, often with the best of intentions. It is of interest that, in 2003, and despite the publication of these new reports, an industry scientist wrote reassuringly in the conclusion to a review article that 'Occupational allergy and asthma to enzymes used in the detergent industry have been successfully controlled'.[40]

How to detect a possible outbreak of asthma

All of these examples show the importance of a low threshold of suspicion. Without this, outbreaks of asthma will not be detected. This alertness must, however, be combined with an appropriate scepticism because, unfortunately, asthma is linked in people's minds with toxic chemicals and potential pollution and this can led to erroneous assumptions that an asthma outbreak has occurred. But such scepticism would be inappropriate in workplaces with a known risk of allergen exposure. In such a setting, if there is a possibility that engineering controls have broken down and there are high air levels of allergen, action must be swift and decisive in order to protect health. Such breakdowns in controls are known to have led in the past to dangerously high levels of airborne allergen and a risk of severe and potentially life-threatening symptoms in sensitized workers who become exposed (Box 12.1).

It is important that the possible cases are evaluated, preferably while still symptomatic, by a doctor with expertise in asthma, so that a correct diagnosis can be made. If asthma is confirmed, the clinical assessment can then include efforts to establish cause, for example, by inhalation challenge tests or immunological tests in specialist settings.

If asthma is confirmed, a decision needs to be made about whether any epidemiological investigation is required. Epidemiology is helpful if the cause is unknown, to better understand exposure-response relationships and the contribution of modifiers and confounders, or to evaluate the effectiveness of preventive measures.

How to investigate a confirmed outbreak of asthma

The first essential is a case definition, which may have more than one level. It is common, for example, to use a sensitive definition based on respiratory symptoms that can

---

Box 12.1 Key factors in detecting a possible outbreak of asthma

- ◆ Low threshold of suspicion.
- ◆ Appropriate scepticism.
- ◆ If an allergen exposure may be high and continuing, rapid and effective action to protect health.
- ◆ Is it asthma? Expert clinical investigation of a sample of cases.
- ◆ If asthma, expert clinical investigation of possible cause in a sample of cases.

Box 12.2 Key factors in investigating a confirmed outbreak of asthma

- Is an epidemiological investigation required?
- Case definition.
- Definition of the study time frame, geographical boundaries, and population.
- Simple epidemiological methods, rigorously applied.
- Multimodal, multidisciplinary team.
- Are the cases actually exposed to the putative cause?
- Does the exposure vary with the symptoms?
- What is the effect of control measures?
- Communications strategy.

be applied using a questionnaire coupled with a specific definition which (depending on the nature of the investigation) may incorporate symptom patterns and severity and the results of other tests, such as of non-specific bronchial responsiveness and, in some circumstances, of specific immunological hypersensitivity. The specific case definition will be more useful than the sensitive in evaluating causal relationships and the effects of preventive measures (Box 12.2).

The investigation must also define its time frame, geography, and population. Without these clear definitions, numerators and denominators may shift. 'Caseness' may vary depending on the prejudices of the various stakeholders: workers, employers, or the investigators. Cases may be incorrectly assigned to work areas deemed to be hazardous or to at-risk time periods. As well as these potential information biases, the investigator must remain aware of the strong workplace selection and 'survival' effects in asthma when symptoms are severe and their relationship to a work exposure is clearly apparent.

Simple 'shoe-leather' methods, rigorously applied, are the key to asthma outbreak investigation. The Barcelona investigators, for example, applied the same methods as are used in communicable disease epidemiology and were able to establish that this was a point-source epidemic. In defined populations, such as a workplace, cross-sectional surveys are the usual design. Case-control methods are more useful where there is a well-defined source of cases, such as emergency departments in thunderstorm-associated asthma and in the Barcelona epidemics. Cohort studies are unusual but, as in the case of enzyme-induced asthma in detergent workers, may be set up to evaluate causal relationships and monitor preventive measures. In some circumstances, routinely collected data may be useful, such as workmen's compensation records.[4]

The advantages of a multidisciplinary, multimodal investigation are clear for asthma epidemics. Epidemiological studies need to be partnered with good clinical investigations, and specialist immunological and exposure assessment expertise may be necessary to support making the link between the hypothesized causal exposure and the epidemic.

Finally, does prevention prevent? Demonstrating that removal of a putative causal agent controls the asthma is a key criterion for a causal association. And, as these examples demonstrate, controls can break down and asthma epidemics recur. There is scope for involving epidemiological expertise in the design of monitoring systems. The Barcelona investigators, for example, proposed the patient panel which is part of the soya bean asthma monitoring programme in the city.[41] Antó has discussed some of these issues and commented on the opportunities for research presented by asthma outbreaks.[42]

Because of the special place of asthma in the public perception of risks from environmental pollution, teams investigating community outbreaks will find it is necessary to have a clear plan for dealing with enquiries and communicating to the public and the media. The Scottish Centre for Infection and Environmental Health has published useful guidance to taking a systematic approach to an investigation, including on communications.[43]

The investigator

Investigating these epidemics is undoubtedly interesting but can also be challenging. Flindt, who initiated the investigations in enzyme detergent workers,[3] has written an illuminating article about his personal experiences: 'It seemed almost as if the discoverer had caused the problem. I had to learn to be philosophical about misrepresentation of my motives and actions, and attempts to belittle the significance of my findings'.[44]

References

1. **Scadding JG.** Meaning of diagnostic terms in broncho-pulmonary disease. *BMJ* 1963;**2**:1425–30.

2. **Porta M, Greenland S, Last JM.** *Dictionary of epidemiology* (5th edn). Oxford: Oxford University Press, 2008.

3. **Flindt MLH.** Pulmonary disease due to inhalation of derivatives of Bacillus subtilis containing proteolytic enzyme. *Lancet* 1969;**293**:1177–81. Reprinted as: Flindt ML, Hendrick DJ. Papers that have changed the practice of occupational medicine: 'Pulmonary disease due to inhalation of derivatives of Bacillus subtilis containing proteolytic enzyme' by M.L.H. Flindt. 1969. *Occup Med (Lond)* 2002;**52**:58–63, discussion 57–8.

4. **Liss GM, Tarlo SM.** Natural rubber latex-related occupational asthma: association with interventions and glove changes over time. *Am J Ind Med* 2001;**40**:347–53.

5. **The Star.** Sheffield residents anger as coal scheme is approved. *The Star*, 9 January 2013. Available at: <http://www.thestar.co.uk/community/green-scene/sheffield-residents-anger-as-coal-scheme-is-approved-1-5293473> (accessed 20 February 2013).

6. **Haahtela T, Lindholm H, Björkstén F, Koskenvuo K, Laitinen LA.** Prevalence of asthma in Finnish young men. *BMJ* 1990;**301**:266–8.

7. **Toelle BG, Ng K, Belousova E, Salome CM, Peat JK, Marks GB.** Prevalence of asthma and allergy in schoolchildren in Belmont, Australia: three cross sectional surveys over 20 years. *BMJ* 2004;**328**:386–7.

8. Latvala J, von Hertzen L, Lindholm H, Haahtela T. Trends in prevalence of asthma and allergy in Finnish young men: nationwide study, 1966–2003. *BMJ* 2005;**330**:1186–7.

9. von Mutius E, Fritzsch C, Weiland SK, Röll G, Magnussen H. Prevalence of asthma and allergic disorders among children in united Germany: a descriptive comparison. *BMJ* 1992;**305**:1395–9.

10. Lane J, Siebers R, Pene G, Howden-Chapman P, Crane J. Tokelau: a unique low allergen environment at sea level. *Clin Exp Allergy* 2005;**35**:479–82.

11. Anderson HR, Gupta R, Strachan DP, Limb ES. 50 years of asthma: UK trends from 1955 to 2004. *Thorax* 2007;**62**:85–90.

12. Gupta R, Sheikh A, Strachan DP, Anderson HR. Time trends in allergic disorders in the UK. *Thorax* 2007;**62**:91–6.

13. Brunekreef B, Holgate ST. Air pollution and health. *Lancet* 2002;**360**:1233–42.

14. Taylor PE, Jacobson KW, House JM, Glovsky MM. Links between pollen, atopy and the asthma epidemic. *Int Arch Allergy Immunol* 2007;**144**:162–70.

15. D'Amato G, Liccardi G, Frenguelli G. Thunderstorm-asthma and pollen allergy. *Allergy* 2007;**62**:11–6.

16. Packe GE, Ayres JG. Asthma outbreak during a thunderstorm. *Lancet* 1985;**326**:199–204.

17. Venables KM, Allitt U, Collier CG, *et al.* Thunderstorm-related asthma—the epidemic of 24/25 June 1994. *Clin Exp Allergy* 1997;**27**:725–36.

18. Thames Regions Accident and Emergency Trainees Association, Davidson AC, Emberlin J, Cook AD, Venables KM. A major outbreak of asthma associated with a thunderstorm: experience of accident and emergency departments and patients' characteristics. *BMJ* 1996;**312**:601–4.

19. Meteorological Office. *Health factsheet: thunderstorm-related asthma.* Available at: <http://www.metoffice.gov.uk/media/pdf/b/s/thunderstorm_asthma_tag.pdf> (accessed 20 February 2013).

20. Ussetti P, Roca J, Agusti AGN, Montserrat JM, Rodriguez-Roisin R, Agusti-Vidal A. Asthma outbreaks in Barcelona (letter). *Lancet* 1983;**322**:280–1.

21. Antó JM, Sunyer J, Asthma Collaborative Group of Barcelona. A point-source asthma outbreak. *Lancet* 1986;**327**:900–3.

22. Antó JM, Sunyer J, Rodriguez-Roisin R, Suarez-Cervera M, Vazquez L, Toxicoepidemiological Committee. Community outbreaks of asthma associated with inhalation of soybean dust. *N Engl J Med* 1989;**320**:1097–102.

23. Sunyer J, Antó JM, Rodrigo MJ, Morell F. Case-control study of serum immunoglobulin-E antibodies reactive with soybean in epidemic asthma. *Lancet* 1989;**333**:179–82.

24. Antó JM, Sunyer J. Epidemiologic studies of asthma epidemics in Barcelona. *Chest* 1990;**98**(5 Suppl):185S–190S.

25. Antó JM, Sunyer J, Newman Taylor AJ. Comparison of soybean epidemic asthma and occupational asthma. *Thorax* 1995;**50**:1101–3.

26. Villalbí JR, Plasencia A, Manzanera R, Armengol R, Antó JM, Collaborative and Technical Support Groups for the study of soybean asthma in Barcelona. Epidemic soybean asthma and public health: new control systems and initial evaluation in Barcelona, 1996–98. *J Epidemiol Community Health* 2004;**58**:461–5.

27. Ordman D. An outbreak of bronchial asthma in South Africa, affecting more than 200 persons, caused by castor bean dust from an oil-processing factory. *Int Arch Allergy Appl Immunol* 1955;**7**:10–24.

28. **Mendes E, Cintrau AU.** Collective asthma, simulating an epidemic, provoked by castor-bean dust. *J Allergy* 1954;**25**:253–9.

29. **Topping MD, Tyrer FH, Lowing RK.** Castor bean allergy in the upholstery department of a furniture factory. *Clin Allergy* 1983;**13**:553–61.

30. **Topping MD, Henderson RT, Luczynska CM, Woodmass A.** Castor bean allergy among workers in the felt industry. *Allergy* 1982;**37**:603–8.

31. **Davison AG, Britton MG, Forrester JA, Davies RJ, Hughes DT.** Asthma in merchant seamen and laboratory workers caused by allergy to castor beans: analysis of allergens. *Br J Ind Med* 1981;**38**:293–6.

32. **Romano C, Sulotto F, Piolatto G, et al.** Factors related to the development of sensitization to green coffee and castor bean allergens among coffee workers. *Clin Exp Allergy* 1995;**25**:643–50.

33. **Chan-Yeung M, Malo J-L.** Tables of major inducers of occupational asthma. In: Bernstein IL, Chan-Yeung M, Malo J-L, Bernstein DI (eds) *Asthma in the workplace* (2nd edn). New York: Marcel Dekker, 1999, pp. 683–720.

34. **Venables KM, Dally MB, Burge PS, Pickering CAC, Newman Taylor AJ.** Occupational asthma in a steel coating plant. *Br J Ind Med* 1985;**42**:517–24.

35. **Walters GI, Moore VC, Robertson AS, Burge CBSG, Vellore A-D, Burge PS.** An outbreak of occupational asthma due to chromium and cobalt. *Occup Med* 2012;**62**:533–40.

36. **Greenberg M, Milne JF, Watt A.** Survey of workers exposed to dusts containing derivatives of Bacillus subtilis. *BMJ* 1970;**2**:629–33.

37. **Newhouse ML, Tagg B, Pocock SJ, McEwan AC.** An epidemiological study of workers producing enzyme washing powders. *Lancet* 1970;**295**:689–93.

38. **Cullinan P, Harris JM, Newman Taylor AJ, et al.** An outbreak of asthma in a modern detergent factory. *Lancet* 2000;**356**:1899–900.

39. **Vanhanen M, Tuomi T, Tiikkainen U, Tupasela O, Voutilainen R, Nordman H.** Risk of enzyme allergy in the detergent industry. *Occup Environ Med* 2000;**57**:121–5.

40. **Sarlo K.** Control of occupational asthma and allergy in the detergent industry. *Ann Allergy Asthma Immunol* 2003;**90**(5 Suppl):32–4.

41. **Soriano JB, Antó JM, Plasencia A, Barcelona Soybean-Asthma Group.** Repeaters count: a sentinel method for asthma outbreaks. *Thorax* 1995;**50**:1101–3.

42. **Antó JM.** Asthma outbreaks: an opportunity for research? *Thorax* 1995;**50**:220–2.

43. **Scottish Centre for Infection and Environmental Health.** *Dealing with assertions of human health risks or effects from environmental exposures: a systematic approach.* Glasgow: Scottish Government, 2000.

44. **Flindt MLH.** Biological miracles and misadventures: identification of sensitization and asthma in enzyme detergent workers. *Am J Ind Med* 1996;**29**:99–110.

Part 5

Using the full potential of epidemiological data

Chapter 13

Occupational risk factors in lung cancer: pooling community-based case-control studies for enhanced evidence

Hans Kromhout, Ann Olsson, Susan Peters, and Kurt Straif

Introduction

Lung cancer is by far the most common cause of cancer death in the world. The incidence rates in men have recently been going down in Europe and North America, while they are still increasing among women. In many other less-developed countries around the world lung cancer incidence is dramatically increasing, both among men and women.[1] Estimates of lung cancer risk attributable to occupational exposures vary considerably by geographical area and depend on study design, especially on the exposure assessment method, but may account for around 5–20% of cancers among men, but less (<5%) among women;[2] among workers exposed to (suspected) lung carcinogens, the percentage will be higher.

Table 13.1 shows confirmed and suspected lung carcinogens as evaluated in the International Agency for Research on Cancer (IARC) Monographs programme on the 'Evaluation of Carcinogenic Risks to Humans' since 1971.[3] From the table it becomes evident that most exposure to known lung carcinogens originates from occupational settings and will affect millions of workers worldwide. Although it has been established that these agents are carcinogenic, only limited evidence is available about the risks encountered at much lower levels in the general population. It could also be that these agents interact with each other and/or with personal habits like smoking. The actual time period in life when the exposure occurs might affect the risk estimate as well, and risk estimates might differ by type of lung cancer. Large (pooled) community-based studies might be better equipped to answer some of these outstanding questions than industry-based studies. The latter will usually have better (more detailed) estimates of exposure but will often lack statistical power, or data on histology of lung cancer or on lifestyle factors, or have only limited information about exposure to other occupational carcinogens to address these outstanding issues in the field of occupational lung cancer.

Table 13.1 List of confirmed and suspected lung carcinogens in the IARC Monographs on the Evaluation of Carcinogenic Risks to Humans, volumes 1–106 (1971–2012)[3]

Carcinogenic agents with sufficient evidence in humans	Agents with limited evidence in humans
1. Aluminium production	1. Acid mists, strong inorganic
2. Arsenic and inorganic arsenic compounds	2. Art glass, glass containers and pressed ware (manufacture of)
3. Asbestos (all forms)	3. Biomass fuel (primarily wood), indoor emissions from household combustion of
4. Beryllium and beryllium compounds	
5. Bis(chloromethyl)ether; chloromethyl methyl ether (technical grade)	4. Bitumens, occupational exposure to oxidized bitumens and their emissions during roofing
6. Cadmium and cadmium compounds	
7. Chromium (VI) compounds	5. Bitumens, occupational exposure to hard bitumens and their emissions during mastic asphalt work
8. Coal, indoor emissions from household combustion	
9. Coal gasification	6. Carbon electrode manufacture
10. Coal-tar pitch	7. Alpha-chlorinated toluenes and benzoyl chloride (combined exposures)
11. Coke production	
12. Engine exhaust, diesel	8. Cobalt metal with tungsten carbide
13. Haematite mining (underground)	9. Creosotes
14. Iron and steel founding	10. Frying, emissions from high temperature
15. MOPP (vincristine-prednisone-nitrogen mustard-procarbazine mixture)	
16. Nickel compounds	11. Insecticides, non-arsenical (occupational exposures in spraying and application)
17. Painting	
18. Plutonium	
19. Radon-222 and its decay products	12. Printing processes
20. Rubber production industry	13. 2,3,7,8-Tetrachlorodibenzopara-dioxin
21. Silica dust, crystalline	14. Welding fumes
22. Soot	
23. Sulphur mustard	
24. Tobacco smoke, second-hand	
25. Tobacco smoking	
26. X-radiation, gamma-radiation	

Source: data from International Agency for Research on Cancer, IARC Monographs on the Evaluation of Carcinogenic Risks to Humans, IARC, Lyon, France, Copyright © IARC 2013. All Rights Reserved. Available at: <http://monographs.iarc.fr/>

Community-based studies, by definition, address a wider range of types of exposure and a much wider range of encountered exposure levels (e.g. relatively high exposures in primary production but often lower in downstream use, or among indirectly exposed individuals). A limitation of single community-based studies is often the relatively low number of exposed individuals. Pooling across studies might therefore be beneficial. Pooling increases the number of individuals exposed to a particular agent and creates exposed population sizes comparable to industry-based studies but with a wider range in (cumulative) exposure levels. Consequently, the increased statistical power will facilitate estimation of lung cancer risk in relatively small subpopulations, like women, never smokers, and other groups unlikely to be studied in industry-based studies.

Pooling community-based case-control studies is also useful to replicate findings from record-linkage studies, like the Nordic Occupational Cancer Study (NOCCA),[4] where census data in the Nordic countries are linked to cancer registry data. NOCCA will be a powerful tool for monitoring cancer risks by occupation in the Nordic countries, but it has limited ability to control for tobacco smoking and other confounders, and has limited detail within its occupational history information.

Pooling is a challenge

Related multicentre studies may have the advantage of being conducted in parallel in different sites at the same time with a common objective, protocol, and questionnaire, and can thereby obtain sufficient power within a reasonable time period. However, large multicentre studies are rare because they are costly to set up. Pooling of community-based case-control studies which have already been conducted can therefore be a good alternative vehicle for studying the outstanding issues in the field of occupational lung cancer.

Pooling projects need careful planning and coordination, because the original studies were conducted for different purposes, at different time periods, using different questionnaires. This heterogeneity is sometimes perceived as a disadvantage but also implies variations that can be studied and thereby provide important insights.

Every pooling project has its own dynamics but there are several general challenges that most pooling projects confront. Creating common variables for all studies can stretch from simple re-naming of variables (e.g. VAR001 → COUNTRY) or recoding of units (e.g. 1 inch → 2.54 cm) to the re-categorization of national educational systems (which even within Europe can be quite different) into years of formal education. Another challenge is to harmonize the different classification systems of, for example, diseases (e.g. International Classification of Disease (ICD)-9 versus ICD-10), occupations (national classifications, International Standard Classification of Occupations (ISCO 1968, 1988, 2008)), and industries (e.g. International Standard Industrial Classification (ISIC)). This requires experts in these respective fields as well as considerable time and money. Harmonization of data may mean losing some information; for example, ISCO-68 contains more detail than ISCO-88, which makes it possible to recode ISCO-68 to ISCO-88 with only a little loss of detail, but it is not possible to recode ISCO-88 to ISCO-68 without losing one or two digits in the job code. Several automatic crosswalks exist between occupational classifications and some perform well in comparison with manual recoding.[5] The website of the International Stratification and Mobility File (<http://home.fsw.vu.nl/hbg.ganzeboom/ismf/ismf.htm>) is useful for finding crosswalks between occupational classifications, and the United Nations Statistical Division website is useful for finding crosswalks between classifications of economic activities (<http://unstats.un.org/unsd/cr/registry/regot.asp>). Sometimes it will be necessary to make compromises when data have been collected in categories and need to be converted into an average number. For example, when this type of questions is asked: 'At age 20, how much did you smoke on average?' and the answers are coded 1 = occasional smoker, 2 = 1–7 cigarettes per day, 3 = 8–15 cigarettes per day, 4 = 16–25 cigarettes per day, 5 = more than 25 cigarettes per day. A common approach is to choose the mid-point value in each category, but alternatives exist, so a decision needs to be taken.

Making the most of the data may imply that not all studies will qualify for all analyses. For example, if a study did not collect data regarding lung cancer cell type, it can contribute to the overall analyses but not to the cell type-specific analyses. It is important to remember that the quality of the original data is critical; poor data do not become better by pooling.

It is often easy to enrol studies into a pooling project because scientists generally wish to advance knowledge and make the best out of their already collected data. For this reason it is wise to define inclusion criteria at the beginning of the project, for example, minimum requirements for variables, or regarding the time period of data collection. It may be more complicated to enrol recent studies because the responsible scientists first need to prioritize and deliver for their funders and institutes, but it is often possible to collaborate because pooled projects usually focus on research questions that cannot easily be addressed at the level of any individual study.

Some scientists may be reluctant to contribute data to pooling projects for fear of losing control of their data. Therefore, it is important to define from the start what objectives should be fulfilled within the project and to have a process in place for approving new ideas because new ideas will emerge as the project goes along. It is also reassuring for data owners if the procedures for pooling are comprehensive and clear, in particular good documentation of each step in the processing and centralization of information about the data, so that scientists know who to contact with questions.

The structure of pooling projects is often composed of a 'steering committee' supported by a 'study coordinator', with the 'study group' including representatives from all studies and other relevant persons, and 'special interest groups' for pooling, exposure assessment, statistical methods, or other specialized work packages. Authorship rules in pooling projects are a common concern for contributing scientists. There is no 'gold standard' but a general approach would be to apply the authorship criteria of the International Committee of Medical Journal Editors (<http://www.icmje.org/>). Furthermore, it is often useful to create a small writing team for each paper and allocate other contributors less prominent places in the author list. It is common within pooling projects that the number of authors per study, and the position in the author list, reflects the size of the original study and/or the level of participation in the study group.

Contributing studies may prefer to adapt their data to the pooled format, or to send their raw data to the coordinating centre; in both cases it is important to have access to the original questionnaires from the study, as well as a code book and a contact person who knows the subtleties of the data. The latter is not necessarily the principal investigator but may be a data manager. Although most of the data have been used previously for their original purposes, quality checks of the pooled dataset are necessary, for example, to ensure that job codes are valid and dates are plausible. Recoding of data should be double-checked, for example by having two persons recode or re-classify the same sample and then comparing the result.

In the analytical phase, sensitivity analyses should be conducted to better understand potential sources of heterogeneity, for example, comparing the risk estimates in hospital-based case-control studies versus population-based studies, old versus recent studies, different geographical areas, or excluding one study at a time to see if any specific study, for whatever reason, has a large influence on the overall result.

In summary, pooling case-control studies is complex and requires considerable effort but it is possible and can greatly contribute to the weight of evidence.

Occupational exposure assessment in community-based studies

One of the major challenges in community-based occupational epidemiological studies has been valid assessment of the occupational exposures experienced by the population at large. Contrary to the detailed information usually available for an industrial population (e.g. in a retrospective cohort study in a large chemical company) that often allows for quantitative exposure estimation, community-based studies (whether cross-sectional, cohort, or case-control designs) have to rely on less precise and less valid estimates. The choice of method of exposure assessment to be applied in an epidemiological study depends on the study design, but it boils down to choosing between acquiring self-reported exposure, expert-based individual exposure assessment, or linking self-reported job histories with job-exposure matrices (JEMs) developed by experts.

Self-reported exposure

Self-reported exposure has the advantage that the exposure is assessed at the individual study subject level. However, differential misclassification can easily occur relating to the health status of the interviewee or questionnaire respondent. This can bias the outcome of cross-sectional and case-control studies in particular,[6] but it has been shown to operate also in a community-based cohort study.[7] The quality of the answers to questions addressing occupational exposures will depend heavily on the format of the questions. Generic questions using brand names might be expected to work better than using the actual chemical name of a substance. Also, prompted exposures and work activities tend to show less differential bias than open-ended questions.[8]

Expert-based individual exposure assessment

With self-reported occupational exposures being more prone to recall bias, expert-based exposure assessment has been promoted as the preferred approach. One or more expert(s), 'blinded' with regard to the subject's case/control status, assess the worker's exposure by looking over the work history, collecting detailed information on tasks performed, products produced, and often answers to detailed job-specific questionnaires or exposure-specific modules.[9] Standardization of these questionnaires has developed considerably in recent decades. Recently a database was developed with standard questionnaires from which to draw.[10] At the same time, decision rules are being elaborated with the aim of making expert assessment more reproducible and, above all, less expensive.[11] Training and standardization are critical in expert-based exposure assessment, especially when more than one expert is used in an international multicentre study.[12,13]

Job-exposure matrices

JEMs have been around for more than three decades[14] Their main distinction from either self-reported or expert-based exposure assessment methods is that exposures are no longer assigned at the individual subject level but at job or task level. As a result, JEMs make no distinction in assigned exposure between individuals performing the same job, or even between individuals performing a similar job in different companies. Assuming no differential recall of jobs performed during a working life, this approach will not suffer from differential misclassification of exposure. With the great majority of occupational exposures having a rather low prevalence (<10%) in the general population it is, however, extremely important that JEMs are developed aiming at a highly specific exposure assessment so that only jobs with a high likelihood (prevalence) and intensity of exposure are considered to be exposed. Aiming at a high sensitivity would be disastrous because a high sensitivity would lead to an enormous number of individuals being assigned an exposure while actually being unexposed; this substantial non-differential misclassification would bias the association between the exposure and health endpoint towards the null.[15]

Combinations of the methods just described exist as well and a good example is the Asthma JEM developed in 2000 by Kennedy and her colleagues.[16] In addition to a JEM, this method foresees the application of an expert step in which mainly incorrectly assigned exposures are reconsidered based on detailed information provided by the interviewed study subject. The expert step will in this way improve sensitivity without compromising the crucial high specificity of the exposure assessment method.[16,17]

Actual exposure measurements in community-based studies are seldom either routinely available or specially collected. A case-control study of leukaemia and brain tumours in the general population in which exposure to extremely low-frequency electromagnetic fields was assessed quantitatively in over 1000 workplaces is one of the few existing examples.[18] A cross-sectional exposure measurement survey might not, however, be any more informative than an expert-based approach or a JEM given the very great variability in measured exposure concentrations in the workplace and the considerable temporal trends.[19–21]

An approach with extensive exposure data mining that might overcome and address the issues of temporal trends in occupational exposures and exposure variability has been carried out in industry-based studies.[22–24] With personal exposure surveys having been performed for more than half a century in industry, and with the existence of large centralized databases, the development of quantitative JEMs for use in community-based studies has been on the horizon for some time.

SYNERGY: the challenges of pooling and quantitative exposure assessment in the study of occupational lung cancer

The SYNERGY project started in 2007 and is a pooling project of 16 case-control studies on lung cancer. To our knowledge it is the largest collection to date of lung cancer cases and control subjects with lifetime occupational and smoking histories. The original studies come from Europe, North America, Hong Kong (China), and

New Zealand and were conducted between 1985 and 2009. The project was initiated to study effect modifications of known occupational lung carcinogens by smoking, but can address many potential occupational risks for lung cancer while adequately adjusting for smoking behaviour. The SYNERGY project brought together scientists in the field of occupational cancer epidemiology and exposure assessment and provided opportunities to study the associations between lung cancer and occupational exposures with precision, in subgroups, and by lung cancer cell type, while adjusting rigorously for smoking or stratifying by smoking status.

Within the 16 case-control studies, as expected, a plethora of exposure assessment approaches had been used, making standardization and consequent pooling of assigned exposures from the individual case-control studies basically impossible. Therefore a decision was made to redo the exposure assessment, based on the recorded occupational histories of all cases and controls (18 000 and 22 000 respectively). Rather than using existing JEMs the project set out to develop a quantitative JEM (SYNJEM) based on collected exposure measurements from national databases (with the acronyms MEGA, NEDB, COLCHIC, EXPO), institutional (chemical- or industry-specific) measurement databases (with the acronyms PAPDEM, EXASRUB, AWE, WOODEX), or from paper records or reports existing in national agencies or research institutes.

A pre-designed protocol with detailed information on auxiliary data to be collected alongside the measured concentration was crucial to be able to make sense of the collected data. Knowledge of measurement strategies, measurement devices, and analytical methods was in order to interpret the reported concentrations. The exposure measurement database developed for SYNERGY (ExpoSYN) incorporated exposure measurement data for five major lung carcinogens (asbestos, respirable crystalline silica, chromium, nickel, and polycyclic aromatic hydrocarbons). Getting access to the data required a considerable amount of effort and time. Confidentiality of measurement data was a major hurdle that was overcome by giving assurances that the individual measurement data would be used only to elaborate the SYNJEM.

Like the occupational histories, the measurement data had to be coded in a similar way to the occupational histories, using the same occupational and industrial codes. Also all identified confounders such as measurement strategy, purpose of the measurement, measurement device (sampler), analytical technique, and limit of detection had to be coded for each and every sample that would enter the database.

Within 2 years more than 350 000 measurements were collected, coded, and incorporated into the ExpoSYN database;[25] 140 000 of these measurements were results of personal monitoring. The measurement data came from 19 countries, all from Europe except for Canada, with Germany (32%), UK (22%), and France (14%) being the main contributors. Crystalline silica accounted for 42% of the data and asbestos for 20%. The time period in which the data were collected covered more than 50 years, but considerable amounts were acquired only after 1970 when personal monitoring became common practice[26] (see Figure 13.1). However, the work history years of cases and controls for which exposures had to be estimated covered more than 80 years, making extrapolation a necessity.

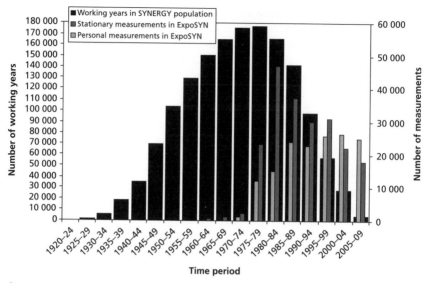

Figure 13.1 Distribution of exposure measurements in the ExpoSYN database over time compared to the working years of the SYNERGY population.

Reproduced with permission from Peters S, et al., Development of an exposure measurement database on five lung carcinogens (ExpoSYN) for quantitative retrospective occupational exposure assessment, *The Annals of Occupational Hygiene*, Volume **56**, Issue, pp. 70–79, Copyright © The Author 2011. Published by Oxford University Press on behalf of the British Occupational Hygiene Society.

The measurement data were consequently modelled using region/country and job titles as random effects in mixed-effect models. Year of measurement, measurement strategy, sampling duration, and an a priori exposure rating for each job from an independently developed semiquantitative job-exposure matrix (DOM-JEM, which assigned none, low, and high exposure to each job code for each carcinogen) were modelled as fixed effects.

For respirable crystalline silica almost 24 000 measurements covered a time period of more than 30 years (1976–2009). A temporal trend indicating a 6% annual decline became apparent. Exposure levels were higher in the UK and Canada and lower in Northern Europe and Germany. Worst-case sampling and sampling duration affected the measured concentrations, necessitating adjustments. Incorporation of the a priori exposure ratings was required in order to override incidental, and therefore heavily biased, measurements among groups normally not assumed to be exposed (e.g. bank directors exposed to respirable crystalline silica) and was also important in order to be able to estimate exposure for assumed exposed jobs where there were not enough measurement results. The resulting model enabled estimation of time-, job-, and region/country-specific exposure to respirable crystalline silica at levels which were plausible when compared to exposure levels described in the literature.[26–28]

SYNERGY: why pooling pays off

As should have become evident from what has been described, pooling community-based (case-control) studies is not easy and requires a lot of input and resources.
Re-doing the exposure assessment and attempting to go beyond semiquantitative
exposure assessment is no sinecure either. However, the SYNERGY project has shown
that pooling is possible, and so is quantitative exposure assessment, for community-
based studies on lung cancer. The idea was that pooling would result in considerably
increased power enabling, for instance, epidemiological analyses by histological sub-
type of lung cancer, and modelling of interactions between smoking and exposure
to five major lung carcinogens, as well as interactions due to simultaneous or serial
exposure to more than one of the five considered lung carcinogens.

The proof will be in the pudding, and only limited results of the SYNERGY project
are available to date. That the SYNERGY mission is paying off, however, can be seen
already from the fact that the data show that smoking exerted a steeper risk gradient
on squamous and small cell carcinoma than on adenocarcinoma.[29]

Analyses by job title have shown no increased risks among cooks and hairdressers, groups for whom increased risks of lung cancer had been reported in the earlier

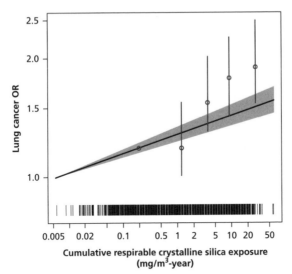

Figure 13.2 Exposure-response relation between respirable crystalline silica exposure
and lung cancer risk obtained with SYN-JEM in the SYNERGY population (straight line,
95% confidence interval (CI) presented by the grey shading). The rug plot indicates the
distribution of cumulative respirable crystalline silica exposure of exposed cases and
controls, the non-exposed group of about 28 000 subjects is represented by a small line
at the far left. Risk estimates from pooled industrial cohort studies[34] are represented by
the dots (with lines for the 95% CI); risk estimates were rescaled to the mid-point of the
reference category (0.2 mg/m³ per year). OR = odds ratio.

literature. Adjusting for smoking, and limiting analyses to never smokers, approaches possible within SYNERGY, clearly indicated a confounding effect from smoking.[30] On the other hand, clear exposure-response associations for lung cancer were seen in subjects occupationally exposed to diesel motor exhaust and organic dusts.[31,32]

The first analyses of the quantitative association between exposure to crystalline silica and lung cancer revealed an exposure-response curve (see Figure 13.2) which was quite comparable to that which had been reported previously based on industrial cohort studies.[33,34] This finding indicated that, with adequate quantitative exposure assessment, it is possible to produce quantitative exposure-response estimates enabling community-based studies to add to the weight of evidence and to contribute to standard setting.

References

1. **Ferlay J, Shin HR, Bray F, Forman D, Mathers C, Parkin DM.** *GLOBOCAN 2008 v2.0, cancer incidence and mortality worldwide: IARC CancerBase No. 10.* Lyon, France: International Agency for Research on Cancer, 2010. Available at: <http://globocan.iarc.fr> (accessed 18 February 2013).

2. **Rushton L, Bagga S, Bevan R, et al.** Occupation and cancer in Britain. *Br J Cancer* 2010;**102**:1428–37.

3. **International Agency for Research on Cancer.** IARC Monographs on the Evaluation of Carcinogenic Risks to Humans (series). Lyon: IARC. (Available at: http://monographs.iarc.fr/> (accessed 17 February 2013).

4. **Pukkala E, Martinsen JI, Lynge E, et al.** Occupation and cancer—follow-up of 15 million people in five Nordic countries. *Acta Oncol* 2009;**48**:646–790.

5. **Koeman T, Offermans SM, Christopher-de Vries Y, et al.** JEMs and incompatible occupational coding systems: effect of manual and automatic recoding of job codes on exposure assignment. *Ann Occup Hyg* 2012;**57**:107–14.

6. **McGuire V, Nelson LM, Koepsell TD, Checkoway H, Longstreth WT Jr.** Assessment of occupational exposures in community-based case-control studies. *Annu Rev Public Health* 1998;**19**:35–53.

7. **de Vocht F, Zock JP, Kromhout H, et al.** Comparison of self-reported occupational exposure with a job exposure matrix in an international community-based study on asthma. *Am J Ind Med* 2005;**47**:434–42.

8. **Teschke K, Kennedy SM, Olshan AF.** Effect of different questionnaire formats on reporting of occupational exposures. *Am J Ind Med* 1994;**26**:327–37.

9. **Stewart PA, Stewart WF, Siemiatycki J, Heineman EF, Dosemeci M.** Questionnaires for collecting detailed occupational information for community-based case control studies. *Am Ind Hyg Assoc J* 1998;**59**:39–44.

10. **Fritschi L, Friesen MC, Glass D, Benke G, Girschik J, Sadkowsky T.** OccIDEAS: retrospective occupational exposure assessment in community-based studies made easier. *J Environ Public Health* 2009;**2009**:957023. doi: 10.1155/2009/957023.

11. **Wheeler DC, Burstyn I, Vermeulen R, et al.** Inside the black box: starting to uncover the underlying decision rules used in a one-by-one expert assessment of occupational exposure in case-control studies. *Occup Environ Med* 2013;**70**:203–10.

12. **Vadali M, Ramachandran G, Banerjee S.** Effect of training, education, professional experience, and need for cognition on accuracy of exposure assessment decision-making. *Ann Occup Hyg* 2012;**56**:292–304.

13. **'t Mannetje A, Fevotte J, Fletcher T,** *et al.* Assessing exposure misclassification by expert assessment in multicenter occupational studies. *Epidemiology* 2003;**14**:585–92.

14. **Pannett B, Coggon D, Acheson ED.** A job-exposure matrix for use in population based studies in England and Wales. *Br J Ind Med* 1985;**42**:777–83.

15. **Kromhout H, Vermeulen R.** Application of job-exposure matrices in studies of the general population: some clues to their performance. *Eur Respir Rev* 2001;**11**:80–90.

16. **Kennedy SM, Le Moual N, Choudat D, Kauffmann F.** Development of an asthma specific job exposure matrix and its application in the epidemiological study of genetics and environment in asthma (EGEA). *Occup Environ Med* 2000;**57**:635–41.

17. **Zock JP, Cavallé N, Kromhout H,** *et al.* Evaluation of specific occupational asthma risks in a community-based study with special reference to single and multiple exposures. *J Expo Anal Environ Epidemiol* 2004;**14**:397–403.

18. **Floderus B, Persson T, Stenlund C, Wennberg A, Ost A, Knave B.** Occupational exposure to electromagnetic fields in relation to leukemia and brain tumors: a case-control study in Sweden. *Cancer Causes Control* 1993;**4**:465–76.

19. **Kromhout H, Symanski E, Rappaport SM.** A comprehensive evaluation of within- and between-worker components of occupational exposure to chemical agents. *Ann Occup Hyg* 1993;**37**:253–70.

20. **Loomis D, Kromhout H.** Exposure variability: concepts and applications in occupational epidemiology. *Am J Ind Med* 2004;**45**:113–22.

21. **Creely KS, Cowie H, van Tongeren M, Kromhout H, Tickner J, Cherrie JW.** Trends in inhalation exposure—a review of the data in the published scientific literature. *Ann Occup Hyg* 2007;**51**:665–78.

22. **de Vocht F, Straif K, Szeszenia-Dabrowska N,** *et al.* A database of exposures in the rubber manufacturing industry: design and quality control. *Ann Occup Hyg* 2005;**49**:691–701.

23. **de Vocht F, Sobala W, Peplonska B,** *et al.* Elaboration of a quantitative job-exposure matrix for historical exposure to airborne exposures in the Polish rubber industry. *Am J Ind Med* 2008;**51**:852–60.

24. **de Vocht F, Sobala W, Wilczynska U, Kromhout H, Szeszenia-Dabrowska N, Peplonska B.** Cancer mortality and occupational exposure to aromatic amines and inhalable aerosols in rubber tire manufacturing in Poland. *Cancer Epidemiol* 2009;**33**:94–102.

25. **Peters S, Vermeulen R, Olsson A,** *et al.* Development of an exposure measurement database on five lung carcinogens (ExpoSYN) for quantitative retrospective occupational exposure assessment. *Ann Occup Hyg* 2012;**56**:70–9.

26. **Cherrie JW.** The beginning of the science underpinning occupational hygiene. *Ann Occup Hyg* 2003;**47**:179–85.

27. **Peters S, Vermeulen R, Portengen L,** *et al.* Modelling of occupational respirable crystalline silica exposure for quantitative exposure assessment in community-based case-control studies. *J Environ Monit* 2011;**13**:3262–8.

28. **Peters S, Kromhout H, Portengen L,** *et al.* Sensitivity analyses of exposure estimates from a quantitative job-exposure matrix (SYN-JEM) for use in community-based studies. *Ann Occup Hyg* 2013;**57**:98–106.

29. **Pesch B, Kendzia B, Gustavsson P,** *et al.* Cigarette smoking and lung cancer—relative risk estimates for the major histological types from a pooled analysis of case-control studies. *Int J Cancer* 2012;**131**:1210–9.

30. **Olsson AC, Xu Y, Schüz J,** *et al.* Lung cancer risk among hairdressers—a pooled analysis of case-control studies conducted between 1985 and 2010. *Am J Epidemiol* (in press).

31. **Olsson AC, Gustavsson P, Kromhout H,** *et al.* Exposure to diesel motor exhaust and lung cancer risk in a pooled analysis from case-control studies in Europe and Canada. *Am J Respir Crit Care Med* 2011;**183**:941–8.

32. **Peters S, Kromhout H, Olsson AC,** *et al.* Occupational exposure to organic dust increases lung cancer risk in the general population. *Thorax* 2012;**67**:111–6.

33. **Peters, S.** *Quantitative exposure assessment in community-based studies.* Thesis. Utrecht University, The Netherlands, 2012.

34. **Steenland K, Mannetje A, Boffetta P,** *et al.* Pooled exposure-response analyses and risk assessment for lung cancer in 10 cohorts of silica-exposed workers: an IARC multicentre study. *Cancer Causes Control* 2001;**12**:773–84. (Correction in: *Cancer Causes Control* 2002;**13**:777.)

Chapter 14

Systematic reviews of occupational safety and health topics

Jos Verbeek and Sharea Ijaz

Introduction

Progress in science is usually considered as a process in which we continuously add small pieces of evidence to a body of knowledge on a specific topic. When we report the results of a scientific study, we usually refer to what is already known on this specific topic and how and what our study will add to this existing knowledge. This model of progress in science requires that we are able to summarize the existing knowledge in a succinct and accessible way. The link between scientific research and professional practice has been reinforced by evidence-based medicine and evidence-based policymaking in the past 20 years. The idea behind evidence-based practice is that underpinning practical interventions and policy measures with evidence from research will lead to a better quality of care and policies.[1–3] This is a strong incentive for providing high-quality research synthesis on concrete and specific questions. There will be few cases in which one study alone would be sufficiently convincing to constitute evidence for changing practice or taking policy measures. Therefore, a review and synthesis of the evidence from more than one study will always be needed.

Evidence-based approach

The evidence-based approach is a sequence involving scoping reviews, clinical studies, systematic reviews, and overviews of reviews. Not all questions can be answered by a single research approach. For example, policy questions can be very broad such as 'How can we best prevent occupational skin cancer?', which implies many sub-questions about the types of outcomes and exposures to be included, each warranting separate systematic reviews. A policymaker might want to know the best intervention to prevent back pain. This will require an overview of several existing systematic reviews each addressing one or more interventions to prevent back pain. Similarly, broad reviews of the literature are also needed to find out what kind of exposures need to be studied in clinical research or which interventions are of interest given the problem at hand. The term 'scoping review' has been coined because it is confusing to also call these broad reviews of the literature systematic reviews.[4] They are thus intended to come before one or more systematic reviews that can answer concrete questions.

Reviews of the literature have long been part of scientific progress although previously they were not highly valued as scientific research. This has changed since the advent of systematic reviews at the end of the 1980s. Systematic reviews are different from narrative reviews in being explicit and specific in their methods in order to find answers to important questions in health care. Chalmers, in the US, was one of the first to advocate systematic reviews in medicine. Based on good systematic reviews, he could show that the harms of lidocaine, which was widely used for treating myocardial infarction at that time, outweighed its benefits, which resulted in its abandonment for this purpose. He also showed the benefits of streptokinase in myocardial infarction and this has been part of treatment since then.[5]

Around the same time, it was recognized that experts very often provide answers that are more based on their personal interests than on the results of research.[6] Following on from this idea, a study in occupational health showed that expert colleagues used for advice by occupational physicians in the Netherlands provided answers that were not in line with the literature in more than 50% of cases.[7] This phenomenon, of experts quite often being wrong, has also been shown in political science and in business management.[8] This provides another strong incentive, when there is an important question to be answered from policy or practice, to systematically search for and synthesize evidence from research.

Often there is confusion about the difference between systematic reviews and meta-analyses. A meta-analysis is a quantitative synthesis of two or more studies, illustrated here (Figure 14.1) by a meta-analysis of ten studies on blunt versus sharp needles for the outcome of surgical glove perforation.[9] A systematic review is a synthesis of evidence on the effects of an intervention or an exposure which may also include a meta-analysis, but this is not a prerequisite. It may be that the results of the studies which have been included in a systematic review are reported in such a way that it is impossible to synthesize them quantitatively. They can then be reported in a narrative manner.[10] However, a meta-analysis always requires a systematic review of the literature. For convenience, we will here refer to both systematic reviews and meta-analyses as 'reviews'.

Reviews and occupational health and safety

Systematic reviews are the ideal instrument to find answers to concrete questions in occupational health and safety, such as:

- Do blunt surgical needles decrease the risk of needle-stick injuries to surgical staff?[9]
- Does exposure to shift work increase the risk of breast cancer?[11]
- Do physical exercise programmes increase the rate of return to work in workers with back pain?[12]

Questions can be about almost any topic, such as the effectiveness of interventions, the effects of exposures or prognostic factors, or about diagnostic problems. One can dream up many different questions about practice or policy, but it is important to translate those questions first to answerable questions. The methods should be adapted to the topic and the type of question, but the overall framework remains the

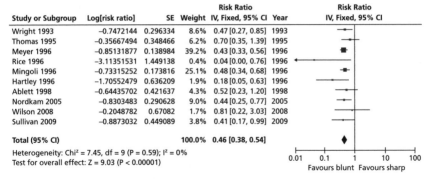

Study or Subgroup	Log[risk ratio]	SE	Weight	Risk Ratio IV, Fixed, 95% CI	Year
Wright 1993	–0.7472144	0.296334	8.6%	0.47 [0.27, 0.85]	1993
Thomas 1995	–0.35667494	0.348466	6.2%	0.70 [0.35, 1.39]	1995
Meyer 1996	–0.85131877	0.138984	39.2%	0.43 [0.33, 0.56]	1996
Rice 1996	–3.11351531	1.449138	0.4%	0.04 [0.00, 0.76]	1996
Mingoli 1996	–0.73315252	0.173816	25.1%	0.48 [0.34, 0.68]	1996
Hartley 1996	–1.70552479	0.636209	1.9%	0.18 [0.05, 0.63]	1996
Ablett 1998	–0.64435702	0.421637	4.3%	0.52 [0.23, 1.20]	1998
Nordkam 2005	–0.8303483	0.290628	9.0%	0.44 [0.25, 0.77]	2005
Wilson 2008	–0.2048782	0.67082	1.7%	0.81 [0.22, 3.03]	2008
Sullivan 2009	–0.8873032	0.449089	3.8%	0.41 [0.17, 0.99]	2009
Total (95% CI)			**100.0%**	**0.46 [0.38, 0.54]**	

Heterogeneity: Chi² = 7.45, df = 9 (P = 0.59); I² = 0%
Test for overall effect: Z = 9.03 (P < 0.00001)

Figure 14.1 A meta-analysis of ten studies on blunt versus sharp needles for the outcome of glove perforation rate. Although the first study showed a statistically significant reduction in exposure incidents, the second was inconclusive. Eight studies followed, six, with varying estimate sizes, favouring blunt needles, but two inconclusive. The meta-analysis showed a clear halving of the risk of exposure incidents, with a tight confidence interval.

Reproduced with permission from Parantainen A et al., Blunt versus sharp suture needles for preventing percutaneous exposure incidents in surgical staff, *Cochrane Database System Review* Issue 11 (CD009170), Copyright © 2011 The Cochrane Collaboration. Published by John Wiley & Sons, Ltd.

same. Here, we describe the most pertinent aspects of reviews of intervention studies and of aetiological studies, and those for which methods are best elaborated.

There is a long history of debate about the value of meta-analysis for occupational cohort studies or other occupational aetiological studies. In 1994, Shapiro argued that 'meta-analysis of published non-experimental data should be abandoned'. He reasoned that 'relative risks of low magnitude (say, less than 2) are virtually beyond the resolving power of the epidemiological microscope because we can seldom demonstrably eliminate all sources of bias'.[13] Because the pooling of studies in a meta-analysis increases statistical power, the pooled estimate may easily become significant and thus incorrectly taken as an indication of causality, even though the biases in the included studies may not have been taken into account. Others have argued that the method of meta-analysis is important but should be applied appropriately, taking into account the biases in individual studies.[14] Long before aetiological reviews became popular, Wong and Raabe[15] advocated rigorous quality assessment and quantitative synthesis of aetiological studies in a systematic review and meta-analysis, an approach which despite their work being opposed at that time has since then become more prevalent.[16] They restricted meta-analysis to cohort studies and used the more biased case-control studies for complementing the results with narrative. They called this approach meta-review. Myers and Thompson criticized the pooling of standardized mortality ratios (SMRs) which are often the outcome parameter in occupational cohort studies.[17] This criticism is, however, related to the complicated concept of a SMR, a ratio that may incorporate standardization on completely different, and therefore non-comparable, standard populations. Dickersin reasoned that some kind of research synthesis is needed in observational epidemiology and that the systematic process of a review would increase the quality of research synthesis of observational studies.[18] She called for more methodological research and international collaboration to undertake reviews of observational studies. Later, McElvenny and colleagues reviewed the practice of meta-analysis in occupational epidemiology and, in addition, called for more attention to the problems with meta-SMRs and the exploration of heterogeneity between the studies included in systematic reviews.[16] We are not aware of additional methodological work on reviews of observational studies since then, so it seems that the calls for more methodological work are still open. We believe that the synthesis of aetiological studies should be based on the same general principles as for intervention studies, and the existing methods adapted to the particular challenges of cohort and case-control studies.

Cochrane Collaboration

The Cochrane Collaboration, an international network of researchers and practitioners, has greatly influenced the practice of systematic reviews of intervention studies. The aim of the Collaboration is to collect, synthesize, and disseminate all available evidence on the effectiveness of health care interventions. The Collaboration started in 1992 on a fairly idealistic basis aiming to become a global network that would cover all health care interventions and that would be open for participation by anyone. Thanks to the development of the Internet and easier international communication, it has been a very fruitful endeavour. At the moment, there are more than 7600 interventions covered in the Cochrane Library (<http://thecochranelibrary.com>) that contains the electronic database of Cochrane Systematic Reviews and Protocols for Reviews. The reviews are highly valued in the medical literature, which is reflected in their scientific impact factor of about 6. The Collaboration is named after the famous British epidemiologist Archie Cochrane, who had a long-standing career in occupational epidemiology. He was most proud of his studies on dust in coal mines that contributed to the decrease in dust levels in British mines.[19] Since 2004, there is a special entity, the Cochrane Occupational Safety and Health Review Group, that is responsible for the preparing and updating of reviews of occupational safety and health interventions (<http://osh.cochrane.org>). There were over 100 systematic reviews on these topics in the Cochrane Library in 2012. The Collaboration has produced a handbook for systematic reviews of interventions that is probably the most comprehensive source of systematic review methods that is regularly updated. It is available both in print and on the Internet at <http://handbook.cochrane.org/>.[20]

Definition and characteristics of systematic reviews

Definition

Egger and colleagues, in their book on systematic reviews, define it as a review that has been prepared using a systematic approach to minimize biases and random errors, which is documented in a materials and methods section.[21] The PRISMA guideline for reporting systematic reviews (Preferred Reporting Items for Systematic

Reviews and Meta-Analyses) defines a systematic review as 'a review of a clearly formulated question that uses systematic and explicit methods to identify, select, and critically appraise relevant research, and to collect and analyse data from the studies that are included in the review. Statistical methods (meta-analysis) may or may not be used to analyse and summarize the results of the included studies'.[22]

Protocol

Being systematic and preventing data-dredging is greatly enhanced by publishing a protocol for the systematic review before the actual project is started. This is a requirement for Cochrane intervention reviews. For non-Cochrane reviews, it is now possible to register a protocol at Prospero, the international prospective register of reviews (<http://www.crd.york.ac.uk/PROSPERO>). This helps to make the review process more transparent, leading to more valid results.

Answerable PICO question

A clear and answerable review question is best formulated using the PICO format (Participants, Intervention/Exposure, Comparison, and Outcome). The PICO for the risk of shift work for breast cancer,[11] for example, can be: P: any female worker, I: exposure to shift work, C: no or lesser exposure to shift work, O: breast cancer. For the needle-stick injuries prevention question[9] the PICO is: P: surgical staff, I: blunt surgery needles, C: sharp surgery needles, O: needle stick injuries, glove perforations. The advantage of using specific questions is that it prevents mixing apples with oranges. It also decreases the differences between studies.[23] Very broad questions naturally lead to greater heterogeneity between studies, which may make it difficult to come to a clear conclusion.

Comprehensive search

A comprehensive search is another key element of a systematic review because it is important to ensure that all available studies are included. A non-random exclusion of studies could easily bias the results. For example, a Cochrane review on occupational stress in health care workers[24] included twice as many studies as those included in a review on the same question carried out at a similar time.[25] The reason for this difference was that the latter review authors did not search Medline, which contains many studies on stress management in health care workers.

Many electronic databases are available that may be general or focused on a specific topic. Medline, accessible through PubMed, is the most comprehensive medical database. However, searching only Medline is rarely enough because bibliographic databases vary in their coverage of occupational health and safety journals. As well as Medline, EMBASE and the Cochrane Occupational Health Review Group's Trials Register are recommended, and other databases should be searched depending on topic. For example, PsychINFO can be relevant for psychological interventions such as stress management, CINAHL is important for the nursing literature, and Econlit, a database of the economic literature, for assessing cost and resource use. Specialist occupational health and safety databases searched for all reviews at the Cochrane Occupational Safety and Health Review Group also include:

- CISDOC—The Health and Safety Information Centre of The International Labour Organization (1974 to present).
- International Bibliographic—produced by Sheila Pantry Associates Ltd.
- HSELINE—UK Health and Safety Executive Information Services (1977 to present).
- NIOSHTIC—US National Institute for Occupational Safety and Health (early 1900s to 1998).
- NIOSHTIC-2—US National Institute for Occupational Safety and Health (1977 to present).
- RILOSH—Ryerson International Labour Occupational Safety and Health (early 1900s to 2004).

For PubMed in particular, researchers have developed strings of search words that have been shown to cover specific topics comprehensively, such as randomized controlled trials (RCTs), occupational health intervention studies, studies on return to work, or aetiological questions.[26–30]

It is important that all studies that exist, published or unpublished, in languages other than English, and from 'grey' literature, are sought. This prevents the bias that exists in scientific research due to 'positive' findings being published more often than 'negative', and usually published in mainstream English-language journals. For example, a search by the authors in the grey literature for studies on shift work and breast cancer identified four unique relevant citations that were not located by searching other databases. One was a recent PhD thesis[31] which would have been omitted had searches been limited to published studies. This would have been unfortunate, because it was of better quality than many published studies and had failed to find an association between shift work and breast cancer. Therefore, electronic database searching should as far as possible be complemented with searches in, for example, book chapters on occupational epidemiology, specialist society archives, university dissertations (available via <http://www.proquest.co.uk/en-UK/>), and specialized conference proceedings (such as ICOH and EPICOH conferences).

Appropriate synthesis

Another important aspect of a systematic review is the method used to synthesize the results of the included studies. Preferably, one would like to see one clear conclusion that the intervention works (or not), with the magnitude and precision of the effect, for example as a relative risk and its 95% confidence interval. The first step is to determine which of the studies identified in the search are sufficiently similar that they can be combined. For intervention studies, this means determining which interventions, controls, outcomes, follow-up periods, and participants are similar enough for a meaningful combination in one comparison.[32]

For aetiological studies, one would prefer to draw a conclusion about a dose-response relation, for example, as risk per unit of exposure and its 95% confidence interval, based on the known or assumed relation between exposure and risk. This relationship may be linear, or based on a log transformation of exposure, or any other model. As in intervention reviews, first the researcher will look at study design, exposure measurement, outcome measurement, type of participants, and adjustment for confounders to assess if the studies can be combined. For example, a study assessing and comparing exposure using job titles (e.g. nurse, paramedic, doctor) is not suitable for combination with a study using exposure duration or quantity as its measure (e.g. years of night work, hours of standing during work, or number of percutaneous exposures to body fluids). Next, the problem is that most studies report relative risks for varying categories of exposure. For example, one study reports a relative risk of 1.4 for 1–2 years of exposure and of 1.6 for over 3 years of exposure. Another study reports a relative risk of 1.018 for 1 year of exposure. Yet another study reports a relative risk of 1.27 for 1–4.4 years and 1.40 for over 4.5 years of the same exposure. The challenge is to combine these risk estimates or dose-response estimates across studies in the most meaningful way. An elegant two-step solution[33] is to first assign a single exposure dose to each category and then convert the category-specific risks into incremental risk ratios per unit of exposure *per study*. The assigned doses can be used in a weighted regression analysis for trend estimation to calculate an incremental risk ratio per unit of exposure for the single studies. In our case, this could yield the following yearly incremental relative risks per study: 1.13, 1.018, and 1.04, which are comparable and combinable risk estimates. The same weighted regression analysis can then be used to combine these studies in a meta-analysis to produce an overall pooled incremental risk ratio.

A review will always use a method to combine the results of studies to arrive at a conclusion about a body of research. One can find many reviews in which the authors state that, because of heterogeneity between studies, they refrained from meta-analysis. This statement is in itself correct but usually the authors then do draw some kind of overall conclusion without explaining how the study results were combined and conclusions drawn. Basically, there are two options for study synthesis: a quantitative meta-analysis or a narrative combination.[15,32] The quantitative meta-analysis is based on a form of weighted pooling of the study results similar to the pooling of results from strata within a study. When the results of studies cannot be pooled, for example because the outcome measures are very different and cannot reasonably be combined, then the preferred method is a description of why and where the studies are similar instead of describing one study at a time. Grouping and presenting studies, for example, by population groups (e.g. children, adults), setting (e.g. hospital based, community based), quality (e.g. blinded, unblinded), or effect direction and size (e.g. 'positive' and 'negative' studies) allows the reader to see patterns in the findings from these varied studies. This also enables the reviewer to draw a conclusion in the absence of a pooled result with confidence intervals. Other methods used frequently include 'vote-counting', a simple summing up of the positive or negative results of studies. It can lead to biased conclusions when, for example, several low-powered studies showing non-significant results outweigh the findings of a small number of large studies. In a meta-analysis, this would not have happened because the large studies have greater weight than the smaller studies.

Risk of bias of included studies

The believability of a systematic review's results depends largely on the quality of the included studies. Therefore, assessing and reporting on the quality of the included studies is important. For intervention studies, randomized trials are regarded as of higher quality than observational studies, and the conduct of the study (e.g. in terms of response rate or completeness of follow-up) also influences quality. A conclusion derived from a few high-quality studies will be more reliable than when the conclusion is based on even a large number of low-quality studies. Some form of quality assessment is nowadays commonplace in intervention reviews but is still often missing in reviews of aetiological studies. 'Risk of bias' has more or less superseded the term 'quality assessment' today. Quality is a more general concept which depends on more than risk of bias. Furthermore, risk of bias puts quality in context: bias may exist in a high-quality study because risk of bias changes from review to review depending on the question. A good example is risk of bias due to the funding source, which is independent from the methodological quality of the study.

Risk of bias assessment in reviews of intervention studies is preferably done at both outcome and study level, and using an instrument that assesses domains, or areas, of bias such as random allocation, blinding, loss to follow-up, and selective reporting.[20,22] In the occupational context the domains should additionally include the methods used for exposure assessment.

It is tempting to use quality scores, such as the Jadad scale for RCTs[34] and the Downs and Black scale for non-RCT intervention studies[35] but these, in their original format, are insensitive to variation in the importance of risk areas for a given research question. The score system may give the same value to two studies (say, 10 out of 12) when one, for example, lacked blinding and the other did not randomize, thus implying that their quality is equal. This would not be a problem if randomization and blinding were equally important for all questions in all reviews, but this is not the case.

For RCTs an important development in this regard has been the Cochrane risk of bias tool.[36] This is a checklist of six important domains that have been shown to be important areas of bias in RCTs: random sequence generation, allocation concealment, blinding of participants and personnel, blinding of outcome assessment, incomplete outcome data, and selective reporting. The tool can be modified as necessary for a given intervention question (adding other important biases) and allows a choice of one of three judgments (high, low, or unclear risk) which can be applied both at domain and study level. It is freely available from the Cochrane Handbook[20] and is fully integrated in the Cochrane free downloadable meta-analysis software RevMan (<http://ims.cochrane.org/revman>).

For the assessment of non-randomized intervention studies, such as cohort studies or controlled before-and-after studies, commonly used tools (Downs and Black checklist[35] and the Newcastle-Ottawa scale[38]) give a total score based on a set of quality criteria. Once again, an overall quality score for a study should not be used because it can be misleading due to the relative equivalence implied for each quality item.

These risks of bias tools developed for intervention studies cannot be used for reviews of aetiological studies without relevant modification. This is because, unlike interventions, exposures are usually more complicated to assess when we want to attribute the outcome to them alone. These scales do not cover all items that may need assessment in an aetiological study, such as confounding and information bias relating to exposures. For example, did the authors adjust for confounding by, say, smoking, and how adequate was the exposure assessment? Surprisingly little methodological work has been done to develop validated tools for aetiological epidemiology and most tools in use are not validated,[38] including the most commonly used Newcastle-Ottawa Scale.[39] Two separate checklists, for observational studies of incidence and prevalence and for risk factor assessment, have been developed and validated recently.[40] Even though their application as developed requires use of Microsoft Access, this is not essential for their use. For practical purposes, any of the bias assessment checklists can (and should) be modified to fit the question asked in an aetiological review. We prefer to apply the Cochrane tool's principles and to judge various items of bias to be at 'high', 'low', or 'unclear' risk.

Finally, the results of risk of bias in the included studies should be incorporated in the analysis and conclusions about the overall quality of the evidence. The GRADE (Grading of Recommendations, Assessment, Development, and Evaluation) working group has proposed a set of decision rules on how to come to a rating ranging from high quality to very low quality.[41] The point of departure for intervention studies is that the evidence is of high quality. Subsequently the evidence rating is downgraded if study limitations are present. The criteria for downgrading used in GRADE are: indirectness, inconsistency, risk of bias, publication bias, and imprecision. For observational studies the point of departure is low quality of evidence and then GRADE uses the following criteria for upgrading the quality of the evidence: a big effect size, a very big effect size, all confounders would work towards the null, spurious factors would work towards the null.

Risk of bias in systematic reviews

This refers to issues in the process and methods used in the systematic review which affect its believability. The characteristics of systematic reviews that we mention here form the most important items of an instrument to assess the quality of reviews called AMSTAR (Assessment of Multiple SysTemAtic Reviews) that has been evaluated and found to be a valid and reliable instrument.[42]

The reporting of systematic reviews is facilitated by using the PRISMA check-list.[22] A separate statement has been made for reporting reviews of observational studies, *M*eta-analysis *Of Observational Studies in Epidemiology* (MOOSE) which is not as well elaborated as PRISMA.[43]

Recent developments and challenges

A policymaker or a patient is less interested in whether an intervention works than in what intervention works best; for example, what is the best way to prevent back pain at work, or what is the best way to treat depression. Such questions can be answered in overviews of reviews that bring together the information from multiple reviews that deal with many interventions. Another way is to use a network meta-analysis, or multiple treatment comparison. This is an analysis using a statistical technique to compare multiple interventions simultaneously and tells us the relative value of each against the rest.[44] In an attempt to bring information conveniently together, the occupational safety and health evidence group of the partnership for European Research in Occupational Safety and Health (PEROSH), started a clearing house. The objective of the clearing house is to bring together all reviews that answer questions pertinent to occupational safety and health (<http://www.perosh.eu>).

For reviews of aetiological studies, many questions are still open. For example, how should we address the inherently greater uncertainty in such reviews? Salanti and Ioannidis[45] proposed calculating the pooled risk estimates based on certainty ceilings (percentage certainty) decided a priori because this shows what happens if uncertainty about the results increases. A certainty ceiling is the probability that the actual effect is not in the direction shown by the observed effect estimate. If the calculated probability is less than the predefined ceiling we inflate the variance of the study before including it in the meta-analysis.

Publication and other reporting bias is probably a much bigger issue for aetiological studies than for intervention studies. This is because, for clinical trials, the introduction of protocol registration, coupled with the regulatory system for new medications, has helped in assessing and preventing publication and reporting bias. No such checks exist for observational studies. It may be relatively easy to explore, say, registry data to see if there is an association between an exposure and an outcome. If the results are interesting, usually meaning a 'positive' association, a study may be set up, but otherwise nothing may be published. This leads to serious publication bias that would

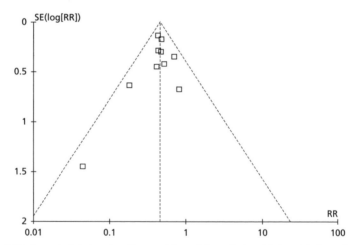

Figure 14.2 Funnel plot showing the precision of the relative risk (y-axis) plotted against the value of the relative risk (x-axis) in a comparison of blunt versus sharp suture needles, for the outcome of glove perforation rate. Note one very small study (lower left corner) with a 'positive' outcome and the absence of a similar study on the opposite side. RR = relative risk; SE = standard error.

be difficult to detect. Ioannidis[46] has proposed tackling the problem by registering research groups or data-sets which may be useful for aetiological studies. Until such systems are in place reviews can benefit from following PRISMA for search methods and by visually inspecting the included studies in a funnel plot (see Figure 14.2, for example).

The quality of the reports of studies in journal articles remains a big challenge for systematic reviewers. In 1996, Wong and Raabe hoped that 'in the future authors will report investigations in a uniform manner...and journal editors will include as part of their decisions the potential contribution of a manuscript to a future meta-analysis of similar studies'.[15] The EQUATOR Network (*E*nhancing the *QUA*lity and *T*ransparency *O*f health *R*esearch, <http://www.equator-network.org/>) has extended the work of guideline development groups into producing and bringing together reporting guidelines for all types of studies.[47] The challenge is to implement these guidelines much more rigorously so that these hopes may be realized in the next decade.

References

1. **Sackett DL, Rosenberg WM, Gray JA, Haynes RB, Richardson WS.** Evidence based medicine: what it is and what it isn't. *BMJ* 1996;**312**:71–2.

2. **European Commission.** Directorate-General for Research. *Scientific evidence for policy-making.* Luxembourg: Office for Official Publications of the European Communities, 2008. Available at: <http://ec.europa.eu/research/social-sciences/pdf/scientific_evidence_policy-making_en.pdf> (accessed 18 February 2013).

3. **Verbeek J.** From evidence to action: how to use evidence in OSH policies. In: Vainio H, Lehtinen S (eds) *Proceedings of the International Forum on Occupational Health and Safety: Policies, Profiles and Services; 2–22 June, 2011; Espoo, Finland.* Helsinki: Finnish Institute of Occupational Health, 2011, pp. 39–45. Available at: <http://www.ttl.fi/en/publications/Electronic_publications/Documents/Forum2011_proceedings.pdf> (accessed 18 February 2013).

4. **Armstrong R, Hall BJ, Doyle J, Waters E.** Cochrane Update. 'Scoping the scope' of a Cochrane review. *J Public Health* 2011;**33**:147–50.

5. **Chalmers TC.** Meta-analysis in clinical medicine. *Trans Am Clin Climatol Assoc* 1988;**99**:144–50.

6. **Oxman AD, Guyatt GH.** Guidelines for reading literature reviews. *CMAJ* 1988;**138**:697–703.

7. **Schaafsma F, Verbeek J, Hulshof C, van Dijk F.** Caution required when relying on a colleague's advice; a comparison between professional advice and evidence from the literature. *BMC Health Serv Res* 2005;**5**:59.

8. **Pfeffer J, Sutton RI.** *Hard facts, dangerous half-truths, and total nonsense: profiting from evidence-based management.* Boston, MA: Harvard Business Press, 2006.

9. **Parantainen A, Verbeek JH, Lavoie MC, Pahwa M.** Blunt versus sharp suture needles for preventing percutaneous exposure incidents in surgical staff. *Cochrane Database Syst Rev* 2011;**11**:CD009170.

10. **Rodgers M, Sowden A, Petticrew M,** *et al.* Testing methodological guidance on the conduct of narrative synthesis in systematic reviews: effectiveness of interventions to promote smoke alarm ownership and function. *Evaluation* 2009;**15**:47–71. doi: 10.1177/1356389008097871.

11. **Ijaz S, Verbeek J, Seidler A,** *et al. Shift work and the development of breast cancer: protocol for a systematic review.* PROSPERO 2012:CRD42012002247. Available at: <http://www.crd.york. ac.uk/PROSPERO/display_record.asp?ID=CRD42012002247> (accessed 18 February 2013).

12. **Schaafsma F, Schonstein E, Whelan KM, Ulvestad E, Kenny DT, Verbeek JH.** Physical conditioning programs for improving work outcomes in workers with back pain. *Cochrane Database Syst Rev* 2010;**1**:CD001822.

13. **Shapiro S.** Meta-analysis/shmeta-analysis. *Am J Epidemiol* 1994;**140**:771–8.

14. **Petitti DB.** Of babies and bathwater. *Am J Epidemiol* 1994;**140**:779–82.

15. **Wong O, Raabe GK.** Application of meta-analysis in reviewing occupational cohort studies. *Occup Environ Med* 1996;**53**:793–800.

16. **Myers JE, Thompson ML.** Meta-analysis and occupational epidemiology. *Occup Med* 1998;**48**:99–101.

17. **Dickersin K.** Systematic reviews in epidemiology: why are we so far behind? *Int J Epidemiol* 2002;**31**:6–12.

18. **McElvenny DM, Armstrong BG, Järup L, Higgins JPT.** Meta-analysis in occupational epidemiology: a review of practice. *Occup Med* 2004;**54**:336–44.

19. **Cochrane AL, Fletcher CM, Gilson JC, Hugh-Jones P.** The role of periodic examination in the prevention of coalworkers' pneumoconiosis. *Br J Ind Med* 1951;**8**:53–61.

20. **Higgins JPT, Green S (eds).** *Cochrane handbook for systematic reviews of interventions* (5.1.0 edn). The Cochrane Collaboration, 2011. Available at: <http://www.cochrane-handbook. org> (accessed 8 February 2013).

21. **Egger M, Davey Smith G, Altman D (eds).** *Systematic reviews in health care: meta-analysis in context* (2nd edn). London: BMJ Publishing, 2001.

22. **Moher D, Liberati A, Tetzlaff J, Altman DG; PRISMA Group.** Preferred reporting items for systematic reviews and meta-analyses: the PRISMA statement. *PLoS Med* 2009;**6**:e1000097.

23. **Guyatt GH, Oxman AD, Kunz R,** *et al.* GRADE guidelines: 2. Framing the question and deciding on important outcomes. *J Clin Epidemiol* 2011;**64**:395–400.

24. **Marine A, Ruotsalainen J, Serra C, Verbeek J.** Preventing occupational stress in healthcare workers. *Cochrane Database Syst Rev* 2006;**4**:CD002892. doi: 10.1002/14651858.CD002892. pub2.

25. **Richardson KM, Rothstein HR.** Effects of occupational stress management intervention programs: a meta-analysis. *J Occup Health Psychol* 2008;**13**:69–93.

26. **Glanville JM, Lefebvre C, Miles JN, Camosso-Stefinovic J.** How to identify randomized controlled trials in MEDLINE: ten years on. *J Med Libr Assoc* 2006;**94**:130–6.

27. **Verbeek J, Salmi J, Pasternack I,** *et al.* A search strategy for occupational health intervention studies. *Occup Environ Med* 2005;**62**:682–7.

28. **Gehanno JF, Rollin L, Le Jean T, Louvel A, Darmoni S, Shaw W.** Precision and recall of search strategies for identifying studies on return-to-work in Medline. *J Occup Rehabil* 2009;**19**:223–30.

29. **Mattioli S, Zanardi F, Baldasseroni A,** *et al.* Search strings for the study of putative occupational determinants of disease. *Occup Environ Med* 2010;**67**:436–43.

30. **Schaafsma F, Hulshof C, Verbeek J, Bos J, Dyserinck H, van Dijk F.** Developing search strategies in Medline on the occupational origin of diseases. *Am J Ind Med* 2006;**49**:127–37.

31. **Li W.** *Magnetic fields, night shift work and the risk of breast cancer among female textile workers in Shanghai, China.* Thesis. University of Washington, Seattle, WA, 2011.

32. **Verbeek J, Ruotsalainen J, Hoving JL.** Synthesizing study results in a systematic review. *Scand J Work Environ Health* 2012;**38**:282–90.

33. **Orsini N, Li R, Wolk A, Khudyakov P, Spiegelman D.** Meta-analysis for linear and nonlinear dose-response relations: examples, an evaluation of approximations, and software. *Am J Epidemiol* 2012;**175**:66–73.

34. **Jadad AR, Moore RA, Carroll D,** *et al.* Assessing the quality of reports of randomized clinical trials: is blinding necessary? *Control Clin Trials* 1996;**17**:1–12.

35. **Downs SH, Black N.** The feasibility of creating a checklist for the assessment of the methodological quality both of randomised and non-randomised studies of health care interventions. *J Epidemiol Community Health* 1998;**52**:377–84.

36. **Higgins JP, Altman DG, Gotzsche PC,** *et al.* The Cochrane Collaboration's tool for assessing risk of bias in randomised trials. *BMJ* 2011;**343**:d5928.

37. **Wells GA, Shea B, O'Connell D,** *et al. The Newcastle-Ottawa Scale (NOS) for assessing the quality of nonrandomised studies in meta-analyses.* Ottawa: OHRI, undated. Available at: <http://www.ohri.ca/programs/clinical_epidemiology/oxford.asp> (accessed 18 February 2013).

38. **Shamliyan T, Kane RL, Dickinson S.** A systematic review of tools used to assess the quality of observational studies that examine incidence or prevalence and risk factors for diseases. *J Clin Epidemiol* 2010;**63**:1061–70.

39. **Stang A.** Critical evaluation of the Newcastle-Ottawa scale for the assessment of the quality of nonrandomized studies in meta-analyses. *Eur J Epidemiol* 2010;**25**:603–5.

40. **Shamliyan TA, Kane RL, Ansari MT,** *et al.* Development quality criteria to evaluate nontherapeutic studies of incidence, prevalence, or risk factors of chronic diseases: pilot study of new checklists. *J Clin Epidemiol* 2011;**64**:637–57.

41. **Guyatt GH, Oxman AD, Schünemann HJ, Tugwell P, Knottnerus A.** GRADE guidelines: a new series of articles in the Journal of Clinical Epidemiology. *J Clin Epidemiol* 2011;**64**:380–2.

42. **Shea BJ, Hamel C, Wells GA,** *et al.* AMSTAR is a reliable and valid measurement tool to assess the methodological quality of systematic reviews. *J Clin Epidemiol* 2009;**62**:1013–20.

43. **Stroup DF, Berlin JA, Morton SC,** *et al.* Meta-analysis of observational studies in epidemiology: a proposal for reporting. Meta-analysis Of Observational Studies in Epidemiology (MOOSE) group. *JAMA* 2000;**283**:2008–12.

44. **Coleman CI, Phung OJ, Cappelleri JC,** *et al. Use of mixed treatment comparisons in systematic review.* Methods Research Report. AHRQ Publication No. 12-EHC119-EF. Rockville, MD: U.S. Department of Health and Human Services, Agency for Health Care Research and Quality, 2012. Available at: <http://effectivehealthcare.ahrq.gov/ehc/products/354/1238/Use-of-Mixed-Treatment_FinalReport_20121004.pdf> (accessed 8 February 2013).

45. **Salanti G, Ioannidis JP.** Synthesis of observational studies should consider credibility ceilings. *J Clin Epidemiol* 2009;**62**:115–22.

46. **Ioannidis JP.** The importance of potential studies that have not existed and registration of observational data sets. *JAMA* 2012;**308**:575–6.

47. **Verbeek J.** Moose Consort Strobe and Miame Stard Remark or how can we improve the quality of reporting studies. *Scand J Work Environ Health* 2008;**34**:165–7.

Chapter 15

Estimating the burden of occupational disease

Lesley Rushton, Sally Hutchings, and Tim Driscoll

Introduction

Epidemiological studies of industrial workforces have played an important role in the identification of environmental hazards, including carcinogens, and the understanding of the aetiology of the adverse health effects these can cause. The risk of disease or injury in the working environment should be minimized, yet many thousands of workers worldwide are exposed to hazardous substances at work every day. There is thus an increasing interest in estimating and comparing burdens of disease generally[1] and for cancer.[2,3] Estimates can identify major risk factors and high-risk populations, support decisions on priority actions for risk reduction, and provide an understanding of important contributions to health inequalities. There have been several studies estimating the burden of disease due to occupational exposures internationally and for specific countries and using a variety of methods. This chapter gives a brief general overview of burden estimation methods, followed by results from selected examples, focusing on carcinogens. Interpretation of these results and their use in policy and decision-making is discussed.

Overview of burden estimation methods

Most ill health that arises from occupational exposures can also arise from non-occupational exposures, and the same type of exposure can occur in occupational and non-occupational settings. With the exception of malignant mesothelioma (which is essentially only caused by exposure to asbestos), there is no way to determine which exposure caused a particular disorder, nor where the causative exposure occurred. This means that usually it is not possible to determine the burden just by counting the number of cases. Instead, approaches to estimating this burden have been developed. There are also several ways to define burden and how best to measure it. A number of commonly used approaches for calculating the burden of ill health arising from occupational exposures are considered here.

Estimation of the population attributable fraction

The population attributable fraction (PAF) is the proportion of cases that would not have occurred in the absence of an occupational exposure. It can be estimated by combining two measures—a risk estimate (usually relative risk (RR) or odds ratio) of the disorder of interest that is associated with exposure to the substance of concern; and an estimate of the proportion of the population exposed to the substance at work (p(E)). This approach has been used in several studies, particularly for estimating cancer burden[4-7] (Table 15.1).

Risk estimates typically come from epidemiological studies of specific industries or occupations. Estimates of the proportions exposed are usually taken from independent sources such as census or national employment data or databases such as the CARcinogen EXposure (CAREX) database.[8] An alternative approach uses estimates of RR from population-based studies, including pooled case-control studies with estimates of the proportion exposed from the distribution of exposures amongst the controls or other cases from the same study.[9] Dose-response risk estimates are often not available in the epidemiological literature, nor are proportions of those exposed at different levels of exposure over time; 'ever/never' exposed categories are therefore often used with a defined ever/never boundary level.[10] There are several possible equations that can be used to calculate the PAF, depending on the available data, the most important of which are Levin's:[11] $PAF = p(E) \times (RR - 1)/\{1 + p(E) \times (RR - 1)\}$ in its simplest form, and Miettinen's:[9] $PAF = p(E|D) \times (RR - 1)/RR$, where $p(E|D)$ is the proportion of cases exposed. Random error confidence intervals can be estimated for the PAFs using Monte Carlo simulations.[12]

For many chronic diseases, such as most cancers, the relevant period for cancer development during which exposure occurred needs to be considered in order to take account of the long latency of these diseases. Earlier studies used estimates of staff turnover to estimate proportions exposed.[5-7,13] More recent estimates have taken account of both turnover of staff and life expectancy during a defined latency period before appearance of disease.[10] This approach was extended to estimate PAFs by age groups for the Global Burden of Disease study, 2010 update.[14]

PAFs cannot in general be combined by summing directly because: (1) summing PAFs for overlapping exposures (i.e. agents to which the same 'ever exposed' workers may have been exposed) may give an overall PAF exceeding 100%, and (2) summing disjoint (not concurrently occurring) exposures also introduces upward bias. Strategies to avoid this include partitioning exposed numbers between overlapping exposures (Hutchings and Rushton[10] provide a good example of this) or estimating only for the 'dominant' carcinogen with the highest risk. Where multiple exposures remain, one approach is to assume that the exposures are independent and their joint effects are multiplicative. The PAFs can then be combined to give an overall PAF for that cancer using a product sum.[15]

Alternative estimates of risk for PAF estimation

Absolute risk measures rather than RRs may be appropriate for some exposures if the PAF is associated with an occupational exposure thought to account for 100% of the risk, for example, mesothelioma and asbestos exposure.[16,17]

Quality of life measures of burden

Attributable fractions and numbers do not address the issue of the relative 'costs' to an individual or society of an occupationally caused disease, such as the potential loss

Table 15.1 Estimates of PAF for occupational causes of selected disease

Location	Lung		Bladder		Skin		Nasal		Leukaemia		All cancers	
	M	**F**	**M**	**F**	**M**	**F**	**M**	**F**	**M**	**F**	**M**	**F**
US[21]	15%	5%	10%	5%	10%	2%	25%	5%	10%	5%	7%	1.2%
Nordic countries[13]	5% asbestos only 13% other exposures	<1% other exposures	2%	<1%	–		30%	<2%	1%	<1%	3%	<0.1%
US[22]	10–33%		21–27%								6–10%[a]	
US[6]	6.3–13.0%[a]		7–19%	3–19%	1.5–6.0%		33–46%		0.8–2.8%[a]		3.3–7.3%	0.8–1.0%
Finland[7]	29%	5%	14%	1%	13%	4%	24%	7%	18%	2%	8%[a]	
World[5]	10%	5%							2%	2%		
Europe[23]				8%[b]			39%[b]	11%[b]				
GB[4]	21.1%	5.3%	7.1%	1.9%	6.9%	1.1%	43.3%	19.8%	0.9%	0.5%	8.2%	2.3%

(Continued)

Table 15.1 (Continued)

Location	Non-malignant disease groups				
	Chronic respiratory	Cardio/cerebrovascular	Nervous system	Renal system	Asthma
New York State extrapolated to US[24]	1–3%	1–3% (included nervous and renal)			
US[22]	10%	5–10% (ages 15–64)	1–3%	1–3%	
US[6]	6–25%	6.3–18.0% (ages 20–69)	8.2–14.5%		
World[5]	12% (18% M, 6% F, COPD mortality)				17% (21% M, 13% F, asthma mortality)
US (NHANES III data)[25]	19.2% overall, 31.1% in never smokers (COPD prevalence in ages 30–75)				
US health maintenance organization[26]	24% (5–39) overall, 43% (0–68) in never smokers (COPD prevalence)				

[a] Male and female, or sex not specified; [b] based on same pooled studies. F, female; M, male.

of life through early death or the cost of ill health in a community. Various measures have been developed to take account of many of these issues. The most widely used measure is the disability-adjusted life year (DALY), which combines the present value of future years of life time lost (YLL) through premature mortality and the present value of years of future life time lived with a disability (YLD), i.e. adjusted for severity of any mental or physical disability caused by disease or injury.[18] YLLs are calculated as the difference between the age at death and the life expectancy at that age. YLDs are calculated by multiplying the years spent with a disability by an appropriate severity weighting, a number between zero (perfect health) and one (death). The number of DALYs for a disorder, or arising from an exposure, is the sum of the YLLs and the YLDs for the condition. DALYs are the main measures used in the Global Burden of Disease studies.[19]

Predicting the future burden of occupational disease

Methods to estimate the future burden of a disease due to occupation include estimating PAFs for a series of forecast target years, accounting for past and projected exposure trends and under targeted exposure reduction scenarios;[20] estimation of the 'lifetime risk' of a cohort of newly exposed workers, based on national incidence rates applied to their future person-years-at-risk and excess risk from their occupational exposure; and estimation of attributable disease directly from projected disease numbers, with the projections based on a structural regression model in which the contributions of non-occupational and occupational risk factors can be estimated separately.

In all approaches, the attributable numbers that could be avoided by reducing occupational exposures can be estimated by comparing estimates made for a baseline (no change) or exposure trend scenario with estimates made for intervention scenarios, the latter being based on targeted reductions in exposure levels.

Selected results from the various studies

Nearly 30 years ago Doll and Peto (1981), in their report[21] to the US Congress, presented a method of estimating the effects of different factors on cancer mortality in the US; their estimate for occupational factors was 4% of all US cancer deaths with an uncertainty range of 2–8%. Since then, several other estimates of burden have been made for a range of occupationally related disease. Table 15.1 presents selected results. The estimates for all cancers are not too dissimilar but those for some of the individual cancers vary considerably between studies. Some of the differences can be explained by differences in the numbers of agents considered or in the occupational situations in which exposures occur in different countries, and by different methodological approaches.

There are fewer estimates for non-malignant disease. Most publications assume that 100% of pneumoconioses are attributable to occupational exposure. Again, there is a range of estimates. Steenland et al. (2003)[6] estimated the separate contribution to cardiovascular burden of noise (0–0.6%), job control (3.8–10.4%), shift work (0–3.4%), and environmental tobacco smoke (4.2–6.8% in non-smokers) and also gave separate estimates for asthma (11–21%), tuberculosis (5–24%), and chronic obstructive pulmonary disease (COPD; 5–6%). Driscoll et al. (2005) for the Global Burden of Disease study estimated global attributable fractions of 21% for men and 13% for women for mortality from asthma and of 18% for men and 6% for women for mortality from COPD;[5] Hnizdo et al. (2002) estimated that 19% of prevalent COPD was due to occupation in a US population-based study, 31% in never smokers.[25]

The British Cancer Burden study is perhaps the most detailed study of occupationally related cancers in that it includes all those relevant carcinogens classified at the end of 2008 (the time of the study) by the International Agency on Research into Cancer (IARC) as group 1 (definite) and group 2A (probable) carcinogens.[4] In the British study the attributable fractions ranged from less than 0.01% to 95% overall, the most important cancer sites for occupational attribution being, for men, mesothelioma (97%), sinonasal (46%), lung (21.1%), bladder (7.1%), and non-melanoma skin cancer (7.1%) and, for women, mesothelioma (83%), sinonasal (20.1%), lung (5.3%), breast (4.6%), and nasopharynx (2.5%). Occupation also contributed 2% or more overall to cancers of the larynx, oesophagus, and stomach, and soft tissue sarcoma with, in addition for men, melanoma of the eye (due to welding), and non-Hodgkin lymphoma.

Figure 15.1 shows the attributable total number of cancer registrations (newly occurring incident cancers) from the British study, for cancer sites with ten or more registrations. Lung cancer (21 carcinogens, especially asbestos, silica, diesel engine exhaust (DEE), mineral oils, polycyclic aromatic hydrocarbons (PAHs), environmental tobacco smoke (ETS) in non-smokers, work as a painter or welder, dioxins, radon, arsenic), non-melanoma skin cancer (solar radiation, mineral oils, coal tars/pitches), breast cancer (shift/night work), mesothelioma (asbestos), and bladder cancer (mineral oils, DEE, work as a painter or hairdresser/barber, aromatic amines, PAHs) are the most

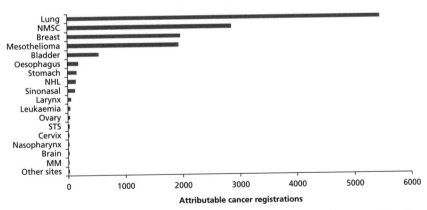

Figure 15.1 Cancer registrations in 2004 attributable to occupation, by cancer site with at least ten total attributable registrations, from the British Cancer Burden study.[4]

Source: data from Rushton L et al., Occupational cancer burden in Great Britain, *British Journal of Cancer* Issue 107, Suppl 1, pp. S3–7, Copyright © 2012 Cancer Research UK. All rights reserved. NMSC = non-melanoma skin cancer, NHL = non-Hodgkin lymphoma, STS = soft tissue sarcoma, MM = multiple myeloma.

prominent cancers. Figure 15.2 shows the attributable registrations for carcinogens resulting in 20 or more registrations a year overall, and for the construction industry. Asbestos is the most important carcinogen, followed by shift/night work, mineral oils, solar radiation, silica, DEE, PAHs from coal tar and pitches, work as a painter, dioxins (2,3,7,8- tetrachlorodibenzo-p-dioxin (TCDD)), ETS, naturally occurring radon, and work as a welder.[4]

The overall results from the occupational risk factors component of the Global Burden of Disease 2010 study illustrate several important aspects of burden studies.[14] Of the estimated 850 000 occupationally related deaths worldwide, the top three causes were: (1) injuries (just over a half of all deaths); (2) particulate matter, gases, and fumes leading to COPD; and (3) carcinogens. When DALYs were used as the burden measure, injuries still accounted for the highest proportion (just over one-third), but ergonomic factors leading to low back pain resulted in almost as many DALYs, and both were almost an order of magnitude higher than the DALYs from carcinogens. The difference in relative contributions of the various risk factors between deaths and DALYs arises because of the varying ages of those affected, and the differing chronicity of the resulting conditions. Both measures are valid, but they represent a different aspect of the burden arising from the hazardous exposures (Table 15.2).

Both the British and Global Burden of Disease studies draw attention to the important issues of: (1) multiple occupational carcinogens causing specific types of cancer, for example, the British study evaluated 21 lung carcinogens; and (2) specific carcinogens causing several different cancers, for example, IARC now defines asbestos as a group 1 or 2A carcinogen for seven cancer sites. These issues require careful consideration for burden estimation and for prioritizing risk reduction strategies.

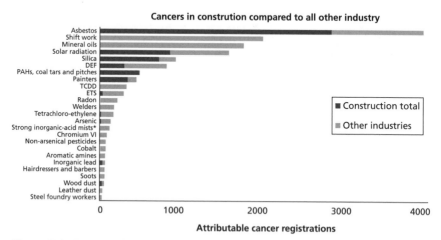

Figure 15.2 Cancer registrations in 2004 attributable to occupation, by exposure with at least 20 total attributable registrations, in construction and in all other industries, from the British Cancer Burden study.[4] * containing sulphuric acid

Source: data from Rushton L et al., Occupational cancer burden in Great Britain, *British Journal of Cancer* Issue 107, Suppl 1, pp. S3–7, Copyright © 2012 Cancer Research UK. All rights reserved.

Table 15.2 Global deaths and DALYS by main occupational risk factor, from the Global Burden of Disease 2010 study[14]

	Deaths	% deaths	DALYs ('000s)	% DALYs
Injuries	481 625	56.5	23 446	37.5
Particulate matter, gases, and fumes leading to COPD	218 904	25.7	9143	14.6
Carcinogens	118 107	13.9	2682	4.3
Asthmagens	33 722	4.0	2020	3.2
Noise	0	–	3451	5.5
Ergonomic factors leading to low back pain	0	–	21 750	34.8
Total	852 358	100.0	62 492	100.0

Source: data from *The Lancet*, Volume **380**, Lim SS et al., A comparative risk assessment of burden of disease and injury attributable to 67 risk factors and risk factor clusters in 21 regions, 1990–2010: a systematic analysis for the Global Burden of Disease Study 2010, pp. 2224–60, Copyright © 2012, published by Elsevier Ltd.

The British study, unlike many other previous studies, estimated burden within industry sectors, with high numbers of attributable cancer deaths and registrations being found in construction, metal-working, personal/household services, mining, land transport, printing/publishing, retail/hotels/restaurants, public administration/defence, farming, and several manufacturing sectors (Table 15.3).[27] Note that, like the Global Burden of Disease results in Table 15.2, the ranking of the industry sectors varies between the burden measures shown in Table 15.3. The majority of industry sectors involve exposure to several carcinogens (many to over ten), with construction and many of the manufacturing sectors involving potential exposure to between 15 and 20 carcinogens. Several key exposures give rise to substantial numbers of registrations across multiple industry sectors, for example see Figure 15.1 for the construction industry and Figure 15.3 for personal and household services (this sector includes repair trades, laundries and dry cleaning, domestic services, hairdressing, and beauty).

Future burden prediction

The current burden results from the British study identified priority carcinogens and industry sectors of concern. An example from the prediction element of the project for respirable crystalline silica and lung cancer illustrates how various reduction strategies can be compared to aid policymakers in choosing a preferred option.[20] The workplace exposure limit (WEL) for respirable crystalline silica at the time of the study (2011) was 0.1 mg/m³. Average exposure levels in the construction industry, where much of the exposure now occurs, were known to be about 0.23 mg/m³, an estimated compliance to the WEL of about 33%. The intervention scenarios tested are described in Table 15.4 together with PAFs and the numbers of attributable cancer registrations for

Table 15.3 Estimates of population attributable fraction (PAF), deaths, and registrations for selected industries with at least 100 attributable cancer registrations, from the British Cancer Burden study[27]

Industry/occupation	No. of agents included in PAF estimate[a]	PAF (%)[b]	Attributable deaths	Attributable cancer registrations
Construction				
Construction	16 (2)	2.30	3457	4668
Painters and decorators (construction)	1 (0)	0.17	254	334
Roofers, road surfacers, roadmen, pavers (construction)	1 (0)	0.00	4	471
Service industry sectors				
Shift work[c]	1 (0)	0.37	552	1957
Personal and household services	17 (2)	0.37	556	670
Land transport	13 (2)	0.28	414	497
Public administration and defence	6 (1)	0.02	31	273
Wholesale/retail trade, restaurants/hotels	9 (1)	0.14	211	246
Manufacturing				
Metal workers	1 (0)	0.19	284	1252
Mining	10 (0)	0.15	228	296
Printing, publishing, allied industries	14 (5)	0.16	243	282
Manufacture of instruments, photographic, and optical goods	13 (5)	0.03	49	206
Manufacture of transport equipment	19 (4)	0.10	155	182
Work as welder	2 (0)	0.10	153	181
Non-ferrous metal basic industries	18 (0)	0.08	119	156
Iron and steel basic industries	17 (1)	0.06	84	135
Manufacture of other chemical products	19 (3)	0.07	103	119
Manufacture of industrial chemicals	23 (3)	0.07	99	116
Manufacture of machinery (not electrical)	18 (5)	0.06	91	111
Painters (not construction)	1 (0)	0.05	79	102

(Continued)

Table 15.3 (*Continued*)

Industry/occupation	No. of agents included in PAF estimate[a]	PAF (%)[b]	Attributable deaths	Attributable cancer registrations
Agriculture, fishing, and forestry				
Farming	5 (1)	0.04	65	220
Total	42 (0)	5.3	8010	13 598

[a] Number of agents with negligible risk in this industry (RR = 1) is shown in brackets. [b] Based on deaths.
[c] Women only.

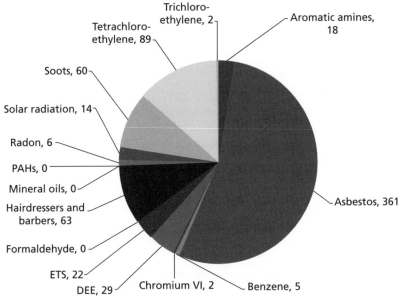

Figure 15.3 Cancer registrations in 2004 by carcinogenic agent in the industry sector Personal and Household Services, from the British Cancer Burden study.[27]

forecast year 2060 when past exposures would no longer have an effect. The reduction in that year is compared with the baseline scenario of no change. Forecast numbers of cancers have been estimated by applying predicted PAFs to future cancer numbers predicted on projected demographic change only, so that future changes due to non-occupational risk factors such as smoking do not affect the estimates.

Table 15.4 Forecast lung cancers for 2060 attributable to occupational exposure to respirable crystalline silica and avoidable numbers for a range of intervention scenarios, from the British Cancer Burden study.[20]

Intervention scenario		PAF (%)	Attributable cancer registrations	Cancer registrations avoided
	Current burden (2010)	2.07	837	
(1)	Current (2005) employment/exposure levels maintained, WEL = 0.1 mg/m³	1.08	794	
To test introduction of a reduced exposure standard, compliance 33%				
(2)	Introduce exposure standard = 0.05 mg/m³ in 2010	0.80	592	202
(3)	Introduce exposure standard = 0.025 mg/m³ in 2010	0.56	409	385
To test timing of introduction of a reduced exposure standard, compliance 33%				
(4)	Introduce exposure standard = 0.05 mg/m³ in 2020	0.90	666	128
(5)	Introduce exposure standard = 0.05 mg/m³ in 2030	1.02	753	42
To test effect of introducing lower exposure standards versus compliance rate				
(6)	Maintain exposure standard = 0.1 mg/m³ in 2010, compliance 90%, all workplaces	0.14	102	693
(7)	Introduce exposure standard = 0.05 mg/m³ in 2010, compliance 90%, all workplaces	0.07	49	745
(8)	Introduce exposure standard = 0.025 mg/m in 2010, compliance 90%, all workplaces	0.03	21	773
To test effect of compliance by workplace size to introduction of exposure standard 0.05 mg/m³ in 2010				
(9)	33% compliance in workplaces employing 0–249, 90% compliance in workplaces employing 250+	0.68	499	295
(10)	33% compliance in workplaces employing 0–49, 90% compliance in workplaces employing 50+	0.61	451	344
(11)	33% compliance in self-employed, 90% compliance in other workplaces	0.35	261	533
(12)	90% compliance in all workplaces	0.07	49	745

Adapted with permission from Hutchings SJ, Rushton L, Towards risk reduction: predicting the future burden of occupational cancer, *American Journal of Epidemiology*, Volume **173**, Issue 9, pp. 1069–1077, Copyright © 2011 Johns Hopkins Bloomberg School of Public Health, published Oxford University Press.

Table 15.4 illustrates that numbers of attributable cancers are forecast to gradually decrease and numbers avoided increase by introducing reduced WELs, even at the current compliance rate of 33% (scenarios 2 and 3 compared to baseline scenario 1 in Table 15.4). However, given the poor compliance to the current standard, policymakers might conclude that this is an impractical option. The effectiveness of enforcement compared to lowering the WEL is shown by comparing scenarios 1 to 3 with scenarios 6 to 8 in which compliance is improved to 90% simultaneously with reduction of the WEL. Retaining the current WEL of 1 mg/m³ and improving compliance to 90% (scenario 6) is forecast to avoid 693 cancers compared with halving the WEL to 0.05 mg/m³ and keeping compliance at 33% (scenario 2) for which only 202 cancers are avoided. These six scenarios are illustrated graphically, in terms of attributable cancers per year and attributable fractions for each prediction year, in Figure 15.4. Numbers of cancers tend to rise from the baseline scenario due to rising numbers of total projected lung cancers caused by an ageing population. An important message from this graph is the lack of any reduction in cancers until after 2030 from any of the interventions, due to the long latency of lung cancer. Other scenarios tested demonstrate the importance of improving compliance in the smaller as well as larger workplaces (745 cancers avoided per year by 2060 if all workplaces are targeted, 295 if only the largest are compliant, scenarios 9 to 12). This highlights the comparative predominance of small enterprises, particularly in the construction industry which is the most important industry sector for potential silica exposure, and of early rather than delayed intervention (scenarios 4 and 5).

Discussion

Burden of disease methods provide a useful means of assessing the absolute and relative contribution of a range of occupational exposures to the ill health of the community. However, they require a number of assumptions. These include, in particular, uncertainties and inaccuracies in the data used, which may introduce bias into the estimates. Potential sources of bias for PAFs include inappropriate choice of risk estimates, imprecision in the risk estimates and estimates of proportions exposed, inaccurate risk exposure period and latency assumptions, and a lack of separate risk estimates in some cases for women and/or cancer incidence. In addition, a key decision is the choice of which diseases and exposures are to be included. Cancer burden studies often use IARC groups 1 and/or 2A carcinogens. The omission of other occupational carcinogens where human studies are defined by IARC as limited (IARC group 2B) may lead to underestimation, but equally their inclusion may lead to an overestimation.

Nevertheless, the results from these studies provide a large amount of information to facilitate development of risk reduction strategies depending on the focus of any proposed intervention. A focus on prevention of deaths might target exposures resulting in potentially fatal diseases, such as myocardial infarction, or poor survival diseases, such as lung cancer and mesothelioma. In contrast, focus on prevention of incidence might target exposures resulting in diseases such as non-melanoma skin cancer which is very common but rarely fatal. Certain diseases might be of national concern, such as COPD, which is common in the general population and a major cost

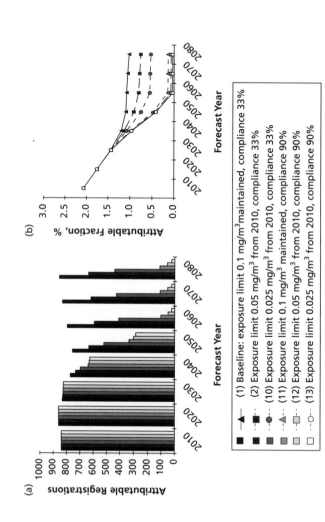

Figure 15.4 Effect of reducing workplace exposure limits and improving compliance for respirable crystalline silica associated with lung cancer, six scenarios (see Table 15.4) from the British Cancer Burden study.[20]

Reproduced with permission from Hutchings SJ, Rushton L, Towards risk reduction: predicting the future burden of occupational cancer, *American Journal of Epidemiology*, Volume **173**, Issue 9, pp. 1069–1077, Copyright © 2011 Johns Hopkins Bloomberg School of Public Health, published Oxford University Press.

to health services. One could target substances with both a high risk and high levels of exposures, or focus on more ubiquitous substances where, although levels of exposure may be low, large numbers of workers are exposed, for example, in service industries. An industry sector approach could be considered where multiple exposures and diseases occur; for example, targeting dusts and fumes as a whole in the construction industry would potentially reduce both respiratory disease and cancers.

The long latency of many cancers means that estimates of current burden are based on exposures occurring in the past, often much higher than those existing today. Many will have been decreasing gradually over time, others have disappeared due to the decline of the industry or the substitution of hazardous substances by other agents. The British study has demonstrated, however, that long latency means that risk reduction measures taken now will take a considerable time to be reflected in reduced disease incidence.

In summary, this chapter has outlined different methods of estimating the burden of occupational disease, illustrated with results from different studies. The potential to be simultaneously exposed to several hazardous substances which may affect multiple diseases has been highlighted. Disease burden methodology has the advantage that it facilitates the evaluation of both high exposures, perhaps only experienced by a few workers, leading to high risks of disease, and also low exposures and low risks experienced by large numbers of workers. The methods have the potential to be adapted for wider use in different occupational circumstances, applied to the general environment, and for extension for social and economic impact evaluation.

References

1. Lopez AD, Mathers CD, Ezzati M, Jamison DT, Murray CJL. Global and regional burden of disease and risk factors, 2001: systematic analysis of population health data. *Lancet* 2006;**367**:1747–57.

2. Brown ML, Lipscomb J, Snyder C. The burden of illness of cancer: economic cost and quality of life. *Annu Rev Public Health* 2001;**22**:91–113.

3. Danaeii G, Vander Hoorn S, Lopez AD, Murray CJL, Ezzati M. Causes of cancer in the world: comparative risk assessment of nine behavioural and environmental risk factors. *Lancet* 2005;**366**:1784–93.

4. Rushton L, Hutchings SJ, Fortunato L, *et al.* Occupational cancer burden in Great Britain. *Br J Cancer* 2012;**107**(Suppl 1):S3–7.

5. Driscoll T, Nelson DI, Steenland K, *et al.* The global burden of disease due to occupational carcinogens. *Am J Ind Med* 2005;**48**:419–31.

6. Steenland K, Burnett C, Lalich N, Ward E, Hurrell J. Dying for work: the magnitude of US mortality from selected causes of death associated with occupation. *Am J Ind Med* 2003;**43**:461–82.

7. Nurminen M, Karjalainen A. Epidemiologic estimate of the proportion of fatalities related to occupational factors in Finland. *Scand J Work Environ Health* 2001;**27**:161–213.

8. Kauppinen T, Toikkanen J, Pedersen D, *et al. Occupational exposure to carcinogens in the European Union in 1990–93. CAREX: international information system on occupational exposure to carcinogens.* Helsinki: Finnish Institute of Occupational Health, 1998. Available at: <http://www.ttl.fi/en/chemical_safety/carex/Documents/1_description_and_summary_of_results.pdf> (accessed 23 February 2013).

9. **Miettinen O.** Proportion of disease caused or prevented by a given exposure, trait or intervention. *Am J Epidemiol* 1974;**99**:325–32.

10. **Hutchings SJ, Rushton L.** Occupational cancer in Britain. Statistical methodology. *Br J Cancer* 2012;**107**(Suppl 1):S8–17

11. **Levin ML.** The occurrence of lung cancer in man. *Acta Unio Int Contra Cancrum* 1953;**9**:531–41.

12. **Greenland S.** Interval estimation by simulation as an alternative to and extension of confidence intervals. *Int J Epidemiol* 2004;**33**:1389–97.

13. **Dreyer L, Andersen A, Pukkala E.** Avoidable cancers in the Nordic countries. Occupation. *APMIS Suppl* 1997;**76**:68–79.

14. **Lim SS, Vos T, Flaxman AD,** *et al.* A comparative risk assessment of burden of disease and injury attributable to 67 risk factors and risk factor clusters in 21 regions, 1990–2010: a systematic analysis for the Global Burden of Disease Study 2010. *Lancet* 2012; **380**:2224–60.

15. **Steenland K, Armstrong B.** An overview of methods for calculating the burden of disease due to specific risk factors. *Epidemiology* 2006;**17**:512–9.

16. **Darnton AJ, McElvenny DM, Hodgson JT.** Estimating the number of asbestos-related lung cancer deaths in Great Britain from 1980 to 2000. *Ann Occup Hyg* 2006;**50**:29–38.

17. **Nelson DI, Concha-Barrientos M, Driscoll T,** *et al.* The global burden of selected occupational diseases and injury risks: methodology and summary. *Am J Ind Med* 2005;**48**:400–18.

18. **Fox-Rushby JA, Hanson K.** Calculating and presenting disability adjusted life years (DALYs) in cost-effectiveness analysis. *Health Policy Plan* 2011;**16**:326–31.

19. **Murray CJL, Vos T, Lozano R,** *et al.* Disability-adjusted life years (DALYs) for 291 disease and injuries in 21 regions, 1990–2010: a systematic analysis for the Global Burden of Disease Study 2010. *Lancet* 2012;**380**:2197–223.

20. **Hutchings SJ, Rushton L.** Towards risk reduction: predicting the future burden of occupational cancer. *Am J Epidemiol* 2011;**173**:1069–77.

21. **Doll R, Peto R.** The causes of cancer: quantitative estimates of avoidable risks of cancer in the United States today. *J Natl Cancer Inst* 1981;**66**:1191–308. (Reprinted: Oxford: Oxford University Press, 1981.)

22. **Leigh JP, Markowitz SB, Fahs M, Shin C, Landrigan PJ.** Occupational injury and illness in the United States. Estimates of costs, morbidity, and mortality. *Arch Internal Med*, 1997;**157**:1557–68.

23. **'t Mannetje A, Kogevinas M, Luce D,** *et al.* Sinonasal cancer, occupation, and tobacco smoking in European women and men. *Am J Ind Med* 1999;**36**:101–7.

24. **Landrigan PJ, Markowitz S.** Current magnitude of occupational disease in the United States. Estimates from New York State. *Ann N Y Acad Sci* 1989;**572**:27–45, discussion 55–80.

25. **Hnizdo E, Sullivan PA, Bang KM, Wagner G.** Association between chronic obstructive pulmonary disease and employment by industry and occupation in the US population: a study of data from the Third National Health and Nutrition Examination Survey. *Am J Epidemiol* 2002;**156**:738–46.

26. **Weinmann S, Vollmer WM, Breen V,** *et al.* COPD and occupational exposures: a case-control study. *J Occup Environ Med* 2008;**50**:561–9.

27. **Hutchings SJ, Rushton L, British Occupational Cancer Burden Study Group.** Occupational cancer in Britain. Industry sector results. *Br J Cancer* 2012;**107**(Suppl 1):S92–103.

Part 6

Applying new concepts to occupational epidemiology

Chapter 16

Biologically based exposure assessment for epidemiology

Thomas J. Smith and David Kriebel

Introduction: surpassing John Snow

John Snow's identification of the link between polluted water and cholera is probably the most famous success story of environmental epidemiology.[1] His work is still cited 150 years later to illustrate the power of epidemiology to detect risks with astute powers of observation, very simple mathematics, and no known causal mechanism (or putting it more plainly, an incorrect causal mechanism). Today, with greatly advanced understanding of disease mechanisms and sophisticated tools for measuring pollutants, epidemiologists should be able to do an even better job than John Snow of identifying environmental health hazards. And while we believe there are many examples of this advance, there is still much to be learned about how best to design studies and analyse occupational and environmental and health data in order to identify hazards sooner and at lower levels of exposure. We believe that in many of the relevant sciences, improvements in our measurement tools have outpaced our understanding of the theoretical framework which underlays efforts to detect small risks to population health. This chapter is a contribution towards building that framework. We believe that exposure-risk relations can best be detected and quantified when the entire enterprise of data gathering and analysis is based on a clearly stated hypothesis about the biological processes which link exposure to disease.

John Snow's ability to detect a link between polluted water and cholera illustrates both a strength and a limitation of epidemiology. The strength is more often discussed—the idea that it is not necessary to have a hypothesis about the mechanism underlying an exposure-disease association in order to detect and prevent a disease. But this strong empiricism is also a limitation because important weak associations may be missed. If, for example, we do not measure the actual causal agent (the *Vibrio cholerae* bacterium in Snow's work) but out of ignorance study a factor which is more-or-less well correlated with it (the private company providing drinking water to the different wells of London), then we run the risk of failing to detect the association through dilution of the true effect (epidemiologists call this misclassification). From this perspective, we would argue that Snow succeeded because the link between *Vibrio cholerae* and water company was very strong—water from the Southwark and Vauxhall Company was very polluted, while that from the competing Lambeth Company was not. Snow would not have been so successful had the difference in cholera contamination been less striking. The modern epidemiologist is often faced with shades of difference in risk—nothing like the stark pattern observed by Snow. We believe that the 'black box' epidemiology inspired by John Snow is reaching its limits, and we propose a systematic approach to pushing back those limits by incorporating biological or toxicological evidence into the design and conduct of exposure assessments and epidemiological investigations.

Inside the black box: exposure, [BLACK BOX], response

When we look inside the black box, we are examining the complex and dynamic biological processes that lead to disease, but do we need the full complexity of the mechanism? The observable quantitative relationship between exposure and disease is a consequence of a series of temporal processes—a chain or web of linked steps occurring through time, such as cell damage and repair. The concentration in the target tissue causes damage, such as cell death or inflammation. If the exposure causes sufficient damage or response, then pre-clinical effects may be detectable by some tests. When sufficient damage has occurred, a clinical disease diagnosis may be detectable. The toxic damage may also trigger secondary processes, such as apoptosis, or repair of the damage. Once exposure stops, some or all of the adverse effects may be repaired, while others once initiated may continue to progress without further exposure. We often move back and forth between description of pathological processes within an individual and the population distribution of some response or disease outcome. At the individual level, the terms 'response', 'outcome', and 'effect' will often be used interchangeably. At the population level, the 'risk' or probability of some particular effect or outcome is most often the object of study.

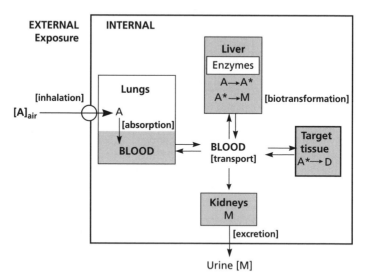

Figure 16.1 Typical example of processes of uptake, transport throughout the body, biotransformation and excretion. Boxes are tissues and arrows are transport or transformation processes. Toxin A enters through inhalation, is transformed into active agent A* in the liver, and leads to tissue damage D in the target tissue. A* is also broken down into a metabolite M which is eliminated through the kidneys.

Reproduced from Ch. 1 *A Biologic Approach to Environmental Assessment and Epidemiology* by Smith, Thomas J. and Kriebel, David (2010). By permission of Oxford University Press, USA.

Exposures and effects are linked by dynamic processes occurring across time. These processes can often be usefully decomposed into two distinct biological relationships, each with several components:

1. The *exposure-dose relationship*, consisting of:

    a. *uptake* of a toxic material from the environment and into the body via one or more of three common routes: inhalation, ingestion, and skin absorption.

    b. *transport* of the agent to the target tissue, and possibly also metabolic activation into a toxic form.

2. The *dose-effect relationship*, consisting of:

    a. the temporal pattern or *time course* of the concentration of the active agent in the target tissue, which is the direct cause of the effect.

    b. *early or intermediate pathophysiological responses*, which are the results of damage processes, that may be repaired or lead to secondary effects.

    c. a *clinical response* detected as signs and symptoms, loss of function, or the onset of disease, once a sufficient dose has been reached.

These two component relationships are sometimes represented by two different mathematical models: a toxicokinetic model (Figure 16.1), and a disease process model (Figure 16.2). Depending on the information available, these models may be relatively simple or highly complex. A disease process model is a description

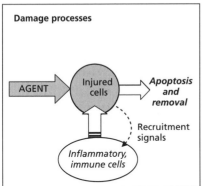
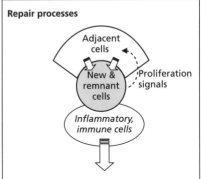

Figure 16.2 Basic damage-repair model. All cellular processes are controlled by cell signalling, which initiates and stimulates them. Feedback signals (not shown) can limit or prevent some damage processes. In the first panel, damage to molecular targets, such as DNA or cell wall proteins, leads to injury or death of cells. Cell injury/death recruits inflammatory cells of the immune system to the area. A strong inflammatory response can directly injure cells and lead to a feedback loop, which can prolong the damage response. The second panel represents the principal repair processes involving cell proliferation and rebuilding of tissue architecture. Inflammatory cells die or leave the area, and repair signalling decreases to normal levels. Misrepair and exaggerated stimulation of cell proliferation are important causes of long-term irreversible effects.
Reproduced from Ch. 1 *A Biologic Approach to Environmental Assessment and Epidemiology* by Smith, Thomas J. and Kriebel, David (2010). By permission of Oxford University Press, USA.

of the pathophysiological mechanisms that lead to the observable adverse effects over time. This biological model will usually have several components, such as damage and death of target cells, and tissue repair that replaces dead cells; the 'damage-repair model' is one common generic type of disease process model. Often the various steps in the disease process do not occur at the same rate, some of these processes are 'fast', such as cell killing, while others are 'slow', such as damage repair. Frequently a few slow steps in a process become limiting to the overall rate, which sets the temporal pattern for the entire exposure-response relationship. We propose a relatively simple but useful disease process model (Figure 16.2) that can be defined from observational data (clinical findings, subject and research reports) just by noting the apparent slow rate-limiting steps, because they define the overall pace of the process.

In this chapter, we argue that formal disease process models have the potential to improve the sensitivity of epidemiology for detecting new and emerging occupational and environmental risks where there is limited mechanistic information. A disease process model is a set of quantitative statements that describe how biological factors are modified over time by processes in response to external and internal characteristics. However, making this potential a reality means explicitly defining exposure-disease hypotheses in simple models as shown here using the example of silicosis:

1. *Biological factors* (quantities)—the quantity of fibrotic tissue, or number of macrophages, or opacity of chest radiographs, inhaled concentration of airborne toxicant, or tissue concentration of signalling proteins or of a toxicant in the tissue.

2. *Processes* (change quantities)—inhalation of particles and their lung deposition, or formation of fibrosis on deposited particles, or kidney clearance of a metabolite.

3. *Process model*—example of a model for forming lung fibrosis by particles:

   total fibrosis (at t + Δt) = total fibrosis (at t) + new fibrosis (during Δt), where new fibrosis forms on the crystalline silica dust deposited in the lungs.

In our approach, these models are often used to create exposure or dose metrics, which are in turn used in epidemiological models to estimate exposure-disease associations.

Suppose, for example, we want to study an acute illness that occurs in response to chemical exposures within the past 24 hours. When exposure ends, this illness also ends and its effects are repaired within 24–48 hours with no further exposure. Knowing this (or correctly hypothesizing it), one would not choose to study the lifetime average exposure, because this will probably show little or no relationship to the risk of the acute effect. However, if each acute illness leaves an undetectable small amount of irreversible damage, then, after many repeated illnesses over a lifetime, lifetime cumulative exposure may be related to the accumulated damage. This is a simple example, but often researchers are not systematic in their choice of metrics, allowing implicit assumptions to guide their choices rather than formal statements of hypothesized mechanisms.

It is not necessary to know the full mechanism of effects to guide selection of an exposure-response model or exposure metric. Because of the strong influence of the rate-limiting steps, often it is only necessary to have observations on the approximate time course of effects. This is true whether the effects appear to be reversible or irreversible, and whether damage progresses proportionately with each unit of exposure (actually dose) or instead occurs suddenly, and seemingly without regard to the amount of exposure, such as an asthma attack. These fairly simple qualitative characteristics of apparent exposure-response relationships can provide useful guidance to the entire investigation of the health effects of an environmental or occupational hazard.

Timing is everything

The responses or effects we observe do not occur instantaneously. They develop over time depending on an agent's specific pathophysiological mechanism. The tissue concentration of the active agent and its variability over time are the causes of those effects. Although timescales for some effects may be measured in seconds, others may be measured in years. The observed response at a point in time (marked on Figure 16.3) is usually the net result of an array of both damage and repair processes, because these generally operate concurrently.[2] We have developed an approach for describing the quantitative relationship between the *observed* response at t_{obs} and the intensity and duration of past exposures. The repair process is critical for the shape of the response time course. For example, if there was no repair, then the response line in Figure 16.3

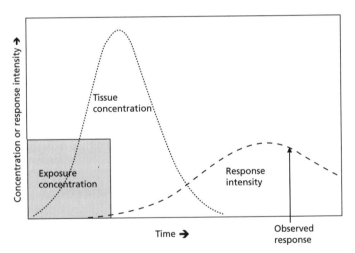

Figure 16.3 Simplified schematic showing how an exposure across time (shaded box = dose) produces a tissue concentration (dotted line), which in turn produces a tissue response (dashed line). Because these are temporal processes, a different exposure-response relationship will be observed depending on when we measure the response.

Reproduced from Ch. 1 *A Biologic Approach to Environmental Assessment and Epidemiology* by Smith, Thomas J. and Kriebel, David (2010). By permission of Oxford University Press, USA.

would plateau after the tissue concentration curve came down to zero again. Thus, the behaviour of the response or disease over time clearly indicates if there is repair or not.

Where these toxicological mechanisms have been studied, research shows them to be quite complex. Another important and useful principle is the independence of local repair processes. For example, consider a small paper cut on your finger; the damage is done in a fraction of a second, while the repair takes a week or longer. If you were unfortunate enough to get a second, similar cut on your finger while the first was healing, the repair of the second one would take about the same time, and would be unaffected by the presence of the first cut, which illustrates the principle of local independence that occurs for many non-systemic processes. If on the other hand (sorry for the pun!), you received a more severe cut, it would probably require more time to repair, and if you get hit by a bus…well,…the damage may overwhelm the repair process. In summary, each instance of damage is repaired independently (when the effects are not overwhelming), and the amount of repair per unit time is roughly proportional to the amount of damage, an approximately fixed percentage. The rate of repair can be estimated from clinical data.

Discrete effects, such as asthma attacks or other immunologically mediated events, are another distinct type of adverse effect. Their temporal dynamics are quite different from the basic damage-repair model we have been discussing. The important characteristic of this type of effect is that once triggered, the strength and duration of response are not determined wholly by the magnitude of the triggering exposure or dose. An asthma attack is triggered by a complex self-propagating cascade of molecular and neural signals, which lead to the response. More generally we observe that the likelihood or probability of a discrete (yes/no) response like an asthma attack is proportional to the magnitude of the initial triggering event or exposure. Thus, the dose-response relationship that defines the *probability* of a response is a quantal relationship, such as a logistic relationship, that is proportional to the magnitude of the triggering dose, such as the exposure multiplied by its duration. Another very important type of discrete response is cancer. The probability of a cancer developing from a chemical exposure will be proportional to some function of the dose of the carcinogen, although the proportionality may be more strongly related to the duration than the intensity of the exposure.

Dynamic versus static models: a key distinction

Our approach develops the idea of using biologically based models of disease processes that occur dynamically through time as the biological system responds to changes in exposure and internal conditions. Like the standard statistical models widely used in epidemiology, our models also are meant to describe relationships between exposure and disease in populations. However, there are important differences in our approach. In general, statistical epidemiological models are not intended to represent disease mechanisms, but to be empirical representations of the 'black box' (unspecified) relationships. In particular, these models implicitly assume that there is a single proportionality constant describing the relationship between exposure and risk or response.

This proportionality is assumed to be invariant over time, static, and the same among all the members of the study population. A relative risk in a case-control study, or a slope parameter in a linear regression model estimating rate of loss of pulmonary function per unit of exposure are examples of such proportionality constants. To distinguish these statistical models from the biological process or dynamic models we are proposing, we call models with invariant proportionality constants linking exposure and response *static*. The word 'linear' is also sometimes used, but static may be more appropriate because linear has many different interpretations and because it is not so much the 'straightness' of the exposure-response relationship that distinguishes these models but the time-invariant nature of the proportionality between exposure and response.

The idea that each pack-year of smoking causes a fixed amount of loss in pulmonary function implies a static exposure-response model, however, long-term studies have shown this is not the case. Models of noise-induced hearing loss are static if they are based only on the assumption that hearing loss is proportional to the number of hours of exposure to noise above 90 dB(A), for example, without considering that your history of noise exposure is a biological process leading to hearing loss. Repeated short periods of intense noise may cause much more hearing loss than a much lower steady exposure. Most models that have been used in cancer epidemiology are static, such as pack-years of smoking cause a fixed amount of risk, with the exception of certain multiple stage models,[3] in which the risk conveyed by a unit of exposure may vary with the stage of the disease process and with the pattern of exposure in earlier time periods.

Biological models

Physiological and toxicological processes, in contrast to epidemiological models, are not static. The degree of response of an individual to a given unit of toxin exposure can vary over time, as a function of past exposure or responses. Models exhibiting this behaviour are dynamic. Epidemiologists are quite familiar with exposure-response relationships that change with age or have secular trends. These could be considered dynamic in one sense, but we reserve the term for models in which the parameter(s) defining exposure are themselves temporal functions of working or other environmental conditions and/or the individual's response to that exposure. Two basic classes can be distinguished: those in which the most recent unit of exposure (dose) carries the same risk to everyone, no matter what the individual's past history of exposure has been, and those in which the entire history or a portion of exposure-response can determine the effect of the next unit of an individual's exposure.

The former is the standard, static, assumption of most epidemiological models. Suppose that an epidemiologist has chosen to summarize each participant's exposure history as 'cumulative exposure' (CE) and is regressing risk on CE with an appropriate multivariate model (a Cox model, for example). Implicit in these choices is the assumption that every individual in the study with the same CE faces the same risk (from exposure)—it matters not whether the pattern of exposure was, for example, many years at low intensity or a few years at very high intensity as shown in Equation 16.1:

$$CE = \sum_{i=1}^{N} C_i \times t_i$$

Equation 16.1 calculation of cumulative exposure, where i counts consecutive time intervals.

The same holds true with other standard summary measures of exposure (average exposure, duration, peak exposure) and other standard exposure-response models.

Now consider that previous exposures inhibit normal toxic agent clearance or repair processes in the target tissue. The result would be to increase the magnitude of the effect of later units of exposure compared to earlier ones. This would violate the assumption underlying the static model. It could also be violated when the toxic agent is a metabolite produced by an enzymatic activation of the agent that is saturable, so that low exposures which do not exceed the saturation level will have a larger effect per unit than exposures that begin to saturate the metabolic system. Asthma is another example where a dynamic model would be more appropriate: the asthmatic subject exhibits an extreme sensitivity to an agent because of an immunological response mechanism not present in that individual before the development of asthma. The incremental response to a unit of the relevant toxic exposure after asthma onset will be much greater than in the same individual before onset. The airway responses to ozone represent another example where a static model may be inappropriate. Ozone causes a 'simple' inflammatory effect in the airways as a result of the oxidation of epithelial cell membranes leading to the leakage of inflammatory mediators and the stimulation of irritant receptors in the airway walls. No immunological mechanisms are believed to be involved, but it is clear that the degree of response to an increment of ozone exposure depends on the recent history of ozone exposure and the degree of inflammation of the airways.[4] Volunteers exposed a few hours each day to a moderately irritating level of ozone (300–600 ppb) show the largest lung function effect on one of the first days of exposure, and by the fourth or fifth day of exposure no drop in lung function is observed between pre- and post-exposure measurements. A change in responsiveness to ozone also occurs: bronchoconstriction seen in pulmonary function tests is often greater on the second than the first day of a week-long protocol of brief (2-hour) exposures. Thus, any dynamic model which seeks to represent the full range of ozone's effects on the airways should be capable of showing both enhanced and diminished responses, depending on the precise timing and intensity of repeated exposures.

As a general principle, we can say that any disease in which repair mechanisms are stimulated by injury would be expected to exhibit dynamic behaviour. Cancer, heart disease, low back pain, neurological or respiratory symptoms, infectious diseases, immunological and inflammatory diseases, are examples of diseases which fall into this category.

Many of the dynamic physiological processes described involve complex interactions between exposure and pathophysiological responses over time. Traditional epidemiological statistical models are structured as if individuals experience just one sudden transition from health to disease, or from alive to dead. The whole history of the individual leading up to the moment of incidence of the disease is summarized in a series of independent variables, some of which may be measures of temporal factors, such as time since first exposure or cumulative exposure. This seems an overly narrow perspective when we realize how fundamental time is to the biological, and especially pathological, processes that we seek to describe with our models. Time is the dimension in which the toxin and the organism interact to produce the disease state. To put it another way, it is the temporal dynamics of exposure and response that must be studied to fully understand a disease process.

Time lags in response

Time lags are common in biological processes, and their existence is well known to epidemiologists and toxicologists. However, time lags resulting from biological processes may lead to far more complex exposure-response patterns than can be accommodated by standard static methods, like ignoring the 10 or 20 years of exposure immediately prior to cancer diagnosis, or associating response at t_1 with exposure at t_{1-lag}. Suppose, for example, that exposure to a respiratory irritant causes an immediate bronchoconstrictive response as well as a delayed recruitment of inflammatory cells into the airway walls from the bloodstream. This latter response also causes bronchoconstriction, but more slowly than the direct irritant effect. Suppose further that the amount of delay between exposure and in-migration of cells into an area of damage is a function of the degree of initial inflammation (an assumption well supported by experimental data).[4] Under these conditions, assessment of the bronchoconstrictive response to brief pulses of exposures might show little or no consistent trend over varying exposure intensities, and a simple lagged exposure variable would not perform well either because the effect is being driven by the intensity of the slow inflammatory response.

A set of graphs may help to contrast alternative ways that time can be handled in occupational and environmental epidemiology (Figures 16.4–16.6). In the standard approach, a summary measure of exposure, CE, for example, is calculated for each subject as in Equation 16.1. At the end of the study period, the moment at which the outcome is evaluated, or the moment of disease onset, subjects are compared to evaluate differences in CE, the summary measure of exposure, between diseased and non-diseased groups. If the summary measures of exposure do not differ between diseased and non-diseased, then it is concluded that exposure is not associated with disease. Figure 16.4 illustrates the standard approach. In this example, the data consist of annual average exposures, so all t_i values are 1 year. The two subjects in Figure 16.4 have identical values of CE, determined at the end of the 10-year time interval shown. Notice though, that subject 1 has a different temporal pattern of exposure than subject 2; the former's early years were rather heavily exposed, while the latter's history is characterized by fairly constant exposures. Do these differences in the pattern of exposure affect the risks faced by these two individuals? Perhaps, and perhaps not—the answer clearly depends on the disease process. But if the investigator chooses to summarize exposure using CE, then implicit in this choice is the assumption that the temporal patterns *do not matter*—only the final value of CE affects risk. Thus the choice of summary measure of exposure carries with it implicit assumptions about the underlying disease process.

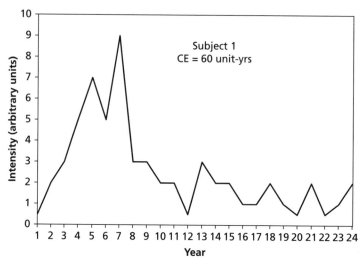

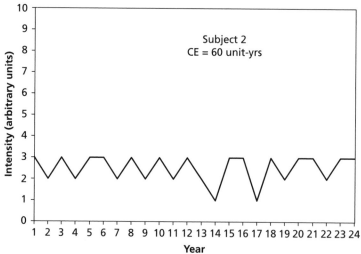

Figure 16.4 Illustration of alternative treatments of the temporal dynamics of exposure and response in epidemiological models. The exposure profiles (arbitrary units) of two subjects with the same cumulative exposures (CE) are shown.

Reproduced from Ch. 1 *A Biologic Approach to Environmental Assessment and Epidemiology* by Smith, Thomas J. and Kriebel, David (2010). By permission of Oxford University Press, USA.

Time windows of susceptibility

This limitation of cumulative exposure is well recognized,[5,6] and 'time windows of exposure' have been advocated as a solution.[6,7] The exposure history of each subject can be partitioned into time windows (usually constructed *backwards* from the time of disease onset), and then the exposure in each window is separately summarized with a summary measure like CE. This approach is illustrated in Figure 16.5. For the two subjects in our example, this has the advantage that in the earliest time window subject 1 has a higher CE than subject 2. Now, instead of one summary measure of exposure there are three, and when these are fitted to the outcome data, the early exposure differences between these two subjects may be found to affect their risks.

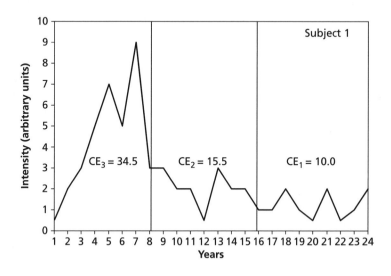

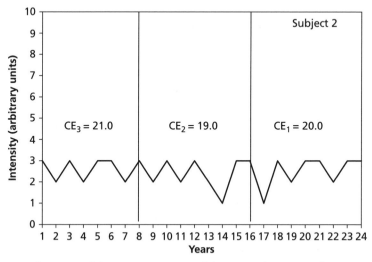

Figure 16.5 Illustration of alternative treatments of the temporal dynamics of exposure and response in epidemiological models. The same cumulative exposure (CE) profiles as in Figure 16.4 are partitioned into three time windows. The first subject has a higher exposure in the early window, while the second subject has fairly constant exposures throughout.
Reproduced from Ch. 1 *A Biologic Approach to Environmental Assessment and Epidemiology* by Smith, Thomas J. and Kriebel, David (2010). By permission of Oxford University Press, USA.

The time windows approach relaxes somewhat the implicit assumptions of a single summary measure like CE, but there are significant limitations as well. How many windows should be used? How should the cut points be determined? Which summary measure of exposure should be calculated within each window? The use of time windows artificially divides a constantly varying lifetime exposure history into 'independent' periods, which carry their own implicit assumption that exposure arriving just prior to a cut-off date for one window may have a very different risk than exposure occurring just a few months later, after the start of the next window.

Exposures in different time windows prior to an outcome are recognized as important for some adverse effects, such as pregnancy outcomes that depend on the temporal development of the fetus. Windows can be defined empirically by dividing a time period into some number of equal periods, or a priori biological data can be used to define the windows of increased or decreased susceptibility. Empirical time windows should be distinguished from the less common practice of separately studying exposures in windows of inherently different susceptibility; as, for example, in different periods of pregnancy, or in life stages like pre- or post-menarche.[8,9]

Time windows defined empirically have another limitation: they do not address the possibility that the risk or effects from a particular unit of exposure may be altered by the pattern of exposure that has preceded it. Suppose that the exposure received by subject 1 in Figure 16.5 in the second time window carries much higher risk because he experienced a period of high exposure in the first time window. The closest we could come to capturing this behaviour using the time windows approach would be to hypothesize that there was a *statistical interaction* between exposures occurring in different windows. This interaction would probably be very difficult to evaluate in regression models, because of the problem of collinearity of the main effects of the time windows with their product term. But even if we could do it, it would likely be an unsatisfactory solution. The standard method of constructing interaction terms captures only one rather simplistic hypothesis for a two-variable interaction.[6,10,11] This pattern may not capture the multiplicity of possible biological interactions, and may miss an important relationship.

Dynamic biological process models

An alternative to the time window approach is a dynamic model in which one or more biological processes operate through time to produce the observed pathology. In the most general case, a disease process operates in response to exposures, and the body responds to the damage with repair processes. As a result, the prior history of exposure affects the response as does the repair process to define what we see and when we see it, by measuring the damage at a point in time (Figure 16.3). The particular pattern of changing response over time will depend on the exposure pattern and on the details of the disease process model. We can test our disease model by comparing its time course with the temporal pattern of a response generated by a disease. An example of a process model driven by the exposure time profiles of Figures 16.4 and 16.5 and the responses are shown in Figure 16.6. This model has two independent opposing

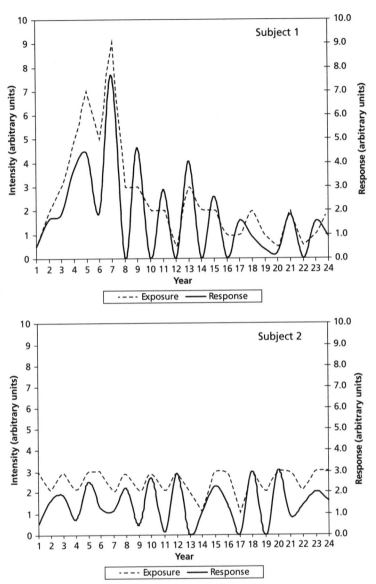

Figure 16.6 Illustration of alternative treatments of the temporal dynamics of exposure and response in epidemiological models. The predicted response from a hypothetical disease process model (shown in Figure 16.7) is shown for the subjects in Figures 16.4 and 16.5. The model predicts different risks for these two, because it is iteratively recalculated over short intervals of time; continually changing the weights on each annual exposure as a function of the previous exposures.

Reproduced from Ch.1 *A Biologic Approach to Environmental Assessment and Epidemiology* by Smith, Thomas J. and Kriebel, David (2010). By permission of Oxford University Press, USA.

proportional processes, a damage process and a repair process, with both operating over short intervals, Δt. The model can be represented as Equation 16.2:

> *Damage $(at\ t + \Delta t) = Damage\ (at\ t) - Repair\ (during\ \Delta t) + Damage\ (during\ \Delta t)$*
> *where*
> *Repair $(during\ \Delta t) = k_{rep}\ Damage\ (at\ t)$*
> *Damage $(during\ \Delta t) = k_{dam}\ Exposure\ (during\ \Delta t)$ and*
> *k_{dam} and k_{rep} are proportionality constants*

Equation 16.2 a dynamic biological model expressed as a difference equation.

Representing the continuous processes as discrete changes over short periods of time (Δt) relative to the process rates makes the mathematics simpler and allows us to use difference equations rather than differential equations. Consider what happens within one time interval: first a portion of the damage at the beginning of the interval is repaired. The amount of damage repaired during the interval is a percentage of the total at the start. A new amount of damage is defined by the average exposure intensity during Δt multiplied by a weighting or conversion factor (the response per unit of exposure) during the interval. At the start of the next interval, the process is repeated. Like an inch worm, the process works its way along the time line of exposure, making a calculation for each interval (Figure 16.7). This biological model has the advantage

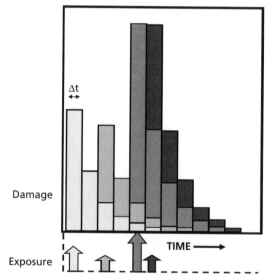

Figure 16.7 Temporal sequence of responses produced by a simple damage-repair model following four short duration exposures—the height of the added damage is proportional to the intensity of exposure. The duration of the time increment, Δt, was chosen to equal the half-time of repair. At each time interval the residual amounts of damage are added to each other. The total damage we would observe is the sum of the new and all residual damage from the prior exposures.

Reproduced from Ch. 1 *A Biologic Approach to Environmental Assessment and Epidemiology* by Smith, Thomas J. and Kriebel, David (2010). By permission of Oxford University Press, USA.

that exposure changes over time do not need to be represented by a smooth function that can be formally integrated, instead the exposures may be random variations measured which can be summed.

In Figure 16.6, the solid line represents the value of a response or effect variable calculated from the damage-repair model for the same exposure histories illustrated in Figures 16.4 and 16.5 (shown as dotted lines). According to the particular disease process acting in this hypothetical example, the effects of high exposures in the early years for subject 1 did not increase his response at the end of the period because those early effects did not carry over but were all repaired. However, ongoing effects for subject 2 (on an arbitrary scale) were nearly twice as large as those of subject 1 at the end of the time interval.

The challenge for those who would like to try this method is the design of the disease process model. Our basic approach is to gather available data about the nature of the exposure agent, observe the time course for the development of the effects or disease, and then develop a disease process model that captures the key temporal patterns of the exposure-response relationship. While detailed biological processes are extremely complex, certain overall basic patterns are common, such as the damage-repair process model, which produce similar time courses for a variety of effects because the pattern is produced by a few rate-limiting steps. These common models can be used to provide the basic structure for a disease process model. We propose that four basic disease process models can represent most of the common diseases and adverse effects caused by environmental exposures. Where more complex behaviour is needed several models can be used in sequence or parallel.

Four disease process models

After examining many different adverse effects and diseases, we have observed that there are two critical elements of the disease process that must be identified (Table 16.1):

1. whether the *time course* of the disease or damage process shows it is reversible (shows evidence of repair) or irreversible, and

2. whether the *type of response* is proportional to the tissue concentration of the toxin or, alternatively, that the adverse effect develops in a discrete step function—from absent to present with the strength of response not proportional to the concentration of the causal agent in the tissue.

These time course and response types define profoundly different pathological processes and exposure-response relationships. Fortunately, these features can often be identified using descriptive and readily observable information about the time course of development and recovery from the adverse effects. As more information is gathered, more complex mechanisms and models can be developed as needed to fit the observed effects. Multistep process models can often be developed by linking together separate basic models, for example, to represent the transition from a reversible effect to one where damage begins to accumulate. Let's look in detail at these two issues.

Table 16.1 The four principal disease process models can be classified based on their time course (reversible or irreversible) and their response (proportional or discrete)

Time course	Response	
	Proportional Pathophysiological responses are proportional to dose	Discrete Pathophysiological responses are quantal, and not proportional to dose
Reversible Damage/repair processes in which there is recovery after exposure ceases	e.g. airway inflammation, gastritis, mechanical injury to musculoskeletal system and skin	e.g. asthma attacks, dermatitis
Irreversible Process with limited repair that leads to the accumulation of effects	e.g. pneumoconioses, hearing loss, macular degeneration	e.g. carcinogenesis, immune sensitization

Reproduced from Ch. 1 *A Biologic Approach to Environmental Assessment and Epidemiology* by Smith, Thomas J. and Kriebel, David (2010). By permission of Oxford University Press, USA

Reversible versus irreversible time course

When a smoker first picks up the habit, smoking produces reversible proportional respiratory airway symptoms. If smoking ceases within a few months or years, all or almost all of the damage may be repaired with no long-term effects. However, if exposure continues, irreversible cell damage accumulates in the small airways, often leading to chronic obstructive pulmonary disease, an example of an irreversible proportional response but associated with a much slower process. Long-term smoking also increases the risk of lung cancer through a series of different types of genetic damage, some of which may be reversible. However, once the final transformation occurs and makes a malignant cell, further cigarette smoke exposure is usually irrelevant and the individual has made the discrete transition to a case of lung cancer; an example of an irreversible discrete response. This illustrates that a single type of exposure (tobacco smoking) may cause several different effects/diseases and each should be represented by its own disease process model, defined by the temporal behaviour of that specific outcome.

It is a matter of considerable importance to know whether the short-term, mostly reversible effects of an agent contribute to long-term irreversible damage, or whether the short-term effects are independent of the irreversible effects. For example, it would be very useful to know if someone who responds acutely to air pollutants that cause short-term airway inflammation is also at higher risk of developing chronic lung disease. Despite considerable research, this question remains largely unanswered.[12] Often the option of detecting a reversible or irreversible time course is made implicitly by the length of the study period: if one is studying the effects of air pollution over a period of hours or days, then necessarily one will be able to detect only those effects that will probably be largely reversible. On the contrary, a study following people for many years usually can detect irreversible effects, although it may also detect short-term reversible effects, confusing the data analysis and its interpretation if care is not taken to separate the two patterns. By explicitly stating in advance what time course we think we are studying, we decrease the chances for confusion and misinterpretation of the results.

Proportional versus discrete response

Whether a response is proportional or discrete may in some cases depend on the time-scale of observation. In many diseases, a very close view of the evolving disease process on a very short timescale (minutes or even seconds) might reveal a 'gradual' development of a response. But when viewed from a timescale of clinical relevance—hours or days for an allergy, or years for a cancer—the response will appear 'instantaneous': one moment the subject was healthy, and the next she was sick.

On the limits of epidemiological data and biological models

Our goal is a methodology to formulate strong tests of our exposure-disease hypotheses in which a hypothesis is developed in as much biological detail as it can be, expressed in a suitable dynamic (temporal) model, and tested by its fit with a rich data set, so that its flaws and misperceptions of reality are fully displayed. Rejecting such a fully developed biological hypothesis is more informative than either rejecting or failing to reject a generic or vaguely defined hypothesis. For example, the hypothesis 'truck drivers have more risk of lung cancer than non-drivers'[13] is of limited usefulness for prevention since truck drivers have many environmental exposures, 'lifestyle' attributes like smoking, diet, and exercise, and socioeconomic characteristics. Hypothesizing that a particular chemical agent in truck exhaust is associated with lung cancer—whether the hypothesis is refuted or supported by data—is more likely to lead to successful prevention activities.

While this biologically based approach is attractive, we must acknowledge some of the challenges that researchers will face. The observational nature of epidemiology and the complexity of pathophysiological processes place limits on the degree to which epidemiological data can directly and confidently be used to quantify environmental health risks. When epidemiologists speak of models, they generally mean empirical statistical models of the population risk, not biological models. Their goal is to find a mathematical relationship between the risk and some set of covariates, such as age, gender, genetics, exposure, etc., that can account for a major part of the variation in risk among the population members. These mathematical models are necessary 'restrictions on the possible states of nature'[14]—restrictions that are needed because epidemiological data can only be expected to distinguish among a very limited set of alternative states.[14,15] While we agree with this rather sobering view of the limits of epidemiology, we believe that the choice of models against which to compare the data should, so far as possible, be guided by explicit hypotheses about the underlying biological processes. In other words, you can get as much as possible from epidemiology by starting from well-thought-out hypotheses that are formalized as mathematical models into which the data will be placed. The disease process models can serve this purpose.

If, as we believe, observational studies are seriously limited by unknown biases and confounders, how should occupational and environmental scientists best contribute to the understanding of disease processes? We could abandon modelling altogether[15] or, the solution we favour, use biologically-based mathematical models with several stated caveats: (1) the modeller's prior beliefs are clearly stated, (2) a range of plausible models are tested, (3) the sensitivity of the results to changes in model parameters is investigated, and (4) the modeller presents as complete a description of the uncertainty in the results as possible.[3,14,15]

Summary

The goal of environmental health is the prevention of disease through identification and elimination of environmental hazards or the reduction of exposures. Exposure assessment and epidemiology can contribute to continued progress in achieving this goal, but we believe that this will not occur without integrated, biologically based methods of study design and analysis. With the rapid proliferation of molecular and cell biology, the mechanisms underlying pathological processes leading to adverse effects are increasingly well understood. This new knowledge should be used more systematically as the theoretical basis of exposure-response modelling. Disease process models can provide a simple but useful starting point and a framework for added complexity as new information is discovered.

Acknowledgement

Extracts from pp. 3–24, including Fig: 1.1–1.7, in *A Biologic Approach to Environmental Assessment and Epidemiology* by Smith, Thomas J. and Kriebel, David (2010) are used by permission of Oxford University Press, USA.

References

1. **Morabia A (ed.).** *A history of epidemiologic methods and concepts.* Basel: Birkhäuser, 2004.

2. **Mehendale HM.** Tissue repair: an important determinant of final outcome of toxicant-induced injury. *Toxicol Pathol* 2005;**33**:41–51.

3. **Thomas DC.** Statistical methods for analyzing effects of temporal patterns of exposure on cancer risks. *Scand J Work Environ Health* 1983;**9**:353–66.

4. **Kriebel D, Smith TJ.** A nonlinear pharmacologic model of the acute effects of ozone on the human lungs. *Environ Res* 1990;**51**:120–46.

5. **Smith TJ.** Occupational exposure and dose over time: limitations of cumulative exposure. *Am J Ind Med* 1992;**21**:35–51.

6. **Checkoway H, Pearce N, Kriebel D.** *Research methods in occupational epidemiology* (2nd edn). Oxford: Oxford University Press, 2004.

7. **Rothman N, Greenland S.** *Modern Epidemiology* (2nd edn). Philadelphia, PA: Lippincott-Raven, 1998.

8. **Thompson D, Kriebel D, Quinn MM, Wegman DH, Eisen EA.** Occupational exposure to metalworking fluids and risk of breast cancer among female autoworkers. *Am J Ind Med* 2005;**47**:153–60.

9. **Agalliu I, Eisen EA, Kriebel D, Quinn MM, Wegman DH.** A biological approach to characterizing exposure to metalworking fluids and risk of prostate cancer (United States). *Cancer Causes Control* 2005;**16**:323–31.

10. **Lewontin R.** The analysis of variance and the analysis of causes. *Am J Hum Genet* 1974;**26**:400–11. (Reprinted in: *Int J Epidemiol* 2006;**35**:520–5.)

11. **Vineis P, Kriebel D.** Causal models in epidemiology: past inheritance and genetic future. *Environ Health* 2006;**5**:21. doi: 10.1186/1476-069X-5-21.

12. **Becklake MR.** Relationship of acute obstructive airway change to chronic (fixed) obstruction. *Thorax* 1995;**50**(Suppl 1):S16–21.

13. **Platt JR.** Strong inference. *Science* 1964;**146**:347–53.

14. **Robins JM, Greenland S.** The role of model selection in causal inference from nonexperimental data. *Am J Epidemiol* 1986;**123**:392–402.

15. **Vandenbroucke JP.** Should we abandon statistical modeling altogether? *Am J Epidemiol* 1987;**126**:10–3.

Chapter 17

Why we should be Bayesians (and often already are without realizing it)

Neil Pearce and Marine Corbin

Introduction

We all live our lives as Bayesians—we always base decisions on past experience (and the theories which shape our perceptions of it), together with any new information that we have. We expect the sun to rise tomorrow much as it did yesterday and today, and most of us have long given up hope of England winning the football World Cup again. Whenever we hear the news we interpret it in light of what we know already. We don't start each day with a clean slate and an empty mind.

Most epidemiologists operate as Bayesians also. We decide what to study based on prior knowledge. For example, we might study pesticides and non-Hodgkin lymphoma because we are aware that there are many studies which have shown an increased risk of this lymphoma in farmers, and that there have been some studies which have specifically linked the increased risk to pesticide use. We may therefore decide to conduct an in-depth investigation into the possible role of some specific pesticides, or classes of pesticide, in causing non-Hodgkin lymphoma. This prior evidence will usually be summarized in the grant application and in the Introduction section of the report from the subsequent study.

When we have finished the study, we also interpret the findings as Bayesians, in the Discussion section of the paper, in light of what the study adds to prior knowledge. Maybe we found an increased risk associated with a particular pesticide. But has anyone studied this before, and what did they find? Is there animal evidence? Is there evidence from geographical or time trends studies? Is it biologically plausible? How does the evidence stack up against the Bradford Hill criteria? So we write our Discussions as Bayesians also.

But what do we do in between? Usually, we write the Methods and Results sections of our papers as if the data we have collected are the only data which exist. We conduct significance tests, attempting to reach a decision solely on the basis of these data. We then second-guess this decision in the Discussion section. Maybe we found a difference which was not statistically significant, but the numbers were small, and the confidence interval was consistent with findings of previous larger studies. Or maybe we found a statistically significant result, but it was an association which had been studied before, and for which no one else had found an increased risk, so maybe it was due to chance even if it was statistically significant. And probably it is biologically implausible anyway. We then feel guilty about 'breaking the rules' and explaining away our results because they are inconsistent with prior knowledge.

So, we write the Introduction and Discussion as Bayesians, and the Methods and Results as frequentists. This is why most epidemiological papers (including our own) are so confused, and written so badly.

In this chapter, we propose that the quality of epidemiological papers can be improved if we consider prior knowledge more formally in the Methods and Results sections of our papers, as well as in the Introduction and Discussion. In other words, we should recognize that we have been thinking like Bayesians all along, even if we have been trying to analyse our data as frequentists.

This chapter is intended as a 'popular' exposition of Bayesian methods and Bayesian ways of thinking. For more formal presentations of these ideas and methods, readers are referred to the series of papers by Greenland.[1–3] By the term 'Bayesian' we refer to any method of analysis which uses prior information. This prior information could be from previous studies or from the current study; the point is that we don't just analyse each exposure-disease association as if it is the only piece of data which exists—we take other data and information into account.

Frequentist and Bayesian statistics

Bayesian methods were used alongside other methods from the eighteenth century until the 1920s.[1] At that time, several influential statisticians (Fisher, Neyman, Pearson) developed the frequentist techniques which form the basis of the orthodox statistics taught on most epidemiology courses today. These analytical methods were developed for large randomized controlled trials and for large agricultural experiments, and generally work well in those situations. They assume that the trial data have been sampled from an infinite population (i.e. that the trial is a sample of an infinite number of possible trials of the same size), and that exposure has been randomized. So, for example, the idea behind the estimation of a 95% confidence interval is that, if we repeated the study an infinite number of times, if exposure had been randomized, there was no confounding, perfect response rates, and no misclassification, then the estimated confidence interval would include the true effect measure 95% of the time.

Epidemiological studies are different. We don't have infinite populations (unless you believe that we are sampling from the multiverse), exposure has not been randomized, we often have poor response rates, and there are serious problems of misclassification. Further uncertainty is introduced when we have to make decisions as to what variables to include in our models, how to categorize them, what form the dose-response should take for a continuous variable, what to do about interactions, and how to assess confounding. But we still estimate confidence intervals (and p-values) as if none of these problems existed, as if we really had data from a perfect randomized trial, sampled from an infinite population. Most epidemiology courses focus ad infinitum on very sophisticated statistical methods to analyse such 'perfect' data while ignoring the elephant in the room, namely that our data are usually not very good, there is always uncontrolled bias, and therefore the frequentist model doesn't fit very well.

It is better to accept that analysing epidemiological data always involves personal judgements, that study samples and exposure status are often markedly non-random, and are not perfectly measured. In this situation, Bayesian methods make these personal judgements more explicit and enable us to assess their validity and to understand how our findings would have been different if we had made different assumptions.

Thus, Bayesian approaches formally take prior evidence into account in the analysis. Unfortunately, these methods have become associated with highly complex approaches, such as Monte Carlo Markov chain methods, while, in fact, most Bayesian methods can be applied using ordinary statistical software packages, or with a hand calculator.[1] Here, we illustrate the use of these methods, both for estimating main effects, and for assessing bias.

Estimation of main effects

One exposure, one outcome

Suppose we have conducted a study where there is one main exposure variable and one main outcome. For example, one of us (NP) conducted a study of dioxin exposure and cancer risk in New Zealand phenoxy herbicide production workers and found a relative risk (RR) for total cancer mortality of 1.24 (95% CI 0.90–1.67). A strict frequentist would interpret such a finding as not statistically significant. On the other hand, we interpreted it as consistent with previous evidence of a small increased total cancer risk. In fact, a very large international study had found a RR of 1.29 (95% CI 0.94–1.76),[4] and there was supporting evidence from animal studies, which had led the International Agency for Research on Cancer (IARC) to classify dioxin as a human carcinogen.[5] So, two reasonable researchers can come to opposite conclusions depending on whether or not they are prepared to take prior evidence into account in the data analysis and in the discussion.

When quantitative prior information is available and the prior data are comparable (in terms of study design, level of exposure, likelihood of residual confounding, etc.) then such prior data can be incorporated formally into the analysis, for example by doing two separate analyses, one based solely on the new data collected for the study and one incorporating the prior data into an expanded meta-analysis. The prior 'belief' is based on the estimates from the previously available data (such as that the RR is 1.29) and this is then updated on the basis of the new data from the study. This updating process essentially yields the same results as if a frequentist had come along at a later date and performed a meta-analysis incorporating all of the available data.

Prior data may not be available in some instances but there is likely to be at least some evidence, or reasonable belief, about the likely effect size. For example, Greenland[1] describes the example of a case-control study in which it is reasonable to assume with 95% certainty that the RR is between ¼ and 4; in this situation, it is not difficult to construct the hypothetical 'prior data' which corresponds to this belief. The analysis of the new study can then be done twice: once with the new data only, and a second time by including the prior data as a separate stratum (e.g. in a Mantel-Haenszel analysis), or as an additional set of records (e.g. in a logistic regression analysis).

This is the classical Bayesian approach. We have a prior belief (perhaps based on prior data, perhaps not) and we then update this belief based on the data newly collected. This approach is straightforward and can be done easily using standard statistical packages. Such analyses can be very useful when we have real prior data in terms of putting the new data into context and updating the historical data in a new meta-analysis. When there are no prior data, the use of data-augmented priors[1] can be helpful conceptually although, in practice, it will usually make little difference to the analysis, since even a sensible prior will carry very little weight compared to the real data collected for the study.

Many exposures, one level of analysis

The situation gets more interesting when we have many exposures to analyse. For example, suppose we are doing a case-control study of occupational risk factors for lung cancer. Typically, we may have a small group of occupations and exposures which are of a priori interest (e.g. asbestos and silica) but we may also collect information on literally hundreds of other occupations and exposures for which there is little or no prior evidence and we are just 'having a look' to see what we find. Of course, if we test hundreds of occupations, and none of them is a cause of lung cancer in reality, then we will get a false association about 5% of the time so that, for example, in a study of 500 occupations we might expect to have 25 'false positive' findings (significantly high or significantly low odds ratios) by chance. The classical solution to this problem is the Bonferroni correction,[6] which adopts more stringent criteria for deciding which p-values will be considered 'significant' depending on the number of tests that we have done (and/or adjusts the confidence interval for each effect estimate to reduce the probability that any individual effect estimate will not include the null value).

The problem with this approach is that in most real-life situations it is complete nonsense. Suppose we do a case-control study of asbestos and lung cancer and along the way we take a complete occupational history, and therefore we are able to 'have a look' at the associations of 500 other occupations with lung cancer risk. Are we really supposed to adjust our asbestos findings because we have also looked at 500 other occupations? Surely, asbestos was the main point of doing the study and there is strong prior evidence that asbestos causes lung cancer. Thus, an association of asbestos exposure with lung cancer is in a completely different league from, for example, a finding that teachers had a higher risk of lung cancer if we had also tested 500 other occupations. For each occupation/exposure, the key issue is not how many other things we tested, but what the prior evidence was before we did the study (very strong in the case of asbestos, non-existent in the case of teachers), and what further evidence the new study adds.

Thus, if we repeated the study in a new population, we would expect the asbestos effect to be replicated whereas chance associations (e.g. with teachers) would be likely to exhibit regression to the mean and usually would not show such strong increased risks again. Bayesian methods can be used to take this likely regression to the mean into account and to shrink our effect estimates, based on how strong the regression to the mean is likely to be. We can do this shrinkage differently for separate groups of exposures. For example, in a case-control study of asbestos and lung cancer, the occupational exposures might fall into three groups: (1) asbestos, the main exposure under study; (2) other exposures/occupations for which there was a priori evidence that they were risk factors for lung cancer; and (3) all other occupations/exposures. For group 1 (asbestos), there is no need to shrink the estimated odds ratio since asbestos essentially forms its own group. For group 3 (other occupations/exposures), the estimated odds ratio for each occupation is shrunk towards the overall mean for these occupations (which will usually be close to 1.0). For group 2, if we consider it reasonable to assume that these a priori high-risk occupations have similar odds ratios (for example, if in previous studies they have generally been found all to have odds ratios of about 2.0), then it is reasonable to consider these occupations as a group. The estimated odds ratio for each occupation is shrunk towards the overall mean for these high risk occupations.

How does the shrinkage work? The basic idea of empirical Bayes (EB) and semi-Bayes (SB) adjustments for multiple associations is that the observed variation of the estimated relative risks around their geometric mean is larger than the variation of the true (but unknown) relative risks. In SB adjustments, an a priori value for the extra variation is chosen which assigns a reasonable range of variation to the true relative risks and this value is then used to adjust the observed relative risks.[7] The adjustment consists in shrinking outlying relative risks towards the overall mean (of the relative risks for all the different exposures being considered). The larger the individual variance of the relative risks, the stronger the shrinkage, so that the shrinkage is stronger for less reliable estimates based on small numbers. Typical applications in which SB adjustments are a useful alternative to traditional methods of adjustment for multiple comparisons are in large occupational surveillance studies, where many relative risks are estimated with few or no a priori beliefs about which associations might be causal.[7]

Table 17.1 shows the findings for a priori high-risk occupations in a New Zealand case-control study of occupational exposures and lung cancer.[8] Cases were all subjects diagnosed with incident lung cancer notified to the New Zealand Cancer Registry during 2007 and 2008 and aged 20–75 years. Controls were recruited from the New Zealand Electoral Roll in two time periods (2003 and 2008) and were frequency matched with the cases for age and gender. The questionnaire included demographic details and information on smoking status, lifetime occupational history, and socioeconomic status, defined using the occupational class of the longest held occupation.

SB estimates were calculated using R (free software for statistical computing and graphics).[9] The input for SB adjustments was the maximum likelihood (ML) estimate of beta (log odds ratio, lnOR) resulting from the multivariate logistic regression for each occupation and industry. The variance of the distribution of the true lnORs was assumed to be 0.25. Assuming a normal distribution of the lnORs, this choice implies that the true odds ratios are within a sevenfold range of each other.[10] Occupations and industries were divided into groups according to the number of digits of the associated codes, and the shrinkage was performed within these groups. For those occupations or industries which were not considered a priori to be at increased risk for lung cancer, estimates were shrunk towards the mean for all such occupations or industries. Similarly, for those occupations or industries which were considered to be at a priori increased risk for lung cancer, estimates were shrunk towards the mean for all such occupations or industries.

Ever being employed in one or more of the a priori high-risk occupations (Table 17.1) was associated with an increased risk of lung cancer ($OR_{\text{a priori occupation}}$ 1.94, 95% CI 1.44–2.61). The SB shrinkage generally resulted in an attenuation of the odds ratios. Only two of the odds ratios for the a priori high-risk occupations remained strongly elevated with reasonable precision after SB adjustment: 8323 Heavy truck drivers (OR_{SB} 1.97, 95% CI 1.13–3.43) and 83231 Heavy truck or tanker driver (OR_{SB} 2.01, 95% CI 1.15–3.50).

The advantage of this approach over classical Bonferroni corrections is that *on the average* it produces more valid estimates of the odds ratio for each occupation/exposure. If we do a study which involves assessing hundreds of occupations, the problem is not only that we get many 'false positive' results by chance. A second problem is that even the 'true positives' tend to have odds ratios that are too high. For example, if we have a group of occupations with true odds ratios around 1.5, then the ones that stand out in the analysis are those with the highest odds ratios (e.g. 2.5) which will be elevated partly because of real effects and partly by chance. The Bonferroni correction addresses the first problem (too many chance findings) but not the second, that the strongest odds ratios are probably too high. In contrast, SB adjustment addresses the second problem by correcting for the anticipated regression to the mean that would have occurred if the study had been repeated, and thereby *on the average* produces more valid odds ratio estimates for each occupation/exposure.

Many exposures, multilevel analysis

In the example presented in Table 17.1, the different occupations/exposures were considered to be independent and to have a similar level of risk. However, in some studies we have more information than this. For example, if we are studying time trends in lung cancer mortality, then we would expect the rate for 2008 to be more similar to the rates for 2007 and 2009 than to earlier or later rates. In classical frequentist statistics we can smooth the data by estimating the rate for 2008 based on a weighted average over several years (e.g. the estimated rate for 2008 might be 0.25×r2007 + 0.5×r2008 + 0.25×r2009).

A more complex example involves spatial analyses. We might expect the rate for a municipality to be more similar to those of the surrounding municipalities than to those for more distant municipalities. For example, Maule et al.[11] analysed data for pleural cancer in 1206 municipalities in Piedmont, north-west Italy, from 1980 to 2000. The Bayesian model allowed for both heterogeneity (through spatially independent random effects) and clustering (through spatially correlated random effects) and, by borrowing information from neighbouring areas, provided stable estimates for areas with sparse data. The aim was to reduce the 'noise' in the disease maps to highlight the true underlying mortality distribution.

A more formal hierarchical approach is illustrated by an analysis which the authors conducted of occupational risks for lung cancer in a case-control study in two areas of Italy.[12] For each occupation, we estimated exposure to three known lung carcinogens

Table 17.1 Odds ratios (OR) and 95% CIs for a priori high-risk occupations: standard analyses and semi-Bayes adjusted analyses

A priori high-risk occupation for lung cancer	Cases/ controls	Not semi-Bayes adjusted		Semi-Bayes adjusted	
		OR	95% CI	OR	95% CI
5151 Fire fighters	3/5	0.76	0.17–3.45	1.20	0.51–2.83
61122 Grape grower and/or wine maker, worker	4/2	4.39	0.68–28.51	1.93	0.74–5.05
61311 Logger	4/3	4.67[a]	0.81–27.03	2.01	0.76–5.28
7112 Carpenters and joiners	25/50	1.07	0.61–1.88	1.16	0.70–1.91
7124 Painters and paperhangers	10/16	0.88	0.37–2.11	1.10	0.55–2.18
722 Blacksmiths, toolmakers, and related workers	7/8	1.79	0.58–5.50	1.51	0.71–3.21
72312 Motor mechanic	17/25	1.22	0.59–2.51	1.32	0.73–2.39
733 Printing trades workers	9/17	0.87	0.36–2.13	1.06	0.53–2.11
73321 Bookbinder	2/4	0.90	0.14–5.56	1.37	0.56–3.33
7411 Butchers	8/1	8.77[b]	1.06–72.55	2.00	0.70–5.73
742 Cabinet makers and related workers	7/7	2.11	0.63–7.09	1.59	0.72–3.54
811 Mining and mineral processing plant operators	6/11	0.98	0.32–3.03	1.16	0.55–2.48
8111 Mining plant operators	5/6	1.93	0.44–8.43	1.58	0.70–3.61
81111 Quarry and mine worker	5/5	1.97	0.44–8.78	1.66	0.73–3.79
8113 Drillers	1/6	0.25	0.03–2.17	1.08	0.38–3.06
8122 Metal casters	3/2	1.82	0.24–13.81	1.52	0.63–3.68
81231 Welder and flame-cutter	12/7	2.50[a]	0.86–7.25	1.92	0.90–4.10
813 Glass and ceramics kiln and related plant operators	7/9	1.60	0.51–5.03	1.44	0.68–3.04
8131 Glass and ceramics kiln operators	4/7	1.15	0.27–4.89	1.35	0.60–3.05
81312 Clay product plant operator	2/3	1.26	0.13–12.40	1.49	0.61–3.69
8132 Other glass and ceramics workers	3/2	2.85	0.40–20.47	1.66	0.67–4.11
8141 Sawmill, wood panel and related wood-processing plant operators	8/5	4.63[b]	1.05–20.29	2.07	0.82–5.23
815 Chemical processing plant operators	8/9	1.43	0.47–4.32	1.37	0.66–2.86
8211 Machine-tool operators	8/2	4.44[a]	0.84–23.63	1.93	0.76–4.93
8212 Cement and other minerals processing machine operators	7/3	3.73[a]	0.87–15.94	1.95	0.80–4.75

(Continued)

Table 17.1 *(Continued)*

A priori high-risk occupation for lung cancer	Cases/ controls	Not semi-Bayes adjusted		Semi-Bayes adjusted	
		OR	95% CI	OR	95% CI
8222 Metal finishers, platers, and coaters	5/6	0.87	0.25–3.03	1.20	0.54–2.65
82221 Electroplater	2/4	0.63	0.11–3.55	1.24	0.49–3.14
8231 Tyre production machine operators	4/2	2.45	0.36–16.65	1.62	0.67–3.94
8232 Other rubber and plastics products machine operators	8/2	6.34[b]	1.08–37.15	2.05	0.76–5.59
8261 Spinning and winding machine operators	3/3	1.77	0.29–11.00	1.52	0.64–3.61
8262 Weaving and knitting machine operators	7/9	1.47	0.49–4.41	1.46	0.70–3.04
82624 Knitter, knitting machinist	2/3	1.63	0.23–11.71	1.56	0.65–3.75
82641 Launderer	9/5	2.29	0.60–8.73	1.77	0.79–3.99
82643 Dry-cleaner	3/4	1.02	0.19–5.38	1.39	0.59–3.28
82644 Presser	6/2	5.74[a]	0.96–34.42	2.09	0.76–5.73
82651 Fibre preparer	2/3	0.75	0.09–6.19	1.36	0.54–3.43
82812 Tanner, splitter, and dyer	3/2	1.15	0.16–8.26	1.46	0.60–3.52
82922 Electric and electronic equipment assembler	7/5	3.61[a]	0.96–13.57	2.08	0.87–5.02
83212 Light truck or van driver	5/11	0.55	0.17–1.81	1.02	0.41–2.49
8322 Bus drivers	5/12	0.46	0.13–1.68	0.96	0.39–2.36
8323 Heavy truck drivers	31/26	2.24[b]	1.19–4.21	1.97	1.13–3.43
83231 Heavy truck or tanker driver	31/26	2.24[b]	1.19–4.21	2.01	1.15–3.50
8331 Motorized farm machinery operators	5/10	0.72	0.22–2.36	1.09	0.49–2.46
8332 Earthmoving and related machinery operators	9/13	1.01	0.37–2.76	1.22	0.59–2.49
83325 Roading and/or paving machine operator	1/9	0.15	0.01–1.48	1.08	0.32–3.62
84117 Roofer	1/4	0.91	0.09–9.47	1.43	0.57–3.58
911 Building caretakers and cleaners	50/50	1.23	0.75–2.00	1.25	0.80–1.93

[a] $p < 0.1$, [b] $p < 0.05$

Reprinted with permission from Marine Corbin et al., Lung cancer and occupation: A New Zealand cancer registry-based case-control study, *American Journal of Industrial Medicine*, Volume 54, Issue 2, pp. 89–101, Copyright © 2010 Wiley-Liss, Inc.

(asbestos, chromium, and silica) under the assumption that occupations with similar exposure characteristics should have similar risks for lung cancer. Table 17.2 illustrates the exposure matrix for selected occupations and shows, for example, that miners and quarrymen are expected, on the basis of prior information, to have medium exposure to asbestos and high exposure to silica. The data were first analysed with a conventional ML estimation analysis (Table 17.3). Hierarchical regression (HR) was then used to attempt to improve on these ML estimates by using a second-stage linear model.[13,14] This regressed lnORs of the occupations against the occupations' estimated exposure levels to asbestos, chromium, and silica. As for the SB analyses, it was necessary to specify an a priori value for the range of the odds ratios (e.g. $\tau = 0.76$ corresponds to a 20-fold range).

Table 17.3 reports the odds ratio estimates obtained through these different methods for the occupations associated with the twenty highest risks of lung cancer in the conventional analysis. Shrinkage is particularly strong for specialized farmers ($OR_{ML} = 3.44$, $OR_{SB} = 1.59$, $OR_{HR}[\tau\, 0.76] = 1.81$, $OR_{HR}[\tau\, 0.23] = 1.00$) and for ships' engine-room ratings, who are highly exposed to asbestos ($OR_{ML} = 5.88$, $OR_{SB} = 1.54$, $OR_{HR}[\tau\, 0.76] = 2.43$, $OR_{HR}[\tau\, 0.23] = 1.78$). This is due to the fact that these two occupations are each held by a small number of subjects and the confidence intervals for the ML estimates are therefore very large. Despite the large confidence intervals, however, the shrunk estimates still indicate that these occupations are associated with an increased risk of lung cancer, and their odds ratios are consistent with those of other occupations which involve exposure to lung carcinogens.

We noted that HR and SB shrinkage had similar effects on the ML estimates. However, since HR uses more detailed prior information than SB, the shrinkage performed by the former method is likely to be more appropriate and specific than the latter

Table 17.2 Exposure matrix for asbestos, chromium and silica

Occupation	Elements of matrix					
	Asbestos (medium)	Asbestos (high)	Chromium (medium)	Chromium (high)	Silica (medium)	Silica (high)
Nursery workers and gardeners	0	0	0	0	1	0
Farm machinery operators	0	0	0	0	0	1
Loggers	0	0	0	0	0	0
Fishermen	0	0	0	0	0	0
Production supervisors	0	0	0	0	0	0
Miners and quarrymen	1	0	0	0	0	1

Source: data from Corbin M et al., Hierarchical Regression for Multiple Comparisons in a Case-Control Study of Occupational Risks for Lung Cancer, *PLoS ONE*, Volume 7, Issue 6, Copyright © 2012 Corbin et al. Licenced under Creative Commons Attribution 2.5.

(provided of course that this prior information is reasonably valid). All the estimates were shrunk towards the null value through SB whereas some of them were pulled in the opposite direction by HR, because of the use of additional prior information (Table 17.3). Thus, both approaches aim at decreasing false-positive findings but HR also mitigates the inherent effect of the shrinkage to increase false-negatives. On the other hand, SB is easier to compute and does not need the manipulation of a second-stage matrix. Therefore the choice between the two methods essentially depends on the availability and reliability of the information included in the second-stage model.

The HR shrinkage we proposed[12] could have two relevant implications when conducting exploratory analyses on risks associated with occupations: (1) it decreases the possibility that an occupation entailing exposure to important known occupational carcinogens is overlooked, and (2) it helps to identify those occupations not entailing exposure to known occupational carcinogens but which should be further investigated and may provide information on new or suspected occupational carcinogens. The findings on construction painters, who had an odds ratio of 1.85 (95% CI 1.09–3.15) in the standard ML approach, are an example of the latter implication. According to the general population job-exposure matrix used in the study (the 'DOM-JEM') construction painters are not exposed to chromium or silica and have a low exposure to asbestos. However, the odds ratio remained elevated after HR even when using a τ of 0.23 (1.23, 95% CI 0.89–1.72), suggesting that any increased risk is due to other exposures. Thus it is worth conducting further studies on painters. Indeed, a recent meta-analysis on 47 independent estimates of the association between employment as a painter and risk of lung cancer calculated an overall relative risk of 1.35 (95% CI 1.29–1.41), which is closer to the HR than the ML estimate.[15] If HR weights information from the DOM-JEM too heavily, we might have incurred the problem that high risks for occupations classified as not exposed to the three considered carcinogens (but likely to be exposed to other carcinogens) were always reduced. Among the twenty occupations with the highest ML odds ratios, six were not exposed to asbestos, chromium, or silica. HR shrinkage was strong for risks based on a small number of subjects but did not nullify those based on larger numbers, such as upholsterers (OR_{ML} 2.27, $OR_{HR}[\tau 0.59]$ 1.62) and tailors/dressmakers (OR_{ML} 2.08, $OR_{HR}[\tau 0.59]$ 1.49).

Estimation of bias

All of the Bayesian methods illustrated attempted to address the problem of random error, particularly in studies making multiple comparisons. All of these involved some type of shrinkage. In this section, we consider Bayesian methods for addressing systematic error, or bias (selection bias, information bias, and confounding). We illustrate these by considering examples of information bias.

Assessment of bias due to misclassification

Information bias in epidemiological studies arises from measurement error, also called classification error or misclassification. Such errors can occur at the design stage (e.g. invalid questions in a questionnaire), at the stage of data collection (e.g. information not accurately reported or recorded), or subsequently (e.g. mistakes in data entry).[16]

Table 17.3 Odds ratios (OR) and 95% CI of lung cancer obtained using maximum likelihood (ML), Semi-Bayes adjustment towards the global mean (SB), and hierarchical regression (HR) for the occupations associated with the 20 highest ORs in the conventional ML analysis

International Standard Code of Occupations	Cases/ controls	ML	SB		HR			Carcinogenic exposure		
			7-fold range	τ 0.76 (20-fold range)	τ 0.59 (10-fold range)	τ 0.41 (5-fold range)	τ 0.23 (2.5-fold range)	Asb[a]	Cr[a]	Si[a]
		OR, 95% CI	OR, 95% CI	OR, 95% CI	OR, 95% CI	OR, 95% CI	OR, 95% CI			
034 Electrical and electronics engineering technicians	5/9	1.61, 0.44–5.88	1.00, 0.45–2.21	1.21, 0.45–3.22	1.12, 0.47–2.66	1.02, 0.51–2.02	0.93, 0.60–1.44	0	0	0
628 Farm machinery operators	9/8	1.62, 0.55–4.81	1.28, 0.62–2.65	1.44, 0.58–3.54	1.38, 0.59–3.22	1.31, 0.61–2.81	1.22, 0.62–2.40	0	0	2
872 Welders and flame-cutters	47/37	1.67, 1.03–2.71	1.53, 0.99–2.36	1.66, 1.06–2.59	1.64, 1.06–2.53	1.60, 1.07–2.41	1.53, 1.06–2.19	0	2	0
039 Engineering technicians not elsewhere classified	7/7	1.71, 0.51–5.72	1.05, 0.49–2.28	1.28, 0.50–3.28	1.18, 0.51–2.72	1.05, 0.54–2.07	0.95, 0.62–1.46	0	0	0
727 Metal drawers and extruders	5/5	1.72, 0.45–6.63	1.24, 0.56–2.76	1.63, 0.66–4.03	1.59, 0.72–3.52	1.54, 0.81–2.91	1.48, 0.94–2.33	0	2	0
725 Metal moulders and coremakers	10/9	1.72, 0.65–4.58	1.35, 0.67–2.70	1.48, 0.70–3.13	1.41, 0.72–2.76	1.32, 0.77–2.28	1.21, 0.83–1.77	0	1	1
952 Reinforced-concreters, cement finishers, and terrazzo workers	13/8	1.78, 0.70–4.56	1.38, 0.70–2.74	1.52, 0.73–3.16	1.44, 0.75–2.78	1.34, 0.78–2.30	1.22, 0.84–1.77	0	1	1
729 Metal processors not elsewhere classified	28/20	1.79, 0.97–3.32	1.54, 0.91–2.61	1.63, 0.95–2.82	1.57, 0.94–2.62	1.45, 0.92–2.28	1.28, 0.91–1.80	0	1	1
931 Painters, construction	42/29	1.85, 1.09–3.15	1.63, 1.02–2.61	1.66, 1.01–2.71	1.57, 0.98–2.52	1.43, 0.93–2.20	1.23, 0.89–1.72	1	0	0

								Asb	Cr	Si
871 Plumbers and pipe fitters	29/22	1.94, 1.03–3.65	1.62, 0.95–2.77	1.90, 1.06–3.43	1.87, 1.05–3.32	1.82, 1.05–3.16	1.76, 1.04–2.98	2	0	0
891 Glass formers, cutters, grinders, and finishers	15/8	1.95, 0.78–4.85	1.46, 0.75–2.87	1.53, 0.72–3.24	1.40, 0.71–2.78	1.24, 0.70–2.19	1.06, 0.71–1.57	0	1	0
751 Fibre preparers	5/5	1.97, 0.48–8.03	1.29, 0.58–2.89	1.31, 0.47–3.64	1.18, 0.48–2.90	1.05, 0.52–2.12	0.94, 0.61–1.46	0	0	0
943 Non-metallic mineral product makers	7/4	2.00, 0.56–7.13	1.34, 0.61–2.92	1.51, 0.64–3.56	1.42, 0.68–2.98	1.31, 0.73–2.35	1.21, 0.82–1.78	0	1	1
723 Metal melters and reheaters	12/6	2.06, 0.75–5.72	1.45, 0.71–2.96	1.84, 0.87–3.90	1.79, 0.91–3.50	1.73, 0.99–3.03	1.70, 1.11–2.61	1	2	0
791 Tailors and dressmakers	14/11	2.08, 0.87–5.00	1.54, 0.79–2.97	1.64, 0.77–3.50	1.49, 0.74–3.01	1.28, 0.71–2.32	1.05, 0.70–1.57	0	0	0
893 Glass and ceramics kilnmen	11/6	2.14, 0.73–6.25	1.45, 0.70–3.01	1.61, 0.76–3.42	1.53, 0.79–2.95	1.44, 0.85–2.45	1.38, 0.95–2.00	1	1	1
796 Upholsterers and related workers	19/11	2.27, 0.99–5.21	1.65, 0.87–3.13	1.79, 0.87–3.69	1.62, 0.82–3.18	1.37, 0.77–2.45	1.08, 0.72–1.62	0	0	0
728 Metal platers and coaters	13/7	3.26, 1.17–9.07	1.81, 0.88–3.72	2.30, 1.05–5.05	2.08, 1.02–4.23	1.82, 1.00–3.29	1.57, 1.01–2.46	0	2	0
612 Specialized farmers	9/3	3.44, 0.90–13.17	1.59, 0.71–3.55	1.81, 0.67–4.93	1.53, 0.63–3.68	1.23, 0.61–2.47	1.00, 0.65–1.55	0	0	0
982 Ships' engine-room ratings	8/2	5.88, 0.94–36.71	1.54, 0.64–3.73	2.43, 0.79–7.46	2.16, 0.82–5.73	1.93, 0.87–4.29	1.78, 0.96–3.32	2	0	0

[a] Asb, asbestos (0 = no exposure, 1 = low exposure, 2 = high exposure), Cr, chromium (0 = no exposure, 1 = low exposure, 2 = high exposure), Si, Silica (0 = no exposure, 1 = low exposure, 2 = high exposure).

Reproduced from Corbin M et al., Hierarchical Regression for Multiple Comparisons in a Case-Control Study of Occupational Risks for Lung Cancer, *PLoS ONE*, Volume 7, Issue 6,

As with all kinds of systematic errors, measurement error can be considered as a missing data problem[3] in that information has been recorded about an imperfect surrogate variable whereas the information is missing for the 'correct' variable. When internal validation data are available, both the misclassified and true values are known for a subsample of the dataset. In this situation, the true values are only partially missing and traditional methods for dealing with missing data can be applied to correct for misclassification e.g. by imputing the missing data.[17] When internal validation data are not available, the values for the 'correct' variable are completely missing and a sensitivity analysis relying on prior information needs to be carried out.

The methods are illustrated with data from the New Zealand population-based lung cancer case-control study.[8] In this, we considered the association between smoking status (ever/never) and lung cancer. In the standard analyses, the odds ratio of lung cancer for ever smokers versus never smokers was estimated using unconditional logistic regression, adjusting for age (5-year age-groups), gender, Māori ethnicity, and socioeconomic status. The crude odds ratio was 7.51 (95% CI 5.41–10.43) and the adjusted odds ratio was 7.74 (5.49–10.91).

We then assumed that the measured smoking status was misclassified and estimated what the 'true' odds ratio for smoking would have been if there had been no misclassification, first using standard sensitivity analysis, and then probabilistic sensitivity analysis.

Table 17.4 shows the findings of the standard sensitivity analysis. It shows, for example, that varying the assumptions about the specificity of the smoking data (i.e. assuming that some non-smokers were randomly misclassified as smokers) had only a moderate effect on the estimated odds ratios. However, even a small change in the sensitivity (e.g. from 1.0 to 0.9) resulted in a very large increase in the 'corrected' odds ratio. Furthermore, some values for sensitivity (e.g. 0.8) yielded impossible results so that the 'corrected' odds ratio could not be estimated. This occurs because if, for

Table 17.4 Estimated 'true' odds ratios based on various assumptions on sensitivity and specificity of the smoking information

Sensitivity	Specificity	Odds ratio
1.0	1.0	7.51[a]
1.0	0.9	8.24
1.0	0.8	9.42
0.9	1.0	83.08
0.8	1.0	NA[b]
0.9	0.9	91.15

[a] Observed odds ratio
[b] Cannot be calculated
Source: data from Marine Corbin et al., Lung cancer and occupation: A New Zealand cancer registry-based case-control study, *American Journal of Industrial Medicine*, Volume 54, Issue 2, pp. 89–101, Copyright © 2010 Wiley-Liss, Inc

example, 95% of cases are smokers, it is not possible to assume that the sensitivity of the smoking questions is only 80%.

This approach can be enhanced by using probabilistic sensitivity analysis, i.e. by specifying a range of possible values or prior distributions for sensitivity and specificity. For example, suppose that each has a minimum of 0.65, a most likely range of 0.85–0.98, and a maximum of 1.0. Lash et al.[16] provide useful Excel spreadsheets to obtain weighted estimates for the 'corrected' odds ratio using aggregate data. For example, Table 17.5 shows that, if we make the above assumptions about the likely range of values for sensitivity and specificity, then the crude odds ratio of 7.51 changes to 17.83 when 'corrected' for misclassification.

These Excel spreadsheets provide valuable estimates of the likely direction and magnitude of bias due to misclassification. However, they do not allow us to control for confounders in the standard way. This can be done applying probabilistic sensitivity analysis to record-level data rather than to summary data. In this approach, we also need to make assumptions about the likely range of possible values for sensitivity and specificity. We then do a random draw of a large number (e.g. 500) of combinations of sensitivity and specificity from these distributions. For each simulation, we can then calculate[18] the positive predictive value and negative predictive value, and then values can be applied to each individual study participant to simulate their 'corrected' exposure status. The association between exposure and outcome can then be estimated in the usual way, adjusting for all covariates. The findings can then be summarized across all 500 simulations. Table 17.5 shows that when this method is applied to the New Zealand case-control data, the adjusted odds ratio of 7.80 for smoking and lung cancer increases to 19.78.

So what is the correct answer? Usually we would wish to do the analysis both ways and estimate the standard (uncorrected) effect estimates but then do a sensitivity analysis to assess how strong the likely bias from misclassification might be, and in what direction. Thus, we can analyse and report the data in the standard way but also include additional paragraphs in the Methods and Results sections.

Table 17.5 Estimated 'true' odds ratios for smoking and lung cancer, corrected assuming misclassification of the smoking information.

Method	Uncorrected odds ratio, 95% CI	Corrected odds ratio, 95% CI
Probabilistic sensitivity analysis—aggregate data	[a] 7.51, 5.41–10.43	17.83, 8.90–288.51
Probabilistic sensitivity analysis—record-level data	[b] 7.80, 5.53–10.85	19.78, 9.50–214.78

[a] Observed crude odds ratio
[b] Observed adjusted odds ratio
Source: data from Marine Corbin et al., Lung cancer and occupation: A New Zealand cancer registry-based case-control study, *American Journal of Industrial Medicine*, Volume 54, Issue 2, pp. 89–101, Copyright © 2010 Wiley-Liss, Inc

Discussion

To summarize, most epidemiologists write their Methods and Results sections as frequentists and their Introduction and Discussion sections as Bayesians. In their Methods and Results sections, they 'test' their findings as if their data are the only data that exist. In the Introduction and Discussion, they discuss their findings with regard to their consistency with previous studies, as well as other issues such as biological plausibility. This creates tensions when a small study has findings which are not statistically significant but which are consistent with prior knowledge, or when a study finds statistically significant findings which are inconsistent with prior knowledge. Thus, in practice, almost all epidemiologists profess to be frequentists, but in practice are qualitative Bayesians.

In some (but not all) instances, things can be made clearer if we include Bayesian methods formally in the Methods and Results sections of our papers, in other words if we act as quantitative, as well as qualitative, Bayesians. In this chapter, we have reviewed and illustrated some of the methods which are currently available, most of which can be done easily with standard statistical analysis packages. One of us (NP) is old enough to remember when logistic regression was regarded as a new and difficult method, but now it has become a routinely used part of the epidemiologist's toolkit. Hopefully, in future years it will become just as routine to use EB and SB adjustments for multiple comparisons, and to conduct sensitivity analyses, using standard statistical packages. In most instances, these will not replace existing methods. Rather, they will supplement them, so that we have an extra paragraph or two in our Methods sections, and an extra paragraph or two, and additional tables, in our Results sections. This will enable us to address the elephant in the room more clearly and to assess problems of multiple comparisons and bias in a quantitative manner. These new methods are applicable to all areas of epidemiology, but particularly to occupational epidemiology, because of the large number of comparisons often involved, the hierarchical nature of much exposure data, and the potential to make a quantitative assessment of bias.

Acknowledgement

We carried out much of this work at the Centre for Public Health Research at Massey University, Wellington, New Zealand, which is supported by a programme grant from the Health Research Council of New Zealand.

References

1. Greenland S. Bayesian perspectives for epidemiological research: I. Foundations and basic methods. *Int J Epidemiol* 2006;**35**:765–75.
2. Greenland S. Bayesian perspectives for epidemiological research: II. Regression analysis. *Int J Epidemiol* 2007;**36**:195–202.
3. Greenland S. Bayesian perspectives for epidemiologic research: III. Bias analysis via missing-data methods. *Int J Epidemiol* 2009;**38**:1662–73. (Correction in: *Int J Epidemiol* 2010;**39**:1116.)

4. **Kogevinas M, Becher H, Benn T,** *et al.* Cancer mortality in workers exposed to phenoxy herbicides, chlorophenols, and dioxins. An expanded and updated international cohort study. *Am J Epidemiol* 1997;**145**:1061–75.

5. **International Agency for Research on Cancer.** *Polychlorinated dibenzo-para-dioxins and polychlorinated dibenzofurans.* IARC Monographs on the Evaluation of Carcinogenic Risks to Humans, Volume 69. Lyon: IARC, 1997. Available at: <http://monographs.iarc.fr/ENG/Monographs/vol69/index.php> (accessed 7 March 2013).

6. **Benjamini Y, Hochberg Y.** Controlling the false discovery rate: a practical and powerful approach to multiple testing. *J R Stat Soc Series B Methodological* 1995;**57**:289–300.

7. **Steenland K, Bray I, Greenland S, Boffetta P.** Empirical Bayes adjustments for multiple results in hypothesis-generating or surveillance studies. *Cancer Epidemiol Biomarkers Prev* 2000;**9**:895–903.

8. **Corbin M, McLean D, 't Mannetje A,** *et al.* Lung cancer and occupation: a New Zealand cancer registry-based case-control study. *Am J Ind Med* 2011;**54**:89–101.

9. *R: A language and environment for statistical computing.* Vienna, Austria: R Foundation for Statistical Computing, 2006.

10. **Greenland S, Poole C.** Empirical-Bayes and semi-Bayes approaches to occupational and environmental hazard surveillance. *Arch Environ Health* 1994;**49**:9–16.

11. **Maule M, Merletti F, Mirabelli D, La Vecchia C.** Spatial variation of mortality for common and rare cancers in Piedmont, Italy, from 1980 to 2000: a Bayesian approach. *Eur J Cancer Prev* 2006;**15**:108–16.

12. **Corbin M, Richiardi L, Vermeulen R,** *et al.* Hierarchical regression for multiple comparisons in a case-control study of occupational risks for lung cancer. *PloS One* 2012;**7**:e38944-e44. doi: 10.1371/journal.pone.0038944.

13. **Chen GK, Witte JS.** Enriching the analysis of genomewide association studies with hierarchical modeling. *Am J Hum Genet* 2007;**81**:397–404.

14. **Witte JS, Greenland S, Haile RW, Bird CL.** Hierarchical regression analysis applied to a study of multiple dietary exposures and breast cancer. *Epidemiology* 1994;**5**:612–21.

15. **Guha N, Merletti F, Steenland NK, Altieri A, Cogliano V, Straif K.** Lung cancer risk in painters: a meta-analysis. *Environ Health Perspect* 2010;**118**:303–12.

16. **Lash TL, Fox MP, Fink AK.** *Applying quantitative bias analysis to epidemiologic data.* New York: Springer, 2009.

17. **Cole SR, Chu H, Greenland S.** Multiple-imputation for measurement-error correction. *Int J Epidemiol* 2006;**35**:1074–81.

18. **Fox MP, Lash TL, Greenland S.** A method to automate probabilistic sensitivity analyses of misclassified binary variables. *Int J Epidemiol* 2005;**34**:1370–6.

Part 7

Making full use of the findings

Chapter 18

Basic principles of economic evaluation of occupational health and safety interventions

Oliver Rivero-Arias, Sue Jowett,
and Marjolein de Weerd

Introduction

Economic evaluation is defined as 'the comparative analysis of alternative courses of action in terms of both their costs and consequences',[1] and is a technique commonly used in the field of health care, in order to determine the cost-effectiveness of an intervention compared with the best available alternative. Economic evaluation of health care technologies will primarily consider differences in health care costs and health outcomes in order to determine whether an intervention is good value for money. The methods for economic analyses in health care are well established and guidelines for conducting economic evaluations are widely available,[1–3] therefore lessons learned in health care can be applied to different disciplines. However, conducting an economic analysis alongside occupational health and safety (OHS) interventions presents a number of interesting challenges, in particular the variety of stakeholders involved with the implications for the definition of the perspective, and the measurement and valuation of costs and consequences associated to the intervention. In addition, economic evaluation of health technologies seeks efficiency in health care decision-making, i.e. maximization of health gains for the population given the scarce resources available. However, the maximization of health gains as a result of the introduction of an OHS intervention is unlikely to be the only or primary objective for a particular company owner or for society as a whole. Maximizing productivity or minimizing sickness absence are also competing objectives across stakeholders when conducting economic evaluations of OHS interventions.

Economic evaluations of OHS interventions are much less common than studies in health, and the slow uptake of economic analysis in OHS is partly due to the lack of expertise or experience of OHS researchers.[4] Recent guidance on good practice in economic evaluation of OHS interventions is contributing to the development of guidelines and shaping up the agenda for a reference case to improve the quality and reporting of these studies in the future.[5,6] This chapter provides an overview of the basic principles of economic evaluation of OHS interventions using an adapted checklist proposed for critical appraisal of economic evaluations of health care technologies,[7] and based on the conclusions of the Panel on Cost-Effectiveness in Health and Medicine.[3] To illustrate the use of this checklist in practice the chapter presents one case study of an economic analysis in an area of high risk of sickness absence.

Principles of economic evaluation of OHS interventions

Economic evaluation of OHS shares similarities with health care in terms of the basic principles of economic evaluation; therefore it is reasonable to consider established guidance. Sections A to D form a 'checklist for critical appraisal' of economic analyses, and provide a standard set of methodologies that a researcher in OHS should seek to improve internal validity and to allow meaningful comparison across studies (see Box 18.1). Briefly, section A concerns the framework of the economic analysis, covering aspects such as the type of analysis conducted, the background of the question that is being addressed, the comparators, and the perspective and time horizon of the analysis. Section B covers the identification, measurement, and valuation of costs and consequences. Section C gives guidance on the presentation of results and putting those results into context, and Section D considers how the findings should be discussed in relation to policy and implementation.

Box 18.1 Checklist for critical appraisal of economic analysis of OHS interventions[7]

A. The framework
1. Justification of type of analysis
2. Addressing the research question, general study design, and target population
3. Definition of the comparator intervention
4. The perspective and time horizon of the study

B. Data and methods
5. Identifying and valuing costs
6. Measuring and valuing consequences
7. Study design and data collection

C. Results
8. Presenting and interpreting the base case results and associated uncertainty
9. Comparison with relevant economic evaluations

D. Discussion
10. Relevance of the study for policy questions, and any ethical or distributive implications

Adapted from Gray A., Economic evaluation, in Dawes M (ed), *Evidence-based practice: a primer for health care professionals*, Second Edition, Churchill Livingstone, London, UK, Copyright © 2005, with permission from Elsevier and Gold MR et al., *Cost-effectiveness in health and medicine*, Oxford University Press Inc., New York, USA, Copyright © 1996, by permission of Oxford University Press.

The framework

Justification of selection of type of analysis

There are three main non-mutually exclusive economic analysis options available to researchers in OHS; the stakeholder and the perspective of importance will drive the choice of analysis type. Cost-benefit analysis, where costs and outcomes are measured in monetary terms, is highly appropriate for those OHS studies where the outcome of interest may be a reduction in absenteeism and/or presenteeism. Economic evaluations in health care commonly use cost-effectiveness analysis, where the outcomes are measured in natural units measuring a clinical or health outcome (e.g. life-years), or cost-utility analysis, where the outcomes are measured in quality-adjusted life years (QALYs), a generic measure which combines information on quality of life and survival. Both types of analyses have their place in OHS if the outcome of interest can be measured in natural units (e.g. days off work), or the health-related quality of life of workers is of importance to the stakeholder. A summary of the three types of economic evaluation with their characteristics is presented in Table 18.1. Whatever the decision, a study should clearly state what type of analysis is being undertaken, and there should be a clear rationale for the choice of evaluation.

Addressing the research question, general study design, and target population

Setting the scene is a key component of any economic evaluation. Firstly, it is essential that the background of the problem being addressed by an intervention is clearly stated, with supporting evidence. This may include information such as the extent of

Table 18.1 Different types of economic evaluations and their characteristics[30]

Type of study	Valuation of consequences	Advantages	Disadvantages
Cost-benefit	Monetary units	Both benefits and costs are valued in monetary units	Objective monetary values for non-monetary consequences may be difficult to obtain
Cost-effectiveness	Natural units (asthma-free days, reduction in sick days, life-years gained, etc.)	Impact of health effects captured through validated instruments and questionnaires	Results from cost-effectiveness studies from different programmes are not easily comparable
Cost-utility	Quality-adjusted life years (QALYs)	Using a QALY metric facilitates comparisons across different programmes	Different methods to estimate QALYs yield different QALY results

Adapted from Hoch JS and Dewa CS, Kind of analysis and decision rule, in Tompa E et al. (eds) *Economic evaluation of interventions for occupational health and safety: developing good practice*, Oxford University Press, Oxford, UK, Copyright © 2008, by permission of Oxford University Press.

the problem (e.g. prevalence of back pain in a particular occupational group), what is already known about interventions for the problem, and why an investigation of the interventions of choice is important. This should then be summarized as a clear and answerable research question, with a primary objective. The design of the research study also needs to be explicitly stated, e.g. is it a randomized controlled trial or an observational study, and how are research participants identified? This allows the reader to critically evaluate the overall methodological quality of the study that the economic evaluation is based upon. Finally, the target population should be described, providing information on which group the intervention should be aimed at, in terms of characteristics such as occupation, age group, gender, and clinical condition (where appropriate). This ensures that the reader can judge whether the target population, and therefore the intervention, is applicable to their own workforce.

Definition of the comparator intervention

A full economic evaluation should be a comparison of two or more courses of action, and it is essential that interventions and comparators are clearly described. Finding an appropriate comparator can be a difficult exercise in OHS studies but, in general, the comparator should be the standard OHS practices currently in place or the status quo in the organization.

The perspective and time horizon of the study

The choice of perspective determines the costs and consequences to be collected and valued within a study, and should always be explicitly stated. The most commonly used perspective in health care is a health services perspective, which takes into account costs that are incurred by the health care provider and benefits in terms of improvement in health. However, health economics textbooks often advocate a societal perspective, where all costs and benefits should be considered, no matter on whom they fall. Within OHS studies, the stakeholder will often determine the perspective, and analyses are often undertaken from the perspective of the employer, taking into account the costs of the intervention and any financial benefits from improved worker performance. However, some OHS research takes a broader perspective and includes costs and benefits to the health care provider, the employer, and the employees. Ideally, an economic evaluation should consider all costs and consequences related to each stakeholder in order to provide results that are meaningful for decision-making. This is important because adopting a narrower perspective in the study can potentially lead to a wrong decision being made. For instance, a company owner who needs to implement a new intervention that improves safety faces the cost of implementing the intervention but most of the benefits are accrued by the employees. The benefits for the owner in terms of productivity improvements may be slim and hence using the sole perspective of the owner in the study may suggest that it is not worth implementing the intervention. However a different decision would be reached if the benefits for the worker (in terms of health improvements) are also included and offset the implementation costs.

A further consideration in an economic evaluation is the time horizon of the analysis, which should be stated and justified. Ideally, a study should have a timeframe which is sufficiently long to observe and capture all the relevant information on costs and consequences. If that time horizon is over a year in length, discounting should be applied to both costs and benefits.[8] The rationale behind discounting is the notion of time preference, whereby benefits are preferred now, and costs later. However, in a study, there may be differential timing of costs and benefits with all the intervention costs upfront and benefits realized later on. Therefore, there is a need to convert all costs and benefits to their present value by applying a discount rate which will be determined by the country in which the study is being conducted and by the decision-maker. Again, the use of discounting and the rate applied should be reported.

Data and methods

Identifying and valuing costs

All resource use and associated costs of both the OHS intervention and any comparator need to be identified and valued. The analysis of costs of a new OHS intervention compared to standard practice provides information about the incremental difference between the costs of the alternatives. Costs should be valued to include their opportunity costs, i.e. the value of the benefits forgone of the best alternative use of the resources.[9] If historical cost information from previous years is used then these data should be inflated to the current price year.

The selection of categories of costs to be included will depend on whether a company or a societal perspective is used. If a company perspective is adopted, then this should differentiate between those categories that relate to the owner of the company and those that relate to the worker. Given that an OHS intervention can affect several stakeholders, it is recommended that a broad perspective that identifies all costs incurred by each stakeholder is followed (see Box 18.2). Box 18.2 identifies the main costs and consequences that may be incurred by stakeholders as a result of a potential OHS intervention. The list should be used as guidance and a starting point as it is by no means exhaustive but it identifies the cost categories that are usually considered important. For an expanded discussion of the identification and valuation of costs see Laporte et al.[10]

After identifying the categories of costs associated to the intervention and the stakeholders involved, a cost estimate needs to be produced. Sources for cost data include administrative records that include payroll information, hours worked, and the value of new/replacement equipment. In addition, these data sources also contain information on the impact of the intervention, for example, a reduction in accidents, or an improvement in productivity. However, it will be unlikely that administrative records include all the relevant cost estimates needed for the study and they will need to be complemented with management and worker surveys. Health care resource use data to explore the impact of an intervention can be collected through questionnaires or national databases that provide patient-level information on hospitalization-related costs.

Measuring and valuing consequences

Figure 18.1 presents the possible relationship of productivity and health as a result of an investment in health and safety.[11] Three types of consequence are identified and

Box 18.2 Categories[a] of costs and consequences of an OHS intervention (adapted from Laporte et al.[10] and reproduced with permission)

Costs of resources consumed

1. Company owner

   Cost incurred to undertake OHS intervention

2. Workers and families

   Out-of-pocket expenditures associated with the intervention

3. Public sector/insurers

   Funds used to support intervention and not paid for directly or indirectly by the company

Consequences of the intervention

1. Company owner

   Productivity consequences of health improvements

   Reduced claims administration, human resources, and insurance costs

2. Workers and families

   Reduced pain, suffering, and loss of enjoyment of life due to prevention initiatives

   Reduced out-of-pocket costs

   Increased time for workers to fulfil domestic, leisure, and community roles

   Increased time for family members to fulfil domestic, leisure, community, and work roles

3. Public sector/insurers

   Reduced programme administration, delivery, and surveillance costs

   Reduced insurance costs not paid by the company

   Reduced health care costs

4. Society

   Productivity consequences of health improvements related to reduced mortality and morbidity

[a] The allocation of costs and consequences to the company owner, public sector, or insurers will depend on the structure and funding of the country's occupational health care system.

Adapted from Laporte A et al., Costs, in Tompa E et al. (eds) *Economic evaluation of interventions for occupational health and safety: developing good practice*, Oxford University Press, Oxford, UK, Copyright © 2008, by permission of Oxford University Press.

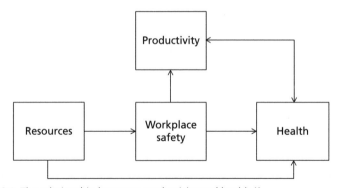

Figure 18.1 The relationship between productivity and health.[11]
Reproduced from Culyer AJ et al., What is a little more health and safety worth?, p. 18, in Tompa E et al. (eds), *Economic evaluation of interventions for occupational health and safety: developing good practice*, Oxford University Press, Oxford, UK, Copyright © 2008, by permission of Oxford University Press.

include improvements in workplace safety, productivity, and health. Improvement in productivity may arise from interventions that address workplace safety or directly impact on health. Similarly, the health of workers can be enhanced by safer workplaces and by improvements in productivity. Finally, health can be directly improved through health care services, including OHS clinical services. This complex scenario presents challenges to researchers deciding which consequences ought to be considered part of the economic evaluation of an OHS intervention. Different types of consequences of an OHS intervention for different stakeholders are presented in Box 18.2. The final decision about what consequences to include will depend on 'the nature of the intervention, context and purpose of the evaluation, perspective taken, projected distribution of benefits across stakeholders, and any consideration to feasibility of data collection and resources likely to be available for the evaluation'.[12]

The choice of consequences for the study will define the type of analysis and, as already introduced in section 1 of this checklist, will include cost-benefit, cost-effectiveness, and cost-utility analyses. Measuring outcomes in monetary terms in cost-benefit analysis is far from straightforward, but methods such as human capital, revealed preference, and stated preference are available.[1,13–15] Natural units for cost-effectiveness analysis, such as number of sick days, are straightforward to collect as part of payroll and administrative records. However, certain natural units, such as asthma-free days or pain levels, to measure the impact on health of a particular OHS intervention need to be collected through disease-specific or generic instruments in surveys using appropriate study designs.[16] QALYs in cost-utility analysis are the combination of survival benefit and quality of life as a result of an intervention. To estimate QALYs, quality of life is estimated using preference-based instruments (e.g. EuroQol EQ-5D[17]) that allow health states to be associated with a valuation of the preference of society for that health state.[18] Cost-benefit and cost-effectiveness analyses are the two most-widely used types of economic evaluation of OHS found in the literature.[4]

Given that productivity consequences are a key outcome of any OHS intervention, it is important to avoid any possible double counting when measuring these consequences. This can happen because productivity consequences of health improvements may already be captured in the measure of health outcome selected. For instance, in cost-benefit analysis productivity implications may be already incorporated in the revealed or stated preference exercises. Similarly, when assessing preference-based valuations to estimate utilities for health states, respondents may incorporate their own productivity implications as part of the valuation exercise.[19,20] Therefore, it is important that revealed preferences, stated preferences, and valuation exercises do not include any productivity implications, and that these consequences should be captured separately. This is the general recommendation in economic evaluation of health care technologies and it is also recommended as good practice in economic analysis of OHS interventions.[12]

Study design and data collection

The study design and how data on costs and consequences are collected need to be clearly reported. Two main types of study design can be found in cost-effectiveness analysis of health care technologies that can be translated to the OHS field: prospective/retrospective data collection, and modelling exercises. Prospective/retrospective data collection, including observational studies and randomized controlled trials, provides detailed worker-level information on the costs and consequences associated to the OHS intervention and any comparator. Randomized controlled trials are the 'gold standard' study design in evaluating the effectiveness of an intervention because they are less subject to biases.[21] Observational studies, such as cohort, before-after, or case-control designs, can also be very useful in gathering information on costs and consequences at worker level when it is not possible or desirable to conduct a randomized trial. Nevertheless, appropriate methods that control for the non-randomized nature of observational studies are needed when estimating the effectiveness of an OHS intervention.[22] Modelling exercises are also a powerful way of estimating the cost-effectiveness of OHS interventions. Evidence from several sources is synthesized in a mathematical model that represents the decision-making problem.[23] The model is informed through parameters that relate to pieces of information on costs and consequences. The sources of information on costs and consequences can include data from the literature, payroll and administrative records, and worker-level data from prospective/retrospective data collection, if available.

Results

Presenting and interpreting the base case results and associated uncertainty

The base case analysis is the original set of results obtained from using methods recommended from a reference case.[3] Costs, consequences, and summary measures of cost-benefit or cost-effectiveness with their associated uncertainty should be presented separately for each stakeholder. If considered appropriate, a final estimate across all stakeholders summarizing the results from the economic evaluation can also be presented. The results of cost-benefit analysis are normally presented using an incremental net present value (INPV), which is simply the difference in net present values between the OHS intervention and the comparator under evaluation. Values of INPV greater than zero represent OHS programmes worth implementing. In contrast, cost-effectiveness and cost-utility analyses are presented using an incremental cost-effectiveness ratio (ICER) which is the difference in costs divided by the difference in effects between the OHS intervention and the comparator. For example, if the effectiveness of a particular OHS programme is measured by the reduction in the number of sickness absence days, the ICER represents the cost per sickness absence day avoided. (A cost-benefit ratio[24] can also be calculated in cost-benefit analysis but it is not recommended so as to avoid confusion with ratios from cost-effectiveness and cost-utility analyses.[10])

It is inherently more difficult to interpret ICERs than the INPV but, to facilitate interpretation, ICERs can be presented on the cost-effectiveness plane (see Figure 18.2).[25] The cost-effectiveness plane (CEP) is an incremental graph, i.e. it expresses differences between the alternatives, which may be positive or negative. The x-axis defines differences in effectiveness while the y-axis defines differences in costs between the alternatives. In discussing the CEP, we assume that the effectiveness of the OHS intervention refers to health improvement. The origin of the plane, where the axes cross, represents the comparator alternative (C) which may be the OHS standard practice or the status quo. Any point plotted in the plane represents an ICER, and any point along a line from the origin has consequently the same ICER. The CEP has four quadrants (represented by compass points) and each quadrant identifies a possible combination of the costs and effectiveness of the alternatives evaluated. In the southeast quadrant, the new OHS intervention 'dominates' the comparator since it is more effective and less costly. In the northwest quadrant of the plane, the comparator

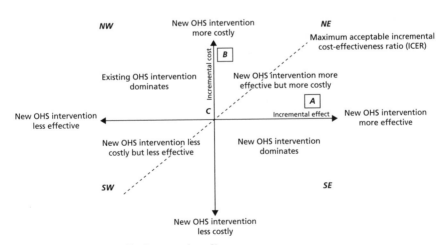

Figure 18.2 The cost-effectiveness plane.[31]
Reproduced from Gray AM et al., *Applied methods of cost-effectiveness analysis in health care*, p. 12, Oxford University Press, Oxford, UK, Copyright ©2011, by permission of Oxford University Press.

dominates because the new OHS intervention is both less effective and more costly. The decision-making process is straightforward in these southeast and northwest quadrants. More interesting are the situations obtaining in the northeast quadrant (where the new OHS intervention is more effective but also more expensive) and the southwest quadrant (where the new OHS intervention is less effective but cheaper than the comparator). In both cases, the decision to adopt will depend on whether the new OHS intervention represents good value for money, i.e. whether the additional effects of the new OHS intervention are worth its additional costs. Point A in the northeast quadrant represents a situation where the new OHS intervention is highly effective and not very much more expensive. Hence, a decision-maker is likely to adopt OHS interventions located near or at point A. However, point B in the same quadrant represents a situation where the new OHS intervention is only marginally more effective than the comparator, but significantly more expensive. In this case, the decision-maker may choose to spend the resources available more efficiently on other OHS programmes that produce more health gains than the OHS intervention which has been evaluated. As a result, points A and B in the same quadrant illustrate clear differences in the decision-making process and an explicit value is needed to determine which situation is the cost-effective alternative. This value should express the maximum amount of money we are willing to pay for health gains (the maximum acceptable ICER). This explicit value or 'threshold' is represented by the dotted line that divides the CEP in Figure 18.2 into two halves. Those interventions that lie below this threshold are said to be cost-effective whereas the interventions located above this threshold are not. What should be the value of the threshold is a subject of much controversy in health care,[26] although guidelines about setting the possible value of this ceiling have been proposed.[27]

The robustness of the base case results should be evaluated using appropriate measures of uncertainty. If worker-level data are available, sampling uncertainty can be assessed using confidence intervals for the differences in costs and consequences, INPV and ICERs. The results of cost-effectiveness and cost-utility analyses can be presented on the CEP with the joint density of differences in costs and consequences. Another useful tool to characterize uncertainty is the use of cost-effectiveness acceptability curves that present the probability of an OHS intervention being cost-effective for different threshold values of willingness to pay.[28] One-way or multi-way sensitivity analysis can be implemented to assess the impact of parameters not subject to sampling uncertainty. Finally, if evidence from different sources has been synthesized in an economic model, probabilistic sensitivity analysis can be used to assess parameter uncertainty and its impact on the base case results.[28]

Comparisons with relevant economic evaluations

The results of the study should be compared with relevant evidence from any previous economic evaluations that have addressed a similar research question. This will help to understand the contribution of the study to current knowledge or evidence. If the study obtains different results from previous similar evaluations, for example because of differences in study methodology, this needs to be clearly reported.

Discussion

Relevance of the study for policy questions, and any ethical or distributive implications

The final area of importance when reporting an economic evaluation is an appropriate discussion of the results. The discussion should consider the generalizability and transferability of the study findings, relevance of results for stakeholders, and whether there are any ethical or distributive implications. An exploration of the generalizability of the findings is essential in research studies, and economic evaluation is no different. The discussion may consider transferability of findings to other settings, for example other workplaces, health care settings, different geographical areas in the same country, or transferability to other countries. Following on from this should be a consideration of how the intervention could be used in practice, implications for policy, and impact on stakeholder groups. The implementation of an intervention may benefit one stakeholder group but with little gain for another. For example, there may be improved health for employees but little change in productivity and an employer may be reluctant to invest with little gain for them, although employee health or well-being is being enhanced.

Case study

The checklist for critical appraisal of economic evaluation is used in this case study to assess the quality of a published example.[29] Taimela et al. used a questionnaire to group workers in a Finnish corporation by their risk of work disability. The high-risk group was randomized into a trial of an intervention consisting of personal feedback about the questionnaire results, coupled with proactive case management by the occupational health service. The intermediate-risk group was also randomized into the trial but with a less intensive intervention consisting of feedback with referral to a telephone counselling service. The investigators conducted a cost-effectiveness analysis to determine whether the intervention was cost-effective in reducing sickness absence when compared with usual occupational health care (no feedback of results and a reactive service).

The framework

Justification of selection of type of analysis

The study was a cost-effectiveness analysis. This study design was selected because consequences were measured using sickness absence days.

Addressing the research question, general study design and target population

Sickness absence places a major economic burden on employers, the health care system, and society as a whole. The objective of this study was to determine whether, from a health care perspective, a specific occupational health intervention is cost-effective in reducing sickness absence when compared with usual occupational health care in workers with high risk of work disability. Subjects were recruited from a corporation in Finland.

Definition of the comparator intervention

The comparator in this case was usual occupational health care which included consultation with an occupational health nurse or physician if the worker requested it.

The perspective and time horizon of the study

The analysis was from a health care perspective, both occupational health care and general health care, and the time horizon of the study was 12 months' follow-up. Because the time horizon of the study did not exceed 12 months, there was no need for discounting.

Data and methods

Identifying and valuing the costs

A detailed costing exercise was conducted and all important categories of health care resource use, both occupational and general, were identified and collected in the study. To avoid double counting the authors did not include productivity costs, because they relate to sickness absence days, which was the primary outcome of the study. All costs were expressed in 2004 euros.

Measuring and valuing consequences

The primary outcome was the difference in sickness absence days at 12 months' follow-up between the intervention and the control group. Such information was collected from Finnish register data on sickness absence.

Study design and data collection

A randomized controlled trial with a 12 months' follow-up was conducted to evaluate the effectiveness of the intervention. Sickness absence data were gathered from register databases whereas health care resource use data were collected using postal surveys.

Results

Presenting and interpreting the base case results and associated uncertainty

A base case analysis was presented which included the reporting of resource use, associated costs, and primary outcome separately by intervention and control group. A summary measure using an ICER and expressed as cost per sickness absence day avoided was also reported. Appropriate characterization of uncertainty of ICERs using the cost-effectiveness plane and bootstrap replicates of difference in costs and effects, and cost-effectiveness acceptability curves were presented. In addition, one-way sensitivity analysis was conducted to evaluate the impact of varying unit costs and resource use parameters on the base case results.

Comparison with other relevant economic evaluations

An explicit detailed comparison with other economic evaluations was included in the discussion section of the study.

Relevance of the study for policy questions, and any ethical or distributive implications

The authors placed the results of the study in context for policymakers and suggested that the study provides robust evidence and support to suggest that proactive case management interventions that target employees who are at high risk of sickness absence and work disability are likely to be cost-effective.

Summary and conclusions

This chapter provides an overview of the basic principles of economic evaluation of OHS interventions using an adapted checklist proposed for critical appraisal of economic evaluations of health care technologies, and based on the conclusions of the US Panel on Cost-Effectiveness in Health and Medicine. The checklist is structured into four main headings that include the framework of the study, data and methods, presentation of results, and discussion and implications of the evaluation. The content in each heading has been adapted to represent aspects of the economic analysis of OHS interventions. This checklist can be used as guidance when preparing proposals for new studies, when reporting the results of economic evaluations of OHS interventions, or when assessing the quality of published evidence.

Acknowledgement

This chapter is based on material presented by the authors during the workshop 'Economic Analyses in Occupational Epidemiology' associated with the 22nd International Conference on Epidemiology in Occupational Health, 6–9 September 2011, Oxford (EPICOH 2011).

References

1. Drummond MF, Sculpher MJ, Torrance GW, O'Brien BJ, Stoddart GL. *Methods for the economic evaluation of health care programmes* (3rd edn). Oxford: Oxford University Press, 2005.
2. National Institute for Health and Clinical Excellence. *Guide to the methods of technology appraisal.* London: National Institute for Health and Clinical Excellence, 2008. Available at: <http://www.nice.org.uk/media/b52/a7/tamethodsguideupdatedjune2008.pdf> (accessed 14 February 2013).
3. Gold MR, Siegel JE, Russell LB, Weinstein MC. *Cost-effectiveness in health and medicine.* New York: Oxford University Press, 1996.
4. Tompa E, Dolinschi R, de Oliveira C, Amick BC 3rd, Irvin E. A systematic review of workplace ergonomic interventions with economic analyses. *J Occup Rehabil* 2010;**20**:220–34.
5. Tompa E, Verbeek J, van Tulder M, de Boer A. Developing guidelines for good practice in the economic evaluation of occupational safety and health interventions. *Scand J Work Environ Health* 2010;**36**:313–8.
6. Tompa E, Culyer AJ, Dolinschi R (eds). *Economic evaluation of interventions for occupational health and safety: developing good practice.* Oxford: Oxford University Press, 2008.

7. **Gray A.** Economic evaluation. In: Dawes M (ed.) *Evidence-based practice: a primer for health care professionals* (2nd edn). London: Churchill Livingstone, 2005, pp. 101–10.

8. **Cairns J.** Discounting in economic evaluation. In: Drummond M, McGuire A (eds) *Economic evaluation in health care: merging theory with practice.* Oxford: Oxford University Press, 2001, pp. 236–55.

9. **Brouwer W, Rutten F, Koopmanschap M.** Costing in economic evaluations. In: Drummond M, McGuire A (eds) *Economic evaluation in health care: merging theory with practice.* Oxford: Oxford University Press, 2001, pp. 68–93.

10. **Laporte A, Dolinschi R, Tompa E.** Costs. In: Tompa E, Culyer AJ, Dolinschi R (eds) *Economic evaluation of interventions for occupational health and safety: developing good practice.* Oxford: Oxford University Press, 2008, pp. 165–77.

11. **Culyer AJ, Amick BC III, Laporte A.** What is a little more health and safety worth? In: Tompa E, Culyer AJ, Dolinschi R (eds) *Economic evaluation of interventions for occupational health and safety: developing good practice.* Oxford: Oxford University Press, 2008, pp. 15–35.

12. **Tompa E, Dolinschi R, De Oliveira C.** Consequences. In: Tompa E, Culyer AJ, Dolinschi R (eds) *Economic evaluation of interventions for occupational health and safety: developing good practice.* Oxford: Oxford University Press, 2008, pp. 179–200.

13. **Sculpher M.** The role and estimation of productivity costs in economic evaluation. In: Drummond M, McGuire A (eds) *Economic evaluation in health care: merging theory with practice.* Oxford: Oxford University Press, 2001, pp. 94–112.

14. **Ryan M, Gerard K, Amaya-Amaya M** (eds) *Using discrete choice experiments to value health and health care.* The Economics of Non-Market Goods and Resources, Volume 11, Bateman IJ (series ed.). Dordrecht: Springer, 2008.

15. **Louviere JJ, Hensher DA, Swait JD.** *Stated choice methods: analysis and application.* Cambridge: Cambridge University Press, 2003.

16. **Gnam W, Robson L, Kohstall T. Study design.** In: Tompa E, Culyer AJ, Dolinschi R (eds) *Economic evaluation of interventions for occupational health and safety: developing good practice.* Oxford: Oxford University Press, 2008, pp. 135–45.

17. **Brooks R.** EuroQol: the current state of play. *Health Policy* 1996;**37**:53–72.

18. **Dolan P, Gudex C, Kind P, Williams A.** The time trade-off method: results from a general population study. *Health Econ* 1996;**5**:141–54.

19. **Luce BR, Manning WG, Siegel JE, Lipscomb J.** Estimating costs in cost-effectiveness analysis. In: Gold MR, Siegel JE, Russell LB, Weinstein MC (eds) *Cost-effectiveness in health and medicine.* New York: Oxford University Press, 1996, pp. 176–213.

20. **Drummond MF, Sculpher MJ, Torrance GW, O'Brien BJ, Stoddart GL.** Cost analysis. In: *Methods for the economic evaluation of health care programmes* (3rd edn). Oxford: Oxford University Press, 2005, pp. 55–101.

21. **Friedman LM, Furberg CD, DeMets DL.** *Fundamentals of clinical trials* (3rd edn). New York: Springer, 1998.

22. **Craig P, Cooper C, Gunnell D,** *et al.* Using natural experiments to evaluate population health interventions: new Medical Research Council guidance. *J Epidemiol Community Health* 2012;**66**:1182–6.

23. **Briggs A, Sculpher M, Claxton K.** *Decision modelling for health economic evaluation.* Handbooks in Health Economic Evaluation, Gray A, Briggs A (series eds). Oxford: Oxford University Press, 2006.

24. **McIntosh E.** Using discrete choice experiments within a cost-benefit analysis framework: some considerations. *Pharmacoeconomics* 2006;**24**:855–68.

25. **Black WC.** The CE plane: a graphic representation of cost-effectiveness. *Med Decis Making* 1990;**10**:212–4.

26. **Donaldson C, Baker R, Mason H,** *et al.* The social value of a QALY: raising the bar or barring the raise? *BMC Health Serv Res* 2011;**11**:8. doi: 10.1186/1472-6963-11-8.

27. **Rawlins M, Barnett D, Stevens A.** Pharmacoeconomics: NICE's approach to decision-making. *Br J Clin Pharmacol* 2010;**70**:346–9.

28. **Briggs AH.** Handling uncertainty in economic evaluation. In: Drummond M, McGuire A (eds) *Economic evaluation in health care: merging theory with practice.* Oxford: Oxford University Press, 2001, pp. 172–214.

29. **Taimela S, Justén S, Aronen P,** *et al.* An occupational health intervention programme for workers at high risk for sickness absence. Cost effectiveness analysis based on a randomised controlled trial. *Occup Environ Med* 2008;**65**:242–8.

30. **Hoch JS, Dewa CS.** Kind of analysis and decision rule. In: Tompa E, Culyer AJ, Dolinschi R (eds) *Economic evaluation of interventions for occupational health and safety: developing good practice.* Oxford: Oxford University Press, 2008, pp. 147–63.

31. **Gray AM, Clarke PM, Wolstenholme JL, Wordsworth S.** *Applied methods of cost-effectiveness analysis in health care.* Handbooks in Health Economic Evaluation, Number 3, Gray A, Briggs A (series eds). Oxford: Oxford University Press, 2010.

Chapter 19

Risk assessment for chemical and physical agents: how does occupational epidemiology contribute?

David Coggon

Introduction

Risk management is the process whereby a choice is made between two or more alternative courses of action according to the benefits that they may confer, their potential to cause harm, and the associated financial costs.

Informal risk management is frequently practised in everyday life. For example, when deciding whether or not to overtake a slower vehicle, a driver weighs up the gains that may accrue from reaching his destination earlier against the possibility of injury and expense if the manoeuvre leads to an accident. Here, the decision-making is rapid and may be based on past experience and practice with minimal thought. However, where circumstances are less familiar and time allows for more lengthy consideration, choices may be more carefully deliberated (e.g. when deciding whether to undergo a major surgical procedure with risk of serious complications).

Some decisions affect large numbers of people (e.g. whether or not to add fluoride to drinking water) and, in this situation, risk management may be carried out at a societal level through a more formalized and systematic process. This is particularly important where the stakes are high (i.e. potential benefits and harms are large), and where impacts differ for different sections of a population. For example, the main benefit from fluoridation of water supplies will occur in children with poor diets and poor oral hygiene, whereas the best established risk (that of dental fluorosis) will apply particularly to children with high intakes of fluoride from sources other than drinking water, such as from the use of fluoridated toothpaste.

One of the major applications of occupational epidemiology lies in formalized assessment and management of the risks from exposure to chemical and physical agents, either in the workplace or in the wider environment. Choices must be made whether to allow exposure to an agent and, if so, whether restrictions should be placed on levels of exposure, or other steps taken to mitigate any associated risks.

This chapter outlines the terminology and methods of formal risk assessment and management for chemical and physical agents, particularly in a regulatory context;

describes the contribution of occupational epidemiology; and explains how that contribution integrates with input from other scientific disciplines.

Definitions of terms

Like many technical activities, formal risk management has its own terminology, in which words are used with a more specific meaning than in common parlance. The definitions that are given in this section are widely applied in regulatory risk assessment for chemicals, and will be used throughout the chapter.

Hazard

The term 'hazard' refers to a potential adverse effect of a chemical or physical agent. It may extend to impacts on the environment or on non-human species but in this chapter will apply particularly to harmful effects on human health. Hazards may be minor (e.g. a transient nasal irritation) or serious, irreversible, and even fatal (e.g. pleural mesothelioma).

Risk

Risk is the probability that a hazard will be realized given the circumstances and extent of exposure to a chemical or physical agent. It is important to appreciate that risk depends crucially on the way in which exposure occurs. Handling a lump of crocidolite asbestos carries no risk of disease if the mineral remains intact, whereas prolonged inhalation of airborne crocidolite fibres at high concentrations leads to a substantial risk of asbestosis and mesothelioma. In addition, the risk from a given exposure may be modified by other factors. For example, the probability that a person working with laboratory animals will develop occupational asthma is higher if they are atopic.

In epidemiology, risk is most often quantified in terms of relative risk—i.e. the ratio of the probability of an adverse outcome in someone with a specified exposure to that in someone who is unexposed, or exposed at a different specified level. However, in the management of risks, individual and population attributable risks are more relevant to decision-making (Box 19.1).

Individual attributable risk is the difference in the probability of an adverse outcome between someone with a specified exposure and someone who is unexposed, or exposed at a different specified level. It is the critical measure when considering the impact of decisions in risk management on individuals. Thus, for example, if faced with a choice between a doubled risk of dying from colon cancer by age 60 and a doubled risk of dying from angiosarcoma of the liver by the same age, a rational person would choose the latter. The relative risk for both diseases would be the same (two), but because angiosarcoma of the liver is extremely rare, the corresponding individual attributable risk for that disease is tiny. In contrast, a doubling of mortality from colon cancer, which is one of the more common malignancies, represents a much larger added chance of death.

Population attributable risk is the difference in the frequency of an adverse outcome between a population with a given distribution of exposures to a hazardous

Box 19.1 Measures of risk and their relevance to risk management

Individual attributable risk

This is the difference in the probability of an adverse outcome between someone with a specified exposure and someone who is unexposed, or exposed at a different specified level. It is the most relevant measure of risk when comparing the impact of decisions in risk management on individuals. The probability of an adverse outcome may be defined in different ways according to circumstances. It might, for example, be the probability of developing a disease during a specified period (corresponding to cumulative incidence rate) or the probability of having a disease at a specified time in the future (corresponding to a prevalence rate). Individual attributable risks may be estimated directly from cohort studies, or indirectly by combining estimates of relative risk with data from other sources on the frequency of the adverse outcome in people with whom the level of risk is being compared (e.g. those with no exposure).

Relative risk

This is the ratio of the probability of an adverse outcome in someone with a specified exposure to that in someone who is unexposed or exposed at a different specified level. Measures such as odds ratios, standardized mortality ratios, and proportional mortality ratios are often used as proxies for relative risks. Relative risks can be estimated from a wider range of study designs than individual attributable risks. They have the advantage that they are often stable across different groups of people (e.g. of different ages, smokers, and non-smokers) which makes them easier to estimate and quantify. Moreover, high relative risks are generally unlikely to be explained by unrecognized bias or confounding. This may be an important consideration in the identification and confirmation of hazards through observational epidemiology. However, individual attributable risks are a more relevant measure by which to quantify the impact of decisions in risk management on individuals.

Population attributable risk

This is the difference in the frequency of an adverse outcome between a population with a given distribution of exposures to a hazardous agent, and that in a population with no exposure or some other specified distribution of exposures. It depends on the prevalence of exposure at different levels within the population, and on the individual attributable risks for each level of exposure. Population attributable risks are highest when a high proportion of a population is exposed at levels which carry high individual attributable risks. On the other hand, an exposure which carries a high individual attributable risk may produce only a small population attributable risk if the prevalence of such exposure is low. Population attributable risk quantifies the impact of an agent at a population level and is relevant to decisions about risk management for populations. For example, a decision on whether to limit concentrations of benzene in petrol might be influenced by the reduction in national incidence of leukaemia (measured in cases per million per year) that could be expected as a consequence.

agent, and that in a population with no exposure, or some other specified distribution of exposures. It depends on the prevalence of exposure at different levels within the population, and on the individual attributable risk for each level of exposure. It is a measure of the impact of the agent at a population level, and is relevant to decisions in risk management for populations. For example, although individual attributable risks from particulate pollution of outdoor air are generally small, large numbers of people are affected and, therefore, in many countries the population attributable risk has been judged sufficient to warrant regulatory controls on emissions of smoke and vehicle exhaust.

Uncertainty

Identification of the hazards that are posed by chemical and physical agents, and quantification of the associated risks, is subject to uncertainty. There may be a lack of relevant scientific information, or the studies which have been conducted may have shortcomings in their design or execution, with limited statistical power or potential for bias.

Some safety professionals conflate uncertainties of this type with risks that are measurable at a population level. It makes for clearer understanding, however, if uncertainty is distinguished from risk. For example, the current balance of scientific evidence does not indicate a hazard of brain cancer from the radiofrequency radiation that is emitted by mobile phones, but there is scientific uncertainty about this, and the possibility of elevated risk after many years of exposure cannot be ruled out (because the technology is novel, such long exposures have not yet accumulated). While it is correct that, because of this uncertainty, a hazard cannot be excluded, a statement that there is a risk of brain cancer from mobile phones might be wrongly misinterpreted as implying that a proportion of users will develop brain tumours because of their exposure.

Statistical uncertainties can be quantified through use of confidence intervals or p-values, but other aspects of uncertainty, such as the potential impacts of bias and confounding, can only be gauged subjectively. Nevertheless, it may be possible to specify a plausible range for an estimate of risk, based on all available evidence, and taking into account confidence intervals and judgements on the possible influence of other shortcomings of study design and execution.

Formal risk management

The process of formal risk management may be broken down into a series of steps (Box 19.2). The first three steps (hazard identification and confirmation, hazard characterization, and exposure assessment and risk characterization) are often grouped together under the heading of risk assessment.

Hazard identification and confirmation

Identification of the hazards associated with an agent may start with prior knowledge of the adverse effects of other similar agents. For example, chemicals with certain features in their molecular structure are more likely to pose a hazard of asthma.[1] Further clues may come from toxicological studies, both *in vitro*, and in whole animals.

Box 19.2 Steps in the formal assessment and management of risk

- Hazard identification and confirmation
- Hazard characterization
- Exposure assessment and characterization of risk
- Risk management
- Checks on the effectiveness of risk management

Collectively, the first three of these steps constitute risk assessment, which is a scientific exercise. Risk management entails the application of subjective value judgements when choosing between alternative policies or courses of action according to estimates of their benefits, risks, and costs, and the associated uncertainties.

Thus, demonstration that a chemical is mutagenic in bacteria may be an alert to a possible hazard of cancer; and a finding that a chemical causes nephrotoxicity in rats may point to a hazard of kidney disease in humans. In addition, hazards from chemical and physical agents have sometimes come to light from human case reports or epidemiological studies.

Where a hazard is suspected on the basis of toxicological studies or human case reports, confirmatory evidence may sometimes be sought through epidemiological research. For example, the carcinogenicity of mustard gas, which was first demonstrated in animal experiments, was subsequently confirmed as a hazard in humans by epidemiology.[2]

Hazard characterization

Hazard characterization entails quantification of risks in relation to routes, levels, and durations of exposure. Most often, and especially for new chemicals, this is based on toxicological studies in whole animals, which combine hazard identification with hazard characterization. When conducted for regulatory purposes, these usually follow standard protocols published by the Organisation for Economic Co-operation and Development (OECD).[3] Animals are exposed using prescribed dosing regimens, by specified routes (e.g. oral, dermal, inhalation, intraperitoneal) at specified life stages, and effects are systematically assessed during and/or after the dosing period. Most study designs entail eventual euthanasia of the test animals, with necropsy and histological examination of tissues. The findings from individual studies are often used to determine a no observed adverse effect level (NOAEL), lowest observed effect level (LOEL), or benchmark dose lower 95% confidence limit (BMDL) for relevant effects (see Box 19.3 for definitions), and this may then serve as a direct comparator for estimated levels of exposure or be used to derive a toxicological reference value for the chemical.

Box 19.3 Outcome measures derived from toxicological studies

No observed adverse effect level (NOAEL)

This is the highest dose or exposure concentration at which there is no discernible adverse effect.

Lowest observed effect level (LOEL)

This is the lowest dose or exposure concentration at which a discernible effect is observed. If comparison with unexposed controls indicates adverse effects at all of the dose levels in an experiment, a NOAEL cannot be derived, but the lowest dose constitutes a LOEL, which might be used as a comparator for estimated exposures or to derive a toxicological reference value, especially if the adverse effects observed at this level were minor.

Benchmark dose lower 95% confidence limit (BMDL)

A BMDL is defined in relation to a specified adverse outcome that is observed in a study. Usually, this is the outcome which occurs at the lowest levels of exposure and which is considered critical to the assessment of risk. Statistical modelling is applied to the experimental data to estimate the dose or exposure concentration which produces a specified small level of effect (e.g. a 5% excess prevalence). The BMDL is the lower 95% confidence limit for this estimate. As such, it depends both on the toxicity of the test chemical (more toxic chemicals will tend to give lower BMDLs), and also on the sample sizes used in the study (other things being equal, larger sample sizes will produce more precise estimates, and therefore higher BMDLs).

In addition to accounting for sample size, BMDLs have the merit that they exploit all of the data points in a study, and do not depend so critically on the spacing of doses that is adopted in the experimental design (by definition a NOAEL or LOEL can only be at one of the limited number of dose levels used in the experiment). On the other hand, BMDLs can only be calculated where an adverse effect is observed. Even if there are no clear adverse effects at any dose level, a NOAEL can be derived (it will be the highest dose administered).

While these measures are used most often to summarize the results of toxicological experiments on animals, corresponding measures may sometimes be derived from human data from epidemiological studies.

A toxicological reference value is the maximum level of exposure over a specified period (e.g. a single day or a lifetime) at which there is reasonable confidence that adverse health effects in humans would not occur. It is based on all studies that are considered relevant to the specified exposure period, and normally the starting point for its derivation is the lowest NOAEL, LOEL, or BMDL from these studies. This 'point of departure' is then divided by an 'assessment factor' (sometimes known as an 'uncertainty factor') to account for various limitations of the available data. Most often, where the reference value is derived from a NOAEL or BMDL, the assessment factor takes a value of 100 (made up of a factor of 10 to allow for uncertainties in extrapolation from animals to humans, and 10 to allow for possible within-species differences in sensitivity). However, additional multiplying factors may be incorporated where the point of departure is a LOEL rather than a NOAEL or BMDL, to account for particular weaknesses of the evidence base, or where the critical health effect is severe (e.g. major birth defects).

Although hazard characterization is usually based on animal toxicology, epidemiology may also contribute. If epidemiological studies are available in which exposures have been assessed with sufficient accuracy to generate quantitative exposure-response relationships, they too can be used to derive a NOAEL, LOEL, or BMDL, and thereby a toxicological reference value. Where this is done, the assessment factor may be smaller because the uncertainty in extrapolation from animals to humans is eliminated.

Exposure assessment and characterization of risk

Occasionally, epidemiology provides direct evidence on the level of risk associated with a particular exposure scenario which can be used when deciding whether action is needed to counter a hazard. More often, however, risks are assessed by collating hazard characterization with estimates of the levels of exposure that would result from a policy or course of action.

In some cases, the management of risk may simply entail specification of an upper limit for permitted exposures (e.g. a maximum time-weighted average exposure to noise in the workplace) which, based on the characterization of hazard, would be expected to prevent unacceptable harm to health. In other cases, however, exposures may be more complex, occurring through multiple pathways and routes.

In this situation, exposure scientists may make an estimate of the realistic upper limit of exposures that an individual might incur if a regulatory decision were implemented. For example, when assessing the potential risk to spray operators from approval of a new pesticide, an estimate is made of the total daily exposure that could reasonably occur if the product were applied according to the proposed conditions of approval. This might include: dermal exposure to pesticide concentrate when mixing and loading; inhalation of, and skin contact with, spray droplets while spraying; and dermal exposures when cleaning and maintaining equipment for spraying. Such exposures are aggregated (taking into account differences in absorption according to the route of exposure) to produce an estimated realistic maximum daily systemic exposure which can then be compared with the relevant toxicological reference value. Similarly, when considering whether interventions are warranted to reduce exposures to lead in the general population of a city or country, it is necessary to estimate the maximum exposure that could realistically occur from consumption of contaminated food and drinking water, combined with inhalation of lead in air, and, in the case of infants and small children, ingestion of lead in soil, dirt, and paint. This can then be set against the hazard characterization for the metal.

Risk management

Once an assessment has been made of the risks that are associated with different policies or courses of action, and also of their benefits and costs and the attendant uncertainties, a decision must be made on which action to follow. This step is termed 'risk management'.

Where risk assessment for a chemical or physical agent gives inadequate reassurance of safety in a particular scenario, strategies to reduce the risk most often entail controls on exposure. In some cases, it may be possible to eliminate the hazardous agent altogether. Thus, in the UK, the risk of bladder cancer in the rubber industry from the aromatic amine, 2-naphthylamine, was addressed by prohibiting use of the chemical. In other situations, however, it may not be possible to remove a hazardous agent completely and instead steps must be taken to ensure that exposures are sufficiently low that any risks to health are minor and acceptable. For example, limits are placed on exposures to ionizing radiation, both through work and in the wider environment.

It should be noted that whereas the assessment of risk is a scientific exercise, the management of risk is not based on science alone. It entails subjective value judgements about the desirability of benefits and the acceptability of risks and costs that are associated with alternative actions or policies, and there is no reason why the values of scientists should prevail over those of other people. For example, many scientists consider that potential health risks from genetically modified foods are of insufficient concern to warrant generic restrictions on their sale or consumption but, in Europe, members of the public worry about the uncertainties associated with this new technology, and its possible adverse effects. Governments have responded to this anxiety by tightly controlling the sale of genetically modified products.

Checks on the effectiveness of risk management

Once a course of action has been adopted on the basis of a risk assessment, it may be prudent to check that the impact is as expected. For example, the effectiveness of controls on occupational exposure to noise could be evaluated by monitoring the hearing thresholds of exposed workers. If results are not as expected, the assessment and control of risk may need to be revisited.

Contribution of epidemiology

Although risk assessment for chemical and physical agents relies heavily on toxicology and exposure sciences, epidemiology makes an important contribution, complementary to that of these other disciplines.

It has the major advantage of providing direct evidence on effects in humans, avoiding the uncertainties in extrapolation from findings in laboratory animals. It allows study of certain health outcomes which at best can only be investigated by proxy in animals. For example, while subtle effects on neuropsychological function may be detectable in humans, the only clue to such a hazard from animal studies may be more severe neurological damage at higher exposures.

Also, because epidemiological studies generally employ much larger sample sizes than animal experiments, they may allow detection of smaller elevations of risk. A good example is the demonstration in multiple epidemiological analyses of small but consistent elevations of cardiorespiratory morbidity and mortality in close temporal relationship to increases in particulate pollution of ambient air.[4] These findings have helped to underpin legislation in many countries to control sources of such pollution.

Against these strengths, there are several important limitations to the use of epidemiology in risk management. It can only provide useful information once sufficient numbers of people have been exposed to an agent. Moreover, if the risk of an adverse effect does not increase until long after first exposure (as is the case for many carcinogens) it may be decades before data are available that allow a hazard to be identified and prevented. By this time, many people may be destined to carry forward a burden of risk from exposures that they have already incurred.

A second weakness is the difficulty in quantifying exposures reliably, especially in retrospective studies. This is less of a problem for hazard confirmation, in which crude ordinal categories of exposure may provide adequate evidence that risk increases monotonically with progressively higher exposures. Nor is it a hindrance where the aim is to test whether restrictions on exposure have been effective in controlling risk. However, it often limits the use of epidemiology to characterize hazards quantitatively.

Thirdly, because epidemiology is largely an observational science and is subject to practical and ethical constraints (for example, subjects cannot be compelled to take part in a study against their wishes), it is susceptible to bias and confounding, leading to uncertainties in interpretation. For this reason, statistical associations that are observed in epidemiological studies must be interpreted in the context of relevant biological knowledge, especially from toxicology, when deciding whether they are likely to be causal. In the case of particulate air pollution, mechanistic studies demonstrating the potential of fine particles to cause inflammation added weight to the epidemiological evidence of a hazard and gave greater confidence in the exposure–response relationships estimated from epidemiological analyses.[4]

Contribution of occupational epidemiology

Within epidemiology more broadly, occupational epidemiology has made a particularly notable contribution to risk assessment for chemical and physical agents. One reason for this is the wider range of harmful agents encountered in the workplace than in other settings. Significant exposures to agents such as vinyl chloride monomer and crystalline silica are almost entirely occupational, and epidemiological evidence for the associated hazards therefore comes from occupational studies. Moreover, since the control of such hazards is implemented in the workplace, that is also where the effectiveness of controls must be demonstrated.

Even where an agent also occurs in the wider environment, exposures in the workplace are often higher (sometimes very much higher), leading to larger risks that are more readily detectable. Examples include formaldehyde and hand-transmitted vibration. In this situation, the information generated by occupational epidemiology may be used in the assessment and management of risk not only in the workplace, but also more widely.

Another strength of occupational epidemiology is that exposures through work can often be determined more reliably than those which occur elsewhere. For example, it is easier to distinguish people with differing exposures to methanol through their employment than through their diet and leisure-time activities.

The case studies that follow exemplify the ways in which occupational epidemiology has informed the different stages of risk management for chemical and physical agents.

Case studies

Hazard identification and confirmation—sino-nasal cancer

During the 1960s, two ear, nose, and throat surgeons became aware of an apparent excess of sino-nasal cancer in and around the English town of High Wycombe, which they suspected might be related to work in the local furniture industry.[2] Subsequent epidemiological investigation confirmed the hazard and demonstrated that it arose from exposure to hardwood dust.[5]

As part of the epidemiological research, Acheson and colleagues mapped out the distribution of cases registered in the Oxford region. As well as confirming the cluster of cases around High Wycombe this exercise revealed a second, unexpected aggregation of cases in the county of Northamptonshire.[6] Further epidemiological research demonstrated that this was attributable to a previously unrecognized hazard from the dust of vegetable-tanned leather used in the manufacture of boots and shoes.

Steps have since been taken to reduce exposure to both of these dusts.

Hazard characterization—coal mine dust and chronic obstructive pulmonary disease

The quantitative relationship between exposure to coal mine dust and risk of chronic obstructive pulmonary disease was investigated in a longitudinal study of British coal miners.[7] As well as informing controls on exposure, the findings were influential in the decision to compensate miners affected by the disease.

Risk characterization—hand arm vibration syndrome in Finnish lumberjacks

During the 1960s, a marked increase was demonstrated in the prevalence of vibration white finger among lumberjacks in Finland. Subsequently, the introduction of chain saws with modified engines and devices to dampen vibration led to a reduction in the prevalence and severity of symptoms.[8]

Risk management—organophosphate sheep dip

Although decisions in the management of risks depend on value judgements and are not primarily a scientific activity, the choice of methods by which to reduce exposures may be informed by scientific evidence. Organophosphate insecticides can cause serious acute toxicity through inhibition of the enzyme acetyl cholinesterase and, during the 1990s, there was concern in the UK about possible overexposure of farmers to organophosphates used in sheep dips. A study by Buchanan and colleagues, which applied epidemiological methods to investigate determinants of systemic dose (measured by assay of excreted metabolites in the urine) found that handling of sheep dip concentrate was the principal source of exposure.[9] This led to re-design of the containers for concentrates, not only of sheep dip, but also of other pesticides, with wider necks to reduce splashing during pouring.

Checks on effectiveness of risk management—proteolytic enzymes and occupational asthma

Research in the late 1960s revealed a substantial incidence of occupational asthma at a factory producing washing-powders.[10] This was caused by sensitization to proteolytic enzymes, which had recently been incorporated into some powders. The problem was addressed by stricter dust controls, improved exhaust ventilation, enclosure of plant, and additional protective clothing for workers. An epidemiological analysis showed that detectable respiratory illness had been successfully eliminated, confirming the effectiveness of the control measures.[11] Subsequently, a further epidemiological study showed that the problem had recurred, for reasons that are not entirely clear.[12] Similar outbreaks have occurred around the world.

Conclusion

The case studies represent just a few examples of the many ways in which occupational epidemiology has contributed to the assessment and management of risks from chemical and physical agents. Controls on exposure prompted or guided by epidemiological research have successfully prevented substantial morbidity and mortality, not only in the workplace, but also more widely. Arguably, this is the most important benefit that occupational epidemiology has generated.

References

1. **Seed M, Agius R.** Further validation of computer-based prediction of chemical asthma hazard. *Occup Med* 2010;**60**:115–20.
2. **Doll R.** Part III: 7th Walter Hubert lecture. Pott and the prospects for prevention. *Br J Cancer* 1975;**32**:263–72.
3. **Organisation for Economic Co-operation and Development.** *OECD guidelines for the testing of chemicals.* Available at: <http://www.oecd-ilibrary.org/environment/oecd-guidelines-for-the-testing-of-chemicals_chem_guide_pkg-en;jsessionid=1ubhypfw5buti.x-oecd-live-01> (accessed 24 January 2013).
4. **Department for Environment, Food and Rural Affairs.** Expert Panel on Air Quality Standards. *Airborne particles: what is the appropriate measurement on which to base a standard? A discussion document.* London: The Stationery Office, 2001. Available at: <http://webarchive.nationalarchives.gov.uk/20060715141954/http://www.defra.gov.uk/environment/airquality/aqs/air_measure/02.htm> (accessed 24 January 2013).

5. Acheson ED, Cowdell RH, Hadfield E, Macbeth RG. Nasal cancer in woodworkers in the furniture industry. *Br Med J* 1968;2:587–96.

6. Acheson ED, Cowdell RH, Jolles B. Nasal cancer in the Northamptonshire boot and shoe industry. *Br Med J* 1970;1:385–93.

7. Marine WM, Gurr D, Jacobsen M. Clinically important respiratory effects of dust exposure and smoking in British coal miners. *Am Rev Respir Dis* 1988;**137**:106–12.

8. Pyykkö I, Sairanen E, Korhonen O, Färkkilä M, Hyvärinen J. A decrease in the prevalence and severity of vibration-induced white fingers among lumberjacks in Finland. *Scand J Work Environ Health* 1978;4:246–54.

9. Buchanan D, Pilkington A, Sewell C, *et al.* Estimation of cumulative exposure to organophosphate sheep dips in a study of chronic neurological health effects among United Kingdom sheep dippers. *Occup Environ Med* 2001;**58**:694–701.

10. Flindt MLH. Pulmonary disease due to inhalation of derivatives of Bacillus subtilis-containing proteolytic enzymes. *Lancet* 1969;1:1177–81.

11. Juniper CP, How MJ, Goodwin BFJ, Kinshott AK. Bacillus subtilis enzymes: a 7-year clinical, epidemiological and immunological study of an industrial allergen. *J Soc Occup Med* 1977;**27**:3–12.

12. Cullinan P, Harris JM, Newman Taylor AJ, *et al.* An outbreak of asthma in a modern detergent factory. *Lancet* 2000;**356**:899–900.

Index

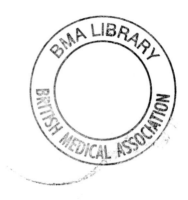